Reperfusion Injuries - Advances in Understanding, Prevention, and Treatment

Edited by Zesergio Melo and Russell E. Peterson

Published in London, United Kingdom

Reperfusion Injuries - Advances in Understanding, Prevention, and Treatment
http://dx.doi.org/intechopen.111320
Edited by Zesergio Melo and Russell E. Peterson

Contributors
Andrew D'Elia, Ashish Patel, Bubul Kalita, Büşra Tuğçe Akman, Cagdas Duru, Cláudio André Martins Roque, Daniya Nawaz, Bhawna Bhimte, Eunice Rut Rodriguez Cornejo, Jerry Toelsie, Johnny Rompis, Marco Ku-Centurion, Maritza G. Verdugo-Molinares, Michael W. Allen, Muhammad Rizwan Khan, Natharina Yolanda, Nina Hadzimustafic, Paul Steels, Pedro José Curi-Curi, Rakesh Jagat, Ranjit Patil, Robbert Bipat, Russell E. Peterson, Shantilal Padhiyar, Siba Haykal, Tejas B. Patel, Thalía Fernanda Camarillo González, Valeria Juarez Garcia, Vashisth Bhavsar, Vipul Prajapati, Zesergio Melo

First published in London, United Kingdom, 2024 by IntechOpen
IntechOpen is the global imprint of INTECHOPEN LIMITED, registered in England and Wales, registration number: 11086078, 167-169 Great Portland Street, London, W1W 5PF, United Kingdom

British Library Cataloguing-in-Publication Data
A catalogue record for this book is available from the British Library

Additional hard and PDF copies can be obtained from orders@intechopen.com

Reperfusion Injuries - Advances in Understanding, Prevention, and Treatment
Edited by Zesergio Melo and Russell E. Peterson
p. cm.

This title is part of the Cardiology and Cardiovascular Medicine Book Series, Volume 4
Topic: Cardiovascular Diseases and Health
Series Editor: Kaan Kırali
Topic Editor: Mahi L. Ashwath

Print ISBN 978-0-85014-153-5
Online ISBN 978-0-85014-154-2
eBook (PDF) ISBN 978-0-85014-155-9
ISSN 3033-361X

For EU product safety concerns:
IN TECH d.o.o., Prolaz Marije Krucifikse Kozulić 3, 51000 Rijeka, Croatia,
info@intechopen.com or visit our website at intechopen.com.

IntechOpen Book Series

Cardiology and Cardiovascular Medicine

Volume 4

Aims and Scope of the Series

Today, since molecular science on structural causes of oncological pathologies and their molecular treatments are developing at an unbelievable rate, the primary medical cause of death in the twenty-first century will be cardiovascular disease. Neither pandemics that threaten all humanity nor deterioration in the ecosystem will be able to change this fact. Especially, this century seems poised to witness an incredible struggle against atherosclerotic disease, which develops in the arterial walls and results in narrowing and occlusion of the arterial lumen. In addition to this disease, there has been an increasing prevalence of heart rhythm problems, deterioration of heart valves due to aging, and heart failure. Serious vascular pathologies such as stenosis and occlusion, dissection and rupture, and aneurysmal enlargement are also major concerns. Medical and invasive treatment methods may work to save human lives, but they will never provide a real solution. All kinds of medical, technological, and genetic engineering developments obtained in these processes have not yet been sufficient to alleviate or eliminate cardiovascular disease. This book series, Cardiology and Cardiovascular Medicine, includes three topics. The first, Cardiovascular Diseases and Health, reviews important cardiovascular diseases and the developments in their prognosis. The second topic, Cardiovascular Electrophysiology, illuminates the abnormal functioning of the cardiac conduction system, which is caused by all heart pathologies and negatively affects prognosis. The third topic in this series, Cardiovascular Surgery, details treatment for cardiovascular pathologies and how to regulate normal physiological functions with percutaneous or extracorporeal interventions.

Meet the Series Editor

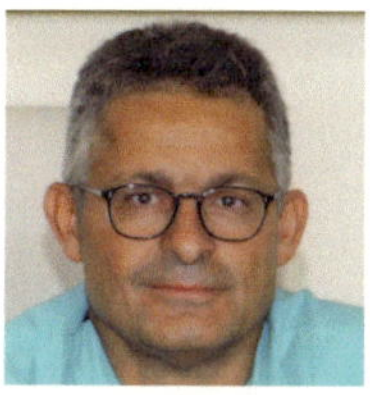

After completing his studies at the Medicine Faculty of Istanbul University in 1990, Prof. Kaan Kırali fulfilled his mandatory medical service and commenced his residency training at Koşuyolu Heart and Research Hospital in 1992. Following five years of assistant education, he pursued further training in England and the USA in 1998. Specializing in laparoscopic and minimally invasive cardiac surgery, he earned the titles of consultant cardiovascular surgeon in 1998, Assistant Professor in 1999, Associate Professor in 2002, and Chief in 2005 at the same hospital. Prof. Kırali also developed an interest in preventive medicine, obtaining an MSc in Public Health from Istanbul University in 2000. Over the past two decades, he has concentrated his scientific pursuits on cardiovascular repairs requiring specialized experience. With his expertise in coronary artery surgery, minimally invasive cardiac surgery, valve repair, and aortic root surgery, he has established new methods for awake coronary bypass revascularization, a new surgical approach for AVR during first and re-operations, aortic valve-sparing procedure, and radiofrequency ablation. Notably, he pioneered awake complete coronary artery bypass grafting (CABG) with bilateral internal mammary arteries (BIMA) and played a crucial role in advancing aortic root surgery with a new aortotomy incision, simplifying aortic valve interventions. Since the year 2000, Prof. Kırali has expanded his interests to heart transplantation, and in recent years, to left ventricular assist devices. He has served as the head of the transplantation department since 2015 and currently continues his work as the director of Koşuyolu High Specialization Education and Research Hospital in Istanbul, Turkey. In his prolific career, he has authored numerous papers in SCI journals, contributed to various book chapters, and served as an editor and reviewer for multiple academic journals. Additionally, he has edited several international books in the field of cardiovascular medicine.

Meet the Volume Editors

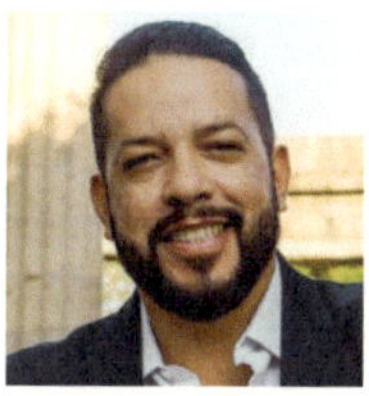

Dr. Zesergio Melo, from Colombia, holds a BSc in Bacteriology from Universidad Industrial de Santander, Colombia, and a Ph.D. in Biochemical Sciences from the National Autonomous University of Mexico (UNAM), specializing in renal salt transport mechanisms. He completed a postdoc at the Instituto de Neurobiología, UNAM, focusing on prolactin variants. He has worked with the Instituto Mexicano del Seguro Social. With more than thirty scientific publications to his credit, Dr. Melo has received awards including the Statal Research Award in Organ and Tissue Donation, Procurement, and Transplantation, the Meritorious Research Award, and the Young Researcher Award. He supervises several theses and leads his research on the regulatory mechanisms of renal ischemia-reperfusion injury.

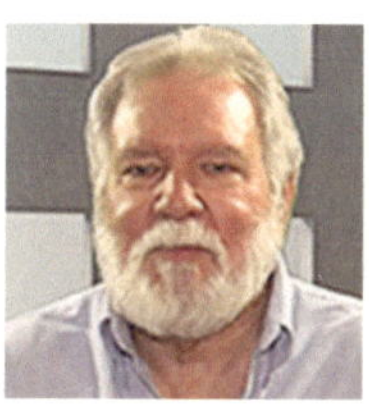

Russell Peterson (REP) received his graduate physiology training under C. J. Lambertsen, MD, head of the Institute for Environmental Medicine, University of Pennsylvania, USA. During this period, Dr. Lambertsen and Dr. James M. Clark were engaged in groundbreaking research on oxygen tolerance. Dr. Peterson's exposure to this latter research enabled him to incorporate oxygen dose parameters into routine and contingency dive procedures he developed over his career. This experience also provided him with insight into using elevated oxygen levels in a variety of new therapeutic situations. Consequently, when Dr. Peterson and his frequent collaborator, Michael W. Allen, were challenged with hyperbaric medical dogma conflicting with their experience in new applications, they set out to understand the reasons for this disparity.

Contents

Preface

This edited volume, *Reperfusion Injuries – Advances in Understanding, Prevention, and Treatment*, brings together innovative research and clinical insights into the complex interplay of oxygen dynamics, biochemical alterations, and ischemic conditions. The chapters within this book offer a comprehensive exploration of therapeutic and pathological phenomena associated with oxygen therapy, hypoxia, and ischemia for a broad audience ranging from researchers and clinicians to students and medical practitioners.

Oxygen applications in therapeutic settings must be carefully balanced. The initial section of this book, "Oxygen Therapy and Biochemical Alterations", examines the delicate relationship between oxygen supplementation and its dose-dependent effects. Chapters 1 and 2, "Dose-Response Relationship of Therapeutic Oxygen: More is Not Necessarily Better and May Be Inferior to No Supplemental Oxygen (Part 1: Proof and Nature) and (Part 2: Implications and Consequences)" scrutinize the optimal use of oxygen therapy and highlights the potential risks of hyperoxia, offering guidelines for its prudent application. Chapter 3, "Biochemical Alterations and Antioxidant Levels in Patients Living with HIV", addresses the metabolic and oxidative challenges faced by HIV patients, emphasizing the critical role of antioxidants in managing the biochemical consequences of the disease.

Understanding the impact of oxygen deprivation, or hypoxia, is crucial for managing many clinical conditions. "Hypoxia and Hemodynamics", the second section, examines the physiological and clinical implications of hypoxia. Chapter 4, "Relationship between Hypoxia and Pulmonary Microcirculation Hemorheology in Pediatric Patients with Patent Ductus Arteriosus Operated on at Moderate Altitude" explores how altitude influences surgical outcomes in pediatric patients, providing insights into managing hypoxia in specialized settings. Chapter 5, "A Severe Clinical Example of Hypoxia: Sickle Cell Anemia" discusses the systemic and cellular effects of hypoxia in sickle cell disease, presenting strategies for effective management of this condition.

Ischemia reperfusion injury, characterized by restricted blood flow, and subsequent reoxygenation, when blood supply returns, are critical areas of concern due to the potential for exacerbated tissue damage. The third section, "Ischemia Reperfusion Injury", addresses these phenomena from cellular mechanisms to advanced clinical practices. Chapter 6, "Cellular and Molecular Effects of Ischemia on Brain Cells" presents an analysis of ischemic damage in the brain and explores potential therapeutic interventions. Chapter 7, "Advances in Ischemia Reperfusion Injury Prevention in Free Flaps and Vascularized Composite Allotransplantation" and Chapter 8, "Advancement in Reperfusion Injury Awareness and Mitigation", extend this exploration to surgical and clinical settings, offering the latest strategies to mitigate reperfusion injury and improve patient outcomes.

Identifying reliable biomarkers and understanding molecular mechanisms are crucial for diagnosing and treating ischemic conditions. The fourth section, "Biomarkers and Molecular Mechanisms", focuses on innovations in this area. Chapter 9, "Perspective Chapter: Role of Caspase-3 as Neonatal Hypoxic Ischemic Encephalopathy Biomarker" highlights the diagnostic potential of Caspase 3 in neonatal care, suggesting novel approaches for managing hypoxic-ischemic encephalopathy. Chapter 10, "Exosomes in Reperfusion Injuries: Role in Pathophysiology and Perspectives as Treatment" investigates the role of exosomes in cellular communication and injury, providing a deep perspective on their therapeutic potential.

The final section, "Renal Ischemia and Hypoxia", emphasizes the importance of understanding the functional differences and clinical implications of renal ischemia and hypoxia. Chapter 11, "Renal Ischemia and Hypoxia: Functional Differences and Possible Clinical and Therapeutic Consequences", provides a detailed comparison, outlining the distinct challenges posed by each condition and potential therapeutic approaches.

In assembling this volume, we aim to provide a resource that not only elucidates the complex dynamics of oxygen, hypoxia, and ischemia-reperfusion injury but also serves as a guide for translating these insights into clinical practice. We hope that this compilation will inspire further research and innovation, contributing to improved patient care and advancing our understanding of these critical areas.

Finally, we extend our gratitude to the contributing authors, whose expertise and dedication have made this volume possible. Their collective efforts offer a valuable resource for all those engaged in the study and treatment of conditions related to oxygen therapy, hypoxia, and ischemic injuries.

Zesergio Melo
CONAHCYT-Western Biomedical Research Center, IMSS,
Guadalajara, Mexico

Russell E. Peterson
NEMO Therapeutics, LLC,
Sarasota, Florida, USA

Section 1

Oxygen Therapy and Biochemical Alterations

Chapter 1

Dose-Response Relationship of Therapeutic Oxygen: More Is Not Necessarily Better and May Be Inferior to No Supplemental Oxygen – Part 1: Proof and Nature

Russell E. Peterson and Michael W. Allen

Abstract

In the early 1990s, the authors had consistently positive experience in the treatment of typical sports injuries and cosmetic surgical wounds with hyperbaric oxygen. These treatments generally consisted of oxygen at 2.0 atmospheres absolute (ATA) for 60 minutes. We were thus surprised to find that recognized experts in the field of hyperbaric medicine did not believe this modality to be effective for such *normal wounds*. Consequently, we asked Eric Kindwall, M.D., a professional acquaintance and published proponent of this prevalent view, what the bases for his beliefs on this matter were. Starting with references provided by Dr. Kindwall, we began an extensive literature review to try to reconcile our practical successes with the prevailing hyperbaric medical dogma. During our analysis, we found that the outcomes of oxygen therapy have a *hormetic* dose-response relationship. This finding explains the mistaken conclusions drawn concerning the treatment of uncompromised or *normal wounds* with hyperbaric oxygen as more oxygen will not provide benefits without limit. At some dose point, even below an inspired partial pressure (P_iO_2) of 3.0 atm, benefits will begin to decline and, in due course, more oxygen will produce negative impact in comparison with no hyperoxic supplementation.

Keywords: dose, dose response, hormesis, hormetic, hyperbaric, hyperoxia, hypoxia, normobaric, oxygen, oxygenation, supplementation, therapy

1. Introduction

This review article concerning oxygen dose response is presented in two parts. In Part 1, we provide evidence for a dose-related response to oxygen therapy and its hormetic nature. In Part 2, we discuss the implications and consequences of dose-response with respect to the use of oxygen as a therapeutic agent. These uses include not only those applications for which it is already employed but also new indications and improved therapeutic strategies for both normobaric and hyperbaric administration.

1.1 Oxygen chemistry, physiology, and pathology

Oxygen is the third most abundant element in the universe. It is nonmetallic and highly reactive forming compounds with almost all other elements. Physiologically, in aerobic organisms, oxygen is essential for producing adenosine triphosphate (ATP), which provides chemical energy for many processes within cells including biosynthetic reactions, motility, and cell division. Further, short-lived free radicals formed from oxygen, *reactive oxygen species (ROS)*, play an important role in many processes including the killing of pathogens by the host's immune system and cell signaling. As a result of its many critical physiological roles, the provision of oxygen to the cells of aerobic organisms in accordance with metabolic and functional demands is a necessity for life.

Because of their reactivity, ROS such as superoxide ($O_2\cdot$), hydroxyl radicals ($OH\cdot$), singlet oxygen ($O_2\cdot$), nitric oxide ($NO\cdot$), and hydrogen peroxide (H_2O_2) have the potential to produce not only beneficial effects but also adverse ones including damage to macromolecules and disruption of cellular metabolism. A number of chemical compounds such as superoxide dismutase, glutathione reductase, catalase, thioredoxins, peroxidases, and antioxidant nutrients (e.g., alpha tocopherol, ascorbic acid, and carotenoids), generally classified as *antioxidant defenses*, minimize free-radical-induced damage in the body and contribute to the repair of such damage when it does occur. Despite this, chronic adverse effects of ROS are believed to play a role in aging, some disease processes, and cell death. Adverse effects from acute overexposure to oxygen (i.e., *oxygen toxicity*) can impact all cells, but have been found to be particularly prominent in the central nervous system, lungs, and eyes of mammalian life forms.

1.2 Clinical uses of oxygen

In medicine, oxygen is commonly administered to:

- Compensate for and/or help correct:
  - Primary delivery insufficiencies (e.g., emphysema, pneumonia, pulmonary embolism, congestive heart failure, carbon monoxide poisoning, and exceptional blood loss anemia);
  - Local delivery insufficiencies (e.g., crush injury, compartment syndrome, and acute arterial insufficiency; non-healing wounds; refractory osteomyelitis; delayed radiation injury; compromised skin flaps and grafts; thermal burns; and frostbite).
- Enhance:
  - Immune system function in bacterial killing (e.g., gas gangrene, necrotizing soft tissue infections, and intracranial abscess);
  - Inert gas elimination and bubble resolution in gas embolic disorders (i.e., arterial and venous gas embolism, and decompression sickness).

1.3 Delivery of hyperoxic gases to patients

In some cases, oxygen is effective when delivered to patients at normal barometric pressure, primarily by mask or nasal cannula. In other cases, to obtain the necessary inspired oxygen pressure, oxygen must be delivered to patients at increased barometric pressure using a whole-body chamber. This is known as *hyperbaric oxygen therapy* (HBO_2). In only two of the conditions listed above for medical oxygen administration is the chamber pressure associated with HBO_2 known with certainty to play a direct role in the therapy. This is in the treatment of gas embolism and decompression sickness, both of which are gas embolic/*bubble* disorders. In these cases, increased hydrostatic pressure reduces the size of any gas phase in closed systems in the body in inverse relationship to the increase in absolute hydrostatic pressure, thus helping to eliminate circulatory blockage and tissue deformation caused by the bubbles. Reducing gas volumes also concentrates the components of the gas phases, thus, hastening their return to solution and the ultimate dissolution of the bubbles.

The explicit details of HBO_2 administration depend on the type of chamber used. In multiplace (i.e., multiple-occupant) chambers, oronasal masks or flow-through hoods are usually used (**Figure 1**). In monoplace (i.e., single-occupant) chambers, the chamber is usually flushed with oxygen so that no special gas delivery apparatus is required (**Figure 2**). The patient simply breathes the chamber atmosphere. Less commonly in monoplace chambers, the patient breathes oxygen by an oronasal mask or flow-through hood, while the chamber is compressed and flushed with air.

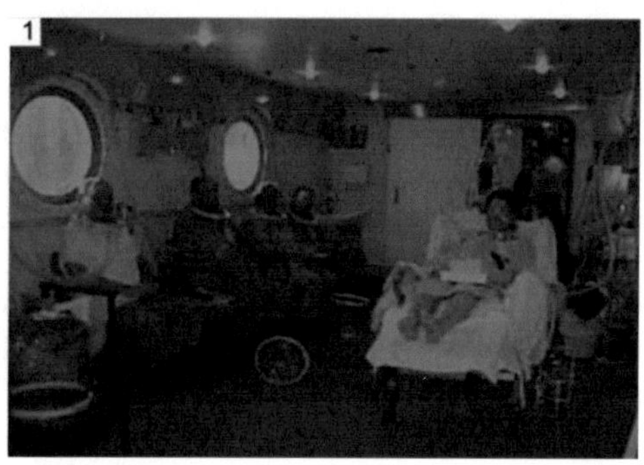

Figure 1.
Clinical multiplace hyperbaric chamber (courtesy of Fink Engineering, Warana, Queensland, Australia).

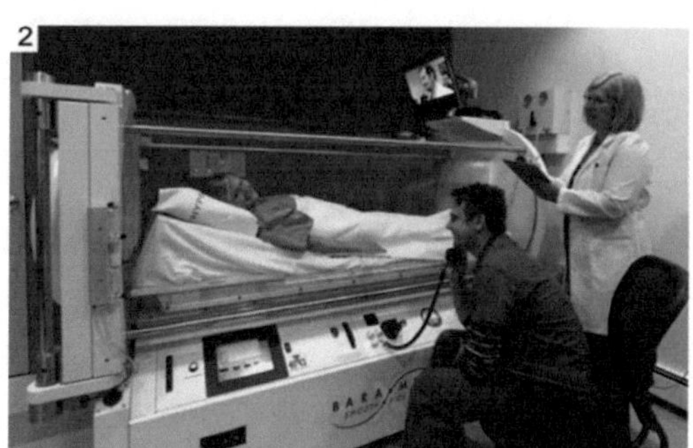

Figure 2.
Clinical monoplace hyperbaric oxygen chamber (courtesy of Environmental Tectonics Corporation, Southampton, PA, U.S.A.).

2. Regulation of clinical uses of hyperoxic gases

In medical applications, oxygen is often considered to be a drug and in many countries is regulated by national healthcare authorities (e.g., the Food and Drug Administration in the United States, Health Canada in Canada, Medicines and Healthcare Products Regulatory Agency (MHRA) in the UK, and the Therapeutic Goods Administration in Australia), and requires the prescription of a licensed physician for its use. Despite this and the fact that dose-response relationships are of fundamental importance to the safe and effective use of pharmaceutical agents, the authors are aware of no broad-scope, in-depth discussion of this aspect of oxygen therapy, either hyperbaric or normobaric, and only a relatively small number of passing references or references severely limited in scope [1–12]. This would seem to go hand-in-glove with the fact that few studies have been conducted to investigate therapeutic outcomes systematically as a function of dose (i.e., *inspired oxygen partial pressure, treatment duration, treatment frequency, total number of treatments, and changes in any of these parameters over time*).

3. Objectives of this review

Since oxygen dose-response relationships are a function of a myriad of both beneficial and detrimental effects of oxygen, the ultimate outcome of any oxygen treatment will be the net result of all these factors acting at the site of interest over the time course of treatment and recovery from the treatment. As such factors are only incompletely understood, even at this time (i.e., March of 2024), establishing any particular dose-response relationship could involve a great many relatively time-consuming hyperoxic treatments. Consequently, comprehensive studies of oxygen dose effects could be difficult to design, and costly and time-consuming to carry out.

The above notwithstanding, we have found that there is information in the scientific and clinical literature sufficient to provide important definitive and practical insights into the basic nature of the oxygen dose-response relationship and some of its clinical implications. This understanding evolved as the result of an extensive literature review we conducted to examine the opinion prevalent in the hyperbaric medical community that HBO_2 is not an effective treatment modality for *normal wounds*.

This opinion runs contrary to our considerable practical experience that HBO_2 can be an effective adjunct for enhancing the healing of so-called *normal wounds* in sports and cosmetic surgery. Our view is supported by not only our own experience in the form of case reports but also by many controlled human and animal studies conducted by numerous investigators over almost 50 years as of the early 2020s. The review and analysis presented here show how the evidence for and against the effectiveness of hyperoxic therapy for normal wounds has been rationalized into a unifying concept of oxygen dose-response. Some important medical implications of this relationship are then discussed.

3.1 Normal wounds and hyperoxic therapy

Margolis et al. [13] provide a definition of *normal wounds*, a "wound that heals normally," which effectively separates this category from others such as delayed effects of radiation, refractory osteomyelitis, and some lower-extremity diabetic ulcers for which special intervention like HBO_2 may be required to produce healing.

Based on this definition, any uncompromised injury, regardless of its origin, whether combat, workplace, domestic, automotive, surgical, sport, recreational, or any other that does not require special intervention for ultimate resolution, would be classified as a *normal wound*.

Even for normal wounds, however, it has been established that oxygen levels resulting from breathing air at one atmosphere absolute (1 ATA) do not fully meet the increased metabolic demand of inflamed and healing tissue. U.S. military studies have shown that the optimal oxygen pressures for fibroblast proliferation and collagen production [14] and for macrophage migration [15] are approximately twice those found in normally oxygenated tissue. These determinations were made with *in vitro* cell cultures having continuous exposure to the given oxygen concentrations. Another study, conducted *in vivo* with rabbits, confirmed that in bone, the optimal oxygen tissue pressure for collagen synthesis is impossible to achieve when breathing air at one atmosphere [16].

Abbot et al. [17] have found that increased oxygen demand resulting from the inflammatory response, together with the effects of associated edema and fibrin in the interstitial fluid, prevent the maintenance of normal tissue oxygen levels despite the hyperemia caused by inflammation. Sheffield [18], through extensive studies of tissue oxygen pressures, has determined that oxygen levels in "normal wounds of any magnitude" are not only suboptimal for healing but are also hypoxic, and the rate at which such wounds heal is oxygen dependent. Hunt et al. [19] measured wound oxygen levels and determined that even for soft-tissue wounds in the early stages of healing under normal circumstances, more oxygen than delivered by the breathing of 100% oxygen at normobaric pressure would be used effectively if it were available at the wound site. Yablon and Cruess [20] and Niinikoski and Hunt [16] have concluded that oxygen is a fundamental and limiting factor in the healing of fractured bones.

Thus, to us, the view that oxygen administration in appropriate dose does not enhance the healing of normal wounds seemed illogical on a first-principle basis. This has, however, been the commonly held opinion, effectively dogma, in the hyperbaric medical community as indicated by clear, emphatic, and unchallenged statements published over almost four decades.

- "In short, hyperbaric oxygen seems to have little role in healing clean, normal, incised wounds. Its role in hypoxic wound healing, however, appears to be established" [21].

- "Hyperbaric oxygen will not heal normal wounds more rapidly but may, under certain circumstances, induce problem wounds to heal more like normal ones" [22].

- "In conclusion, HBO_2 can significantly improve the healing of ischaemic incisional wounds if the treatment takes place during the first few days of wound healing. In contrast, HBO_2 therapy has no effect on the healing of normal wounds" [23].

- "HBO_2 may not speed healing in normal wounds, but it proves particularly useful when an injury occurs in an area of local hypoxia or decreased blood flow" [13].

- "Current evidence suggests that popular alternative therapies such as massage, cryotherapy, and hyperbaric oxygen exposure as currently practiced on humans have little effect on recovery from minor muscle damage such as induced by exercise. While further research is still needed, hyperbaric oxygen exposure shows clear promise for potentially being a successful adjunct treatment for enhancing muscle repair and recovery from more severe crush or contusion injury in humans" [24].

Despite this prevalent view, interest in HBO_2 to treat normal wounds was stimulated when some professional sports teams began this practice in the early-to-mid 1990s. The first reported studies of HBO_2 as an adjunctive therapy for sports injuries were conducted by professional *football* (i.e., soccer) teams in Scotland beginning in the late 1980s. These studies, uncontrolled except for the teams' *physios' extensive past experience* with similar cases, showed that HBO_2 when added to their standard treatment regimens, significantly accelerated recovery from typical injuries without increased risk of relapse [25].[1] Following this research and an accumulation of related anecdotal experience, a number of professional sports teams in the United Kingdom and North America began the routine use of hyperbaric oxygen therapy to treat injured athletes. This in turn fostered research intended to explore, confirm, or perhaps in some cases, to refute [26–28] the efficacy of this application.

At present, controlled animal and human studies with uncompromised trauma to ligaments, tendons, muscles, and bone support the fact that hyperoxic therapy can significantly enhance the healing of normal wounds. A study of cutaneous wound healing using an animal model also attests to this fact, as do several reports on the practical application of HBO_2 to cosmetic surgery and research related to its use in uncompromised reconstructive surgery.

3.2 Enhanced and diminished healing

In the sections below, *enhanced healing* and *diminished healing* are critical aspects in discussing the outcomes of hyperoxic therapy regimens. By *enhanced healing*, we are referring to an outcome that is either significantly better in an absolute sense and/or has occurred significantly faster, temporally, than the outcome of some alternate therapy regimen or no therapy, whatsoever. By *diminished healing*, we are referring to an outcome that is either significantly inferior in an absolute sense and/or has occurred significantly slower, temporally, than the outcome of some alternate therapy regimen or no therapy, whatsoever.

While the superiority of a better absolute outcome (e.g., greater wound bursting strength, greater ligament stiffness, less scaring, greater survival of transferred autologous fat, and/or transplanted hair follicles) is obvious, the importance of faster healing of a normal wound may not be so apparent. After all, by definition, at some point in time, the outcomes of different therapy regimens for normal wounds should be identical [29]. There are, however, circumstances where faster healing can be of considerable importance.

As an example, if a surgeon suffers a severe knee injury while skiing and this prevents him from working until his injury has effectively healed, an actual situation we were approached about by an American surgeon seeking treatment with hyperbaric oxygen, a significantly faster recovery could reduce the work and income he would lose because of his accident. Likewise, in U.S. workers' compensation cases, if the cost of hyperoxic therapy to return an injured employee to work more quickly were more than offset by the reduction in the temporary total disability payments to the employee, then the insurance company would have a net reduction in its costs. At the same time, the employee would more quickly return to earning his or her full income. Thus, if the economics were born out in practice, this would be a win-win situation

[1] James PB. Hyperbaric oxygen in soft tissue injury. Report to the Directors of Dundee United F.C, 1989.

for both the injured employee and the worker's compensation insurer or equivalent in countries with different (e.g., national) healthcare management programs. Multiplied many times over, the amount that might be saved by insurance companies or national healthcare programs in such cases could be quite substantial.

An obvious situation for the benefit of faster recovery is in athletics. More rapid recovery from injury with the attendant reduction in deconditioning over the healing period translates into less lost competitions. In the case of professional sports where some athletes can make amounts as much as US$1M or even more per event, enabling that individual to compete through use of adjunctive HBO_2 when he would not have been able to do so otherwise could, in some cases, have profound financial impact and greatly influence the outcome of a season for the individual and/or his team. In many such cases, the cost of administering hyperbaric oxygen therapy would be moot. Consequently, the speed of recovery as well as the extent of recovery can be an important aspect of an outcome. Research that demonstrates the enhanced healing of normal wounds by hyperbaric oxygen therapy is summarized below.

3.3 Supporting evidence for treatment of normal wounds with HBO_2

Connective Tissue Healing: A prospective, randomized, double-blind study of the effects of HBO_2 on the healing of second-degree (Grade 2) medial collateral ligament sprains of the human knee demonstrated statistical differences in measured parameters and the way these values changed over time during the first 3 weeks of recovery [30]. In particular, range of motion, maximum flexion, reduction of edema determined by MRI, and functional running were significantly better in the HBO_2-treated subjects than in the control subjects.

In another human study of HBO_2 treatments for Grade 2 medial collateral ligament injuries of the knees of rugby players [31], visual analog scales done on the same day immediately before and after HBO_2 showed significant improvement when walking and jogging ($p < 0.001$ in both cases). Further, the mean time to return to competition was significantly reduced by 12.5 days in comparison with untreated (with HBO_2) control subjects ($p < 0.05$).

In a third human study of HBO_2 treatments for connective tissue involving Grade 2 ankle sprains, thirty-six patients were divided evenly into three groups (A, B, and C) and received seven treatments over 5 days breathing 100% oxygen in a multiplace chamber, each treatment with a duration of 90 minutes [32]. Two treatments per day were received on Days 1 and 2, and one treatment per day was received on Days 3, 4, and 5. Group A received treatments at 1.0 ATA; Group B received treatments at 2.0 ATA; and Group C received treatments at 2.5 ATA. At the end of the course of treatments, edema in the injured ankle of Group C was reduced by 97%, in Group B by 80%, and in Group A by only 30%. At the same point, Groups B and C had no pain in their injured ankle and Group A had reduced pain [32].

These three human studies have been complemented by a number of animal studies in which significant differences between HBO_2-treated and control animals in the healing of ligaments and tendons, assessed morphologically, histologically, biochemically, and mechanically were consistent with more rapid healing in the HBO_2-treated human groups.

- HBO_2 significantly enhanced recovery in the stiffness of experimentally lacerated medial collateral ligaments in rat knees and produced a strong tendency for ligament strength to recover more quickly, as well [33, 34].

- HBO_2 resulted in the more rapid increase of pro-a1 (I) mRNA assessed biochemically and the more rapid formation of collagen fibers assessed histologically following experimental laceration of the patellar tendons of rat knees [35].

- The healing of experimentally lacerated ligaments in the hind limbs of rats with HBO_2 treatments at 2.0 ATA for 60 minutes, 2.0 ATA for 30 minutes, and 1.5 ATA for 30 minutes were assessed morphologically, histologically, and biochemically and found to be enhanced when compared to controls breathing air at 1.0 ATA. Of the three HBO_2 conditions, 2.0 ATA for 60 minutes produced the best outcome [36].

- HBO_2 accelerated the healing of knee ligaments of rats from which a 2-mm segment was surgically removed [37]. Comparisons with controls included the formation of scar tissue assessed by macroscopic inspection, Type I procollagen gene expression assessed histochemically, and tensile strength and stiffness assessed mechanically.

- HBO_2 enhanced the outcome of anterior cruciate ligament reconstruction in a rabbit model [38]. Blindly assessed parameters including histological (i.e., fibrocartilage formation, new bone formation, tendon graft bonding to adjacent tissue, and the number of blood vessels in the area of tendon-bone junction); biomechanical (i.e., tensile strength of tendon and failure modes including graft pullout from the bone tunnel, graft rupture, and avulsion fracture of the tendon-bone junction); electron microscopic (i.e., nature and organization of regenerated collagen fibers).

Soft Tissue Healing: A study using a well-defined, blunt trauma model of skeletal muscle injury (i.e., contusions) in rats showed that HBO_2 inhibits the muscle wasting normally associated with such injuries [26]. A complementary study of muscle contusions in rats showed that HBO_2 accelerates the recovery of muscle function (i.e., twitch and tetanic force) in response to electrical stimulation [39].

Another study using calf muscle contusion in rats as a skeletal muscle injury model [40] found that among other effects, HBO_2 in the acute phase suppressed elevation of circulating macrophages and reduced both lower limb volume and the wet weight of the contused muscles. It also increased the amount of regenerated muscle fibers and, at 7 days, promoted isometric muscle strength. Thus, HBO_2 reduced early inflammation and accelerated myogenesis in muscle contusion injuries [40].

A fourth study investigating the effects of HBO_2 on reproducible muscle tears in rats found significantly increased hydroxyproline levels in the urine of treated rats compared to untreated control rats at 1- and 2-weeks post-injury [41]. It was concluded that HBO_2 enhances collagen metabolism which may be helpful for muscle healing.

A fifth study using a rabbit model to investigate the effects of HBO_2 on the healing of muscle stretch injuries showed highly significant functional (i.e., ankle isometric torque) and marked morphological differences (i.e., inflammation and damage around the muscle-tendon junction) between the HBO_2-treated and untreated control groups, with the HBO_2-treated group recovering more quickly [42].

Three other studies investigated the effects of HBO_2 on the functional and morphological properties of rat muscles regenerating from myotoxic injury. Two found significantly increased force-producing capacity and larger regenerating muscle fibers in the extensor digitorum longus [43] and the soleus [44], respectively, in HBO_2-treated animals compared to untreated control animals. In the soleus muscles, the difference between test and control muscles was significant at 14 days but not at 25 days [44].

The third study investigated recovery with HBO_2 from injury to the tibialis anterior muscles of rats induced by injecting cardiotoxin (CTX) into them [45]. The HBO_2 treatments consisted of 120 minutes of oxygen at 2.5 ATA once a day, 5 days per week for 2 weeks. In addition to untreated controls, other post-injury management utilized air at 2.5 ATA and oxygen at 1.0 ATA with the other treatment parameters similar to those for the HBO_2-treated subjects. Assessments comparing the HBO_2-treated rats to untreated controls, normobaric oxygen-treated animals, and hyperbaric-air-treated animals included histological analyses and measurement of the maximum force-producing capacity of the regenerating muscle fibers. The results showed that HBO_2 treatments accelerated satellite cell proliferation and myofiber maturation in rat muscle that was injured by a CTX injection, particularly at the end of the 2-week course of treatments. This suggested to Horie and associates [45] that HBO_2 treatments accelerate the healing and functional recovery of skeletal muscle after injury.

Finally, two studies evaluated the efficacy of HBO_2 for treating human muscle injuries. The first involved 20 patients who had sustained sports-related muscle injuries and were admitted to the hospital of Tokyo Medical and Dental School in Tokyo, Japan for therapy [46]. There, they received daily sessions of HBO_2 for 60 minutes at 2.8 ATA for 1 to 7 days. These treatments significantly improved before- and after-course-of-therapy results of visual analog scales (VAS) for resting pain and motion pain, the patient's subjective evaluation of edema, muscle stiffness measured with a muscle tonometer, and leg volume measured with a water-filled volumetric gauge for patients with gastrocnemius muscle injury [46].

The second was a blinded study of recovery from exercise-related (i.e., baseball) first-degree strains to skeletal muscles of the extremities [47]. This was conducted with HBO_2-treated human subjects compared to sham-treated control subjects. The HBO_2 treated subjects received 10 sessions of HBO_2 administered at 2.5 ATA twice per week for 5 weeks. Their hyperbaric oxygen treatments were given for 70 minutes at maximum pressure with two 5-min air breaks included in those periods. The control subjects breathed air at 1.3 ATA for 70 minutes with the same frequency. Significant reduction in levels of serum creatine phosphokinase, glutamic oxaloacetate transaminase, myoglobin, and other muscle enzymes were found in the HBO_2-treated subjects at the end of the course of therapy and persisted for the next 2 weeks over which they were monitored. No such changes were found in the control subjects. At the end of therapy, the Brief Pain Inventories for the HBO_2-treated subjects demonstrated significant reductions in the pain intensity subscale not found in the control subjects. It was concluded that the HBO_2 treatments accelerated recovery of humans from routine, sports-related muscle injuries.

The enhanced healing of normal wounds has also been reported outside the sphere of sports-type musculoskeletal injuries. The healing of a standardized wound to the ears of homozygous hairless mice was used to investigate the effect of HBO_2 on the reepithelialization and microvascular perfusion in normal and ischemic skin tissue [48]. It was found that HBO_2 at the dose employed significantly accelerated healing in normal tissue as well as ischemic tissue, though the relative improvement in healing was greater for ischemic wounds. As final examples of enhanced healing in normal soft-tissue and connective-tissue wounds, HBO_2 has been effectively utilized to improve outcomes in uncompromised reconstructive surgery [49, 50] and in laser face resurfacing by cosmetic surgeons [51–53].

Fracture/Bone Healing: With respect to bone repair/fracture healing, a number of studies have shown that hyperbaric oxygen enhances the various processes involved. In addition, anecdotal results of the benefits of HBO_2 for fracture healing in professional athletes have been noted [54], though literature surveys to support such application of HBO_2 have not produced formally reported findings to the standards of evidence-based medicine [54–56]. Despite this, a number of research publications have reported statistically significant enhanced bone repair in comparison with controls for fracture/bone damage properly classified as *normal*.

- Coulson et al. [57] produced closed fractures in one femur of rats and found that daily HBO_2 increased Ca^{++} deposition in the fracture callus and increased the breaking strength of the healing bone relative to that of the other, uninjured femur.

- Yablon and Cruess [20] studied the healing of experimental fractures of the femurs of rats. While no difference in healing between the HBO_2-treated and control animals was shown by standard X-rays after 9 days, significant differences in the time course of events were evident after 22 and 40 days with the HBO_2-treated animals healing more quickly.

- Natiella et al. [58] found that the healing of experimentally produced cryogenic injuries to the femurs of dogs was accelerated by HBO_2 though the 2 months this therapy was administered but did not produce a different long-term outcome.

- Wilcox and Kolodny [59] conducted a study on the effects of HBO_2 on the healing of mandibular and maxillary osteotomies in humans. Controls were retrospectively paired with untreated cases, and outcomes were assessed by two experienced surgeons. It was found that HBO_2 hastened the decrease in fracture mobility, thus reducing the need for post-immobilization retainers and training elastics. Wilcox and Kolodny [59] concluded that "hyperbaric oxygen augments clinical bone healing subsequent to osteotomy procedures."

- Karapetian et al. [60] reported that the healing of non-inflamed mandibular fractures in rats was enhanced by HBO_2 at 2.0 ATA.

- Barth et al. [61] found that holes drilled in the proximal and distal metaphyses of rat femurs filled in 4 weeks through enchondral ossification (i.e., differentiation to cartilage than bone) without HBO_2 and in 3 weeks through primary ossification (i.e., direct differentiation to bone) with a course of 20 HBO_2 treatments administered once a day 5 days per week.

- Johnsson et al. [50] found that a 21-day course of HBO_2, once a day at 2.8 ATA for 90 minutes, significantly increased the interface strength of a bone-titanium implant, both following irradiation and with no irradiation. The benefit was relatively larger in the case of irradiation, however.

- Ehler et al. [29] studied the effects of HBO_2 on autogenous cancellous bone graft healing in the canine femur. The breaking strength of the bones was assessed over time, and it was found that HBO_2 improved the outcomes early but produced no different result over the long term.

- Kitakoji et al. [62] studied the effects of HBO_2 on a lengthened callus model in rabbits. It was found that bone mineral density was significantly greater in the

HBO_2-treated animals than in the control animals after 1, 2, 3, and 4 weeks, with these differences tending to normalize after 5 and 6 weeks.

- Kawada et al. [63] studied the effect of HBO_2 on the healing of an open fracture model in mice. At 2 weeks post-fracture, the callus was significantly larger in the HBO_2-treated group than the control group. At four- and six-weeks post-fracture, radiographic findings showed accelerated healing in the HBO_2-treated group. At 6 weeks, bone stiffness and maximum load were significantly higher in the HBO_2-treated group. These results suggested that HBO_2 enhances bone anabolism and accelerates fracture healing.

In view of such factors as the recognized essential role of oxygen in all aspects of bone healing [16, 20], the substantial evidence for oxygen's enhancement of the healing of uncompromised trauma such as that cited in the approximately 30 studies above, and the considerable positive practical experience in the application of HBO_2 to actual sports injuries and cosmetic surgery cases[2] (e.g., [47, 51–53, 64–70]), understanding the basis for what we believed to be the hyperbaric medical community's mistaken dogma that hyperbaric oxygen therapy has no efficacy for normal wounds was of considerable interest to the authors. Consequently, an investigation was begun with several references suggested by a professional acquaintance, Dr. Eric Kindwall[3] who was a recognized expert in the field of hyperbaric medicine and a published proponent of the prevailing view on the treatment of normal wounds Kindwall et al. [22]. These citations were provided by Dr. Kindwall when he was asked about the foundation of his opinion on this specific issue. The analysis of these references led the authors to review other reports and the eventual *formation and validation* of a hypothesis concerning the general nature of oxygen dose-response described below.

3.4 Case against effectively treating normal wounds with HBO_2

In addition to the three references suggested by Dr. Kindwall (i.e., [1, 71, 72]), two similar references (i.e., [2, 73]) were discussed by Hunt et al. [21] in a chapter on the effects of oxygen in wound healing in an early text on hyperbaric oxygen therapy [74]. Because of the findings of the latter two research reports, particularly those of Penttinen et al. [73], Hunt and his associates concluded that hyperbaric oxygen therapy has no role in the healing of normal wounds [21]. This would seem to be the origin of the dogma in question that has persisted from 1977 to the present time (i.e., about 47 years as of early 2024).

As noted, the references listed immediately above would appear to have formed the foundation of the view that hyperbaric oxygen therapy is not of benefit for the treatment of normal wounds. Through critical analysis of these reports and their comparison to similar research conducted with different partial pressures of oxygen, we determined that oxygen has a biphasic dose-response relationship which impacts some outcomes of oxygen therapy differently than envisioned by its practitioners. So that readers may more easily understand the conclusion we reached in this endeavor, the references below are presented in greater detail than those discussed in the prior section of this report.

[2] Peterson RE, Allen MW. The adjunctive use of Hyperbaric Oxygen Therapy for the treatment of sports injuries. Hyperbaric Medicine 1995, Columbia, South Carolina, March 20-22, 1995.

[3] Peterson RE. Personal communication with Dr. Eric Kindwall, June 1996.

Lundgren and Sandberg [1]: A study to determine the effects of HBO_2 on the tensile strength of the healing skin of rats was conducted by Lundgren and Sandberg [1]. Incisions long enough to facilitate measuring the force required to rupture the healing wound three times were made on one side of a rat's back. The animal was then allowed to heal for 5 days, either with or without receiving HBO_2. After measuring the rupture force three times on that side, a similar procedure was performed on the other side of each rat's back with healing taking place in the manner opposite to that of the first case (i.e., with HBO_2 if HBO_2 were not administered initially; without HBO_2 if HBO_2 were administered initially). This permitted each rat to be its own control in the study. Five groups (i.e., A–E) of 7–8 animals, each, were included in the study.

- Group A received oxygen at 2.0 ATA for three, 120-minute sessions each day for 5 days. The tensile strength of the wound was 43% less with HBO_2 than without it, but three animals died from what was likely oxygen toxicity. Thus, this difference was not statistically significant due to the small group size of the treated animals, though in view of the results of Group B, the difference would certainly have been significant had there been more HBO_2-treated subjects alive at the end of the oxygen treatments.

- Group B received oxygen at 2.0 ATA for two, 120-minute sessions each day for 5 days. The tensile strength of the wound was 27% less with HBO_2 than without it. This difference was statistically significant ($p < 0.01$).

- Group C received oxygen at 1.5 ATA for two, 120-minute sessions each day for 5 days. The tensile strength of the wound was 6% less with HBO_2 than without it. This difference was not statistically significant.

- Group D received oxygen at 2.0 ATA for two, 120-minute sessions each day from Day 2 through Day 5 (i.e., a total of 4 days). The tensile strength of the wound was 2% more with HBO_2 than without it. This result was not statistically significant.

- Group E had the primary artery to the wound area ligated, reducing local blood flow, and received oxygen at 2.0 ATA for two, 120-minute sessions each day for 5 days as with Group B. The tensile strength of the wound was 8% less with HBO_2 than without it. This result was not statistically significant.

Clearly, these results indicate that HBO_2 in the higher doses administered in this study impedes healing in comparison with no HBO_2. This would superficially support the contention that HBO_2 is not efficacious for normal wounds.

It is also clear, however, that as the dose of inspired oxygen was progressively reduced, the experimental outcome (i.e., wound tensile strength) progressively improved. Further, a comparison of Groups B and E, which had the same HBO_2 treatment schedule, shows that a lower dose of oxygen local to the wound site, caused by ligation of the primary artery, improved the outcome.

In discussing their results, Lundgren and Sandberg [1] observed that the outcomes appeared *dose-dependent* (**Figure 3**). In view of the outcome for Group E and since oxygen delivery to the wound sites in Groups A, B, C, and D would be directly related to the oxygen doses of the hyperbaric oxygen treatments, it appears that the outcomes of this study were inversely related to the oxygen dose at the wound site. Thus, the lower the dose of oxygen used of those included in this study local to the wound, the better the outcome.

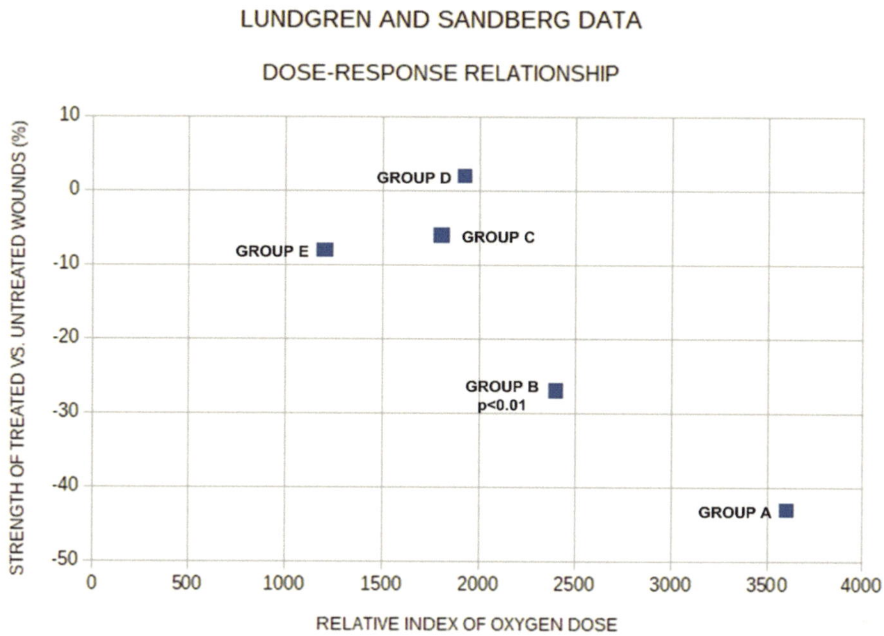

Figure 3.
*Data for Lundgren and Sandberg's [1] five groups showing a decline in outcomes as the dose of oxygen was increased. What we shall call the relative index of oxygen dose was calculated as the PO_2 of treatment (Tx) * duration of Tx * frequency of Tx * days of Tx for Groups A, B, C, and D. Group E, with the ligated primary artery to the wound region impacting negatively on healing, it was arbitrarily assumed that the dose index was reduced by ½ after calculation as described for the other groups, above.*

As a final point, some of the doses of oxygen used in the Lundgren and Sandberg study [1], particularly for Group A, were greater than is typical for clinical cases involving the treatment of tissues with impaired oxygen delivery. The fact that three of the seven HBO_2-treated animals in this group died after 3 days of treatment from what could readily be construed to be oxygen poisoning strongly suggests that this dose of oxygen was excessively high [1].

Kulonen and Niinikoski [71]: Research was conducted by Kulonen et al. [2] on the impact of hyperoxic therapy at normobaric pressure on normal wound healing. They found significantly positive impacts of normobaric hyperoxygenation in direct relation to the PO_2 (i.e., 35 and 70% oxygen in comparison with 21% oxygen Kulonen et al. [2]). Kulonen and Niinikoski [71] then wished to extend these findings to hyperbaric oxygen conditions. In this latter study, the tensile strengths of healing skin wounds and granulomas were determined for groups of HBO_2-treated rats and control animals that did not receive HBO_2. Hyperbaric oxygen was administered at 2.0 ATA for two, 120-minute sessions each day with a 120-minute interval between them. These treatments started in the morning immediately after wounding and extended for 3 days or 9 days. Assessments were made the day after treatment ended (i.e., Days 4 and 10 for the two groups, respectively). The tensile strength of the healing skin wounds and the granulomas were significantly less in the HBO_2-treated rats than in the control animals ($p < 0.0005$) at both 4 and 10 days. All animals gained weight normally over the course of the study and there were no signs or symptoms of oxygen poisoning (i.e., convulsions) in the treated groups. Considering their positive outcomes with hyperoxic breathing gas at 1 atm, Kulonen and Niinikoski [71] concluded that the optimal concentration of oxygen for healing had been exceeded in this hyperbaric oxygen study.

Wray and Rodgers [72]: A study to determine the effects of HBO_2 on the breaking load of tibial fractures in rats was conducted by Wray and Rodgers [72]. Fractures were produced with a rotary saw, and HBO_2 at 2.0 ATA was administered 6 hours a day for from 20 to 26 days starting 1 day after a fracture. A control group received no HBO_2.

Results showed that despite increased callus activity on histological examination, the breaking loads for healing fractures with HBO_2 were lower than those in the untreated control group. This result was not statistically significant but was strongly suggestive ($0.05 < p < 0.07$). The authors concluded that their hyperbaric oxygen regimen produced local tissue oxygen levels that were too high and resulted in adverse (i.e., toxic) effects on the cells, perhaps altering the lysosomal membrane [72].

Other notable points included that the HBO_2-treated rats gained less weight than the control rats over the study period, though this difference was not statistically significant; and nine HBO_2-treated rats died from "pulmonary complications" when one of the 6-hour treatments was inadvertently allowed to overrun by about 14 hours.

Niinikoski [3]: In this report, Niinikoski comprehensively covers material addressed in a number of prior publications [2, 71, 75–77]. The latter of these Kulonen and Niinikoski (i.e., [71]) was one of the reports cited by Kindwall and has been discussed above. As the pertinent information from Niinikoski [3] concerning the impact of HBO_2 on normal wounds has, therefore, already been presented in detail, it will not be repeated here.

Penttinen et al. [73]: The effects of HBO_2 on fracture healing in rats were assessed. Both tibias of the subject rats were broken in the middle of the diaphysis by manually bending them to an angle of 90° under anesthesia. HBO_2 was begun immediately and administered at 2.5 ATA for 120 minutes twice daily until sacrifice [73].

In comparison with untreated control animals 11–21 days post-fracture, the healing fractures of the HBO_2-treated animals had significantly greater collagen formation and accumulation of minerals. The tensile strength of the calluses of the HBO_2-treated fractures, however, were not different from those of untreated control fractures, nor were the RNA/DNA ratios of callus cells as reported in a related publication different than those of untreated control fractures [78]. These results suggested to Hunt and associates [21] that hyperbaric oxygen by itself does not accelerate bone healing in normal wounds.

3.5 Further consideration of oxygen dose response

In contrast to the results of Lundgren and Sandberg [1] and Kulonen and Niinikoski [71] in which the bursting force for healing skin wounds was generally less for HBO_2-treated rats than control animals, Meltzer and Myers [79] reported greater bursting strength for healing incisional skin wounds in HBO_2-treated rats than in untreated controls at 3 days and 7 days post-wounding. In Meltzer and Myers' study, however, HBO_2 was administered at 2.5 ATA for 120 minutes only three times, once a day at 0-, 24-, and 48-hours following creation of the experimental incisions.

In comparison, Lundgren and Sandberg [1], at the extreme (i.e., Group A), administered HBO_2 at 2.0 ATA for 120 minutes three times daily for 5 days. In the next most extreme case of oxygen exposure (i.e., Lundgren and Sandberg Group B), HBO_2 was administered at 2.0 ATA for 120 minutes twice daily for 5 days. As noted above, the wound bursting strength of this latter group was significantly lower than for wounds healing in the untreated (i.e., without HBO_2) control animals and the wound bursting strength for the former (i.e., A) group was only insignificantly lower than the untreated controls because of the subject fatalities almost certainly due to oxygen toxicity.

Likewise, Kulonen and Niinikoski [71] administered greater doses of oxygen than Meltzer and Meyers [79]. Their exposures were comparable to Lundgren and Sandberg's Group B, 2.0 ATA for 120 minutes twice daily for 3 or 9 days. As with Lundgren and Sandberg's Group B outcome, the bursting strength of the healing wounds in Kulonen and Niinikoski's study was significantly lower for the HBO_2-treated rats than for the untreated controls.

Parallel results have been reported for HBO_2 administered for bone repair. Wray and Rodgers [72] found decreased breaking force (not quite statistically significant) in HBO_2-treated animals in comparison to their control animals for the healing fractures. Penttinen et al. [78] found unchanged tensile strength in the healing fractures of the femurs of rats for HBO_2-treated animals in comparison to untreated controls. Wray and Rodgers sectioned one tibia of each subject rat with a rotary saw and administered HBO_2 at 2.0 ATA for 6 hours a day for from 20 to 26 days to the test group. The rebreaking loads for the healing fractures of the test and control groups were then compared to the breaking load for the animals' uninjured tibias. The HBO_2-treated animals were found to have lower relative rebreaking loads than the untreated controls. Penttinen et al. [78] administered HBO_2 to their subject rats at 2.5 ATA for 120 minutes twice daily from the fracture creation until sacrifice and found no difference in the rebreaking load compared to the untreated controls.

In contrast, Coulson et al. [57] administered HBO_2 at 3.0 ATA for 120 minutes to rats once daily from the time a 3/32-inch defect was created in the rats' left femurs with a dental drill until sacrifice at 2 weeks. With this reduced therapy regimen, the strain necessary to break the healing femur was found to be 93% of that of the uninjured right femur, on average, for the HBO_2-treated rats, and only 82% of the uninjured right femur, on average, for the untreated control rats.

A study supplementing the bone repair findings summarized above was conducted by Barth et al. [61]. As noted previously, they found that HBO_2 at 2.0 ATA for 120 minutes once a day for 20 days significantly accelerated bone repair in rats and resulted in notably greater blood vessel in-growth into the new bone than that occurring in untreated control animals. In contrast, HBO_2 administered at 2.0 ATA for 120 minutes twice a day for 10 days significantly retarded bone repair and blood vessel in-growth into the holes compared to untreated controls. In the case of the rats treated twice a day with HBO_2, the holes were filled by enchondral ossification in 5 weeks, a full week (i.e., 25%) longer than the untreated control animals and two full weeks (i.e., 67%) longer than the animals treated only once per day with HBO_2. Further, at 5 weeks, there were still islets of cartilage in the forming plugs of the animals treated twice per day.

While the studies summarized immediately above do show that HBO_2, under certain circumstances, can produce healing of normal wounds not better than or even inferior to that without adjunctive HBO_2, there is a consistent pattern through all of them. When healing in either soft tissue, connective tissue, or bone was adversely affected by hyperoxic therapy, the doses of oxygen were high, either in absolute terms or relative to other experimental protocols which produced the opposite (i.e., beneficial) outcomes. In other words, *higher doses of oxygen hindered healing for*

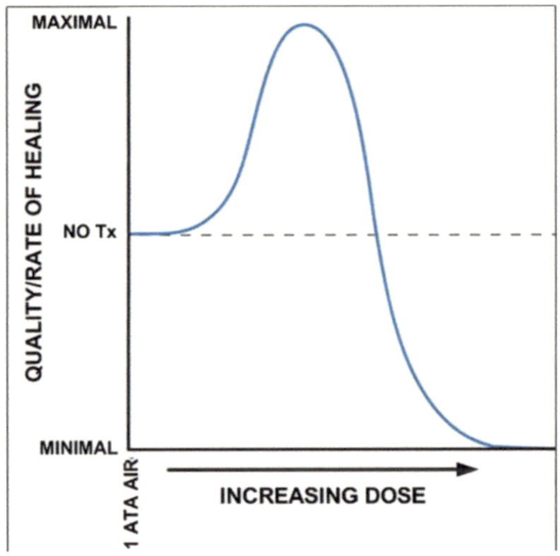

Figure 4.
Oxygen dose-response relationship envisioned by the authors circa 2000 to illustrate the understanding they had evolved through extensive research and analysis of the scientific and medical literature on hyperoxic treatments of a variety of wounds to soft tissues, connective tissues, and bones [80, 81].

uncompromised wounds! In support of the Barth and associates' findings, Karapetian et al. [60] reported that while the healing of non-inflamed mandibular fractures in rats was enhanced by HBO_2 at 2.0 ATA, it was hindered by HBO_2 administered at 2.5 ATA.

This insight suggested to the authors that the oxygen dose-response relationship has a descending limb at high doses. Thus, we developed the biphasic dose-response relationship shown in **Figure 4** which at the high dose end eventually goes below the level of response to normal conditions (i.e., no supplemental oxygen administration, whatsoever).

4. Is hyperoxic therapy dose dependent?

4.1 Common dose-response relationship

When dealing with therapeutic drugs, the most common dose-response relationship considered seems likely to be the one that is for a substance that has only beneficial effects or that is used at dose levels where only beneficial effects occur. After reaching a threshold for effects to begin to take place, the response increases until a maximum level is reached. Then, the response goes no higher. This type of pharmaceutical agent has the typical sigmoidal response when the dose is plotted on a logarithmic scale (**Figure 5**).

In view of absolutely no mention of a different type of dose-response relationship, this must certainly be the one most healthcare professionals and researchers are familiar with and/or think of when considering higher doses of oxygen. Clearly, without statements to the contrary, when considering hyperbaric oxygen doses in the treatment of normal (i.e., uncompromised) wounds, Hunt et al. [21] could not have imagined there to be a biphasic oxygen dose-response relationship with a down-side at higher doses (**Figure 4**). Nor could Margolis et al. [13]; Kindwall et al. [22]; Quirinia and Viidik [23]; nor Tiidus [24] have considered such a dose-response relationship when they published their statements about HBO_2 and normal wounds. It seems that they all

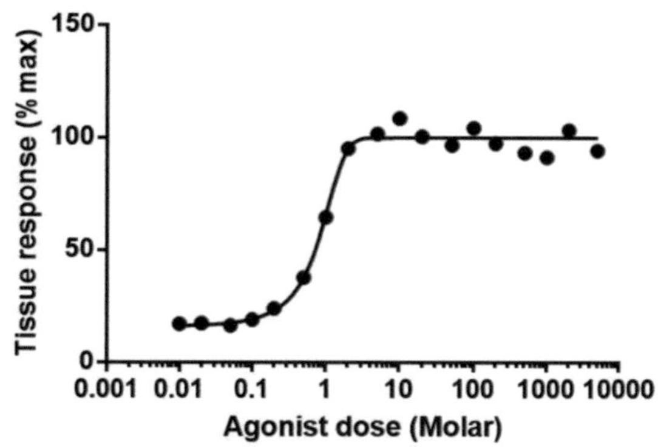

Figure 5.
A simulated dose-response curve for the stimulation of a tissue by an agonist with a $\log_{10}$ (EC50) of 0.70. This curve was generated in GraphPad Prism with a randomized relative error of 5% and with a fitted curve following the Hill Equation. This shows a typical, sigmoidal dose-response relationship with low doses insufficient to generate a response while higher doses ultimately reach a maximum response and go no higher (JM Goodman 17 July 2019. Licensed by Wikipedia under the Creative Commons Attribution-Share Alike 4.0 international (https://crelativecommons.org/licenses/by-sa/4.0/deed.En) license).

had lost sight of the fact that unlike most pharmaceuticals where amount (equivalent to the partial pressure of a gas (oxygen) and frequency of administration) is the critical aspects of dose, hyperoxic treatments are also dependent upon the duration of exposure. Thus, any given P_iO_2, and most especially higher values within the 2.0 to 3.0 atm envelope can span values across the entire dose-response range with longer and longer treatments Clark et al. [82]. In addition to Lundgren and Sandberg's [1] observation that their results of utilizing hyperbaric oxygen therapy to treat cutaneous wounds in rats appeared to demonstrate dose dependence, though it was not stated that this relationship was the inverse of how dose-response is routinely thought of (**Figure 3**). Barr and Perrins [4] made a similar general observation for human patients:

> *"The response to HBO_2 is clearly dose-dependent. Some ulcers (i.e., non-healing wounds) respond to 1.5 ATA while others require up to 3.0 ATA. Some fail to respond to 2 hours a day, while others heal with less than 1 hour a day. This anomaly probably results from differing vascularity in the affected limbs and how late HBO is applied in the destructive phase."*

In view of the conflicting research outcomes that have led to the belief that hyperbaric oxygen therapy is not effective for normal wounds, if hyperoxic therapy is dose-dependent, then this relationship must be along the lines of that shown in **Figure 4** which was constructed by the authors in the early 2000s [80, 81]. This relationship has a progressively increasing benefit over the lower range of doses, then at higher doses, has a progressively decreasing or negative impact, ultimately falling below the no-hyperoxic-therapy-at-all response, as per the Lundgren and Sandberg [1] findings (**Figure 3**).

In considering this hypothesis from a superficial standpoint, it seemed to fit our practical experience in treating sports injuries and cosmetic surgery cases. At the outset, the chamber most frequently used for these treatments was the HYOX HTU (**Figure 6**). This chamber has an upper pressure limit of 2.0 ATA, and the treatments conducted in it were usually only an hour in duration once a day, though some treatments for fractures were 90-minutes long, and occasionally, serious injuries occurring during sports

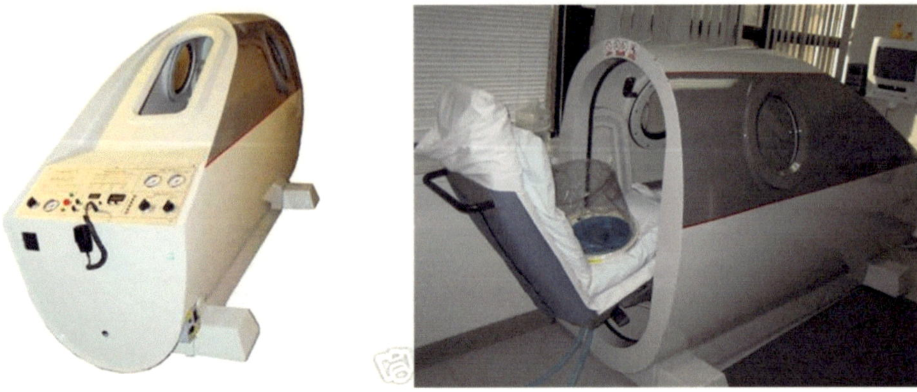

Figure 6.
HYOX HTU is the 2.0 ATA monoplace chamber used in many treatments of athletes and cosmetic surgery cases. The chamber is compressed with air and oxygen is breathed by mask or hood. The gas exhaled by the patient is dumped overboard.

competition were treated twice a day, but only for a day or two. Thus, the doses used to treat uncompromised sports injuries and cosmetic surgery wounds were, in our experience, typically lower than those administered in routine clinical HBO_2.

With this view in mind, we set out to determine if there were sufficient data in the scientific and clinical literature to conclusively establish that the oxygen dose-response relationship is of the general nature as shown in **Figure 4**. Fortuitously, the literature from the 1960s into the 2000s is rife with research relevant to this inquiry, including the data already presented, which concerns a variety of tissues, wound types, and methods of assessment.

As a critical test, we determined if the hyperbaric oxygen doses administered in the treatment of normal wounds which produced negative outcomes were significantly greater in comparison with those hyperbaric oxygen therapy doses which produced positive outcomes with normal wounds. To do this, we utilized both the human and animal data described previously in this report computing a parameter we have called the *mean relative index of oxygen dose per day* (i.e., Tx PO_2 * Tx duration * #Tx/day) as the values to compare.[4] These data include a variety of soft tissue wounds (e.g., muscle and skin), connective tissue wounds (e.g., ligaments and tendons), and bone breaks/injuries. In addition, the research consisted of many different approaches to assessing healing including morphological, histological, mechanical, biochemical, radiological, and functional. Of the data related to positive outcomes for the treatment of normal wounds with hyperbaric oxygen therapy, thirty-six reports with forty-one different outcomes have been used in the analysis presented here [20, 26, 29–34, 37–44, 46, 48–53, 57–63, 71, 79, 83–86]. Regarding the negative outcomes, 10 reports with thirteen different outcomes have been utilized [1, 60, 61, 71–73, 78, 85, 87–89]. The statistical parameters calculated and included in this comparison are given in **Table 1**. The oxygen doses producing negative outcomes when treating normal wounds were very significantly higher than those oxygen doses which produced positive outcomes

[4] While a published calculation for some specific aspect of oxygen toxicity could be used for this calculation (e.g., Cumulative Pulmonary Oxygen Dose) Peterson [83], these tend to weigh higher pressures of oxygen and/or longer exposure durations to oxygen more heavily. Since it was our objective to determine if unweighted exposures to oxygen were different, we used the straightforward computation described above in this report.

Parameter	Negative outcomes	Positive outcomes
Number of samples	13	41
Mean dose/day	805.4	222.0
Standard deviation	233.5	107.2
One-tailed t-value	8.722	
Degrees of freedom	52	

Table 1.
Statistical comparison of mean relative index of oxygen dose per day for hyperbaric oxygen treatments that produced negative outcomes with normal wounds to hyperbaric oxygen treatments that produced positive outcomes with normal wounds [90]. The number of degrees of freedom was computed with this same data [90]. A table of one-tailed t-test values was used to determine the statistical significance of the amount by which the mean index of oxygen dose per day for the negative outcomes exceeded the mean index of oxygen dose per day for the positive outcomes (Table of Critical Values) [91].

(i.e., $P < 0.00005$). Thus, we conclude that the outcomes of oxygen treatments are definitely dose-dependent with significant relative overdose producing inferior outcomes to those achieved with lower doses.

4.2 Oxygen dose-response relationship

In 2011, while researching general references related to dose-response on the Internet, the authors encountered the term, "hormesis" [92]. In toxicology, hormesis is a dose-response phenomenon typically characterized by low-dose stimulation and high-dose inhibition [93–95]. This relationship produces a biphasic dose-response curve [94] as shown in **Figure 7**. This matched almost exactly the dose-response relationship the authors had independently derived for oxygen therapy, **Figure 4**, which underlays the hormetic curve below. Upon further investigation, we found that oxygen was already on lists of hormetic agents [97], though not for the same reason as our independent development of an hormetic dose-response relationship.

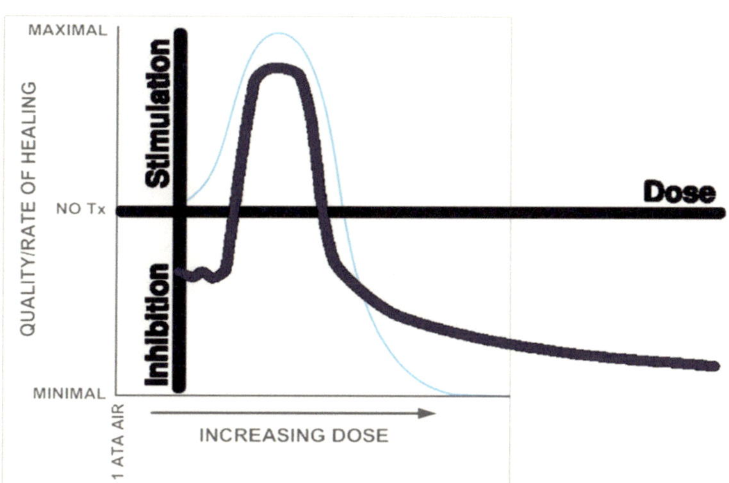

Figure 7.
*Example of hormetic dose-response relationship from Wikipedia article circa April 2021 "Hormesis", which is released under the Creative Commons Attribution-Share-Alike License 3.0 [96]. Our independent derivation of the dose-response relationship for oxygen (i.e., **Figure 4**) is shown in the background [80].*

An important aspect of hormesis is that agents which exhibit it are likely to produce preconditioning to stressful situations with exposures in the lower-dose range. For this reason, hormesis is also referred to by a number of different terms such as preconditioning, conditioning, pretreatment, cross-tolerance, adaptive homeostasis, and rapid stress hardening (mostly low temperature rapid cold hardening) [94].

Oxygen, however, is outside typical patterns for hormesis as we are routinely exposed to a finite level (i.e., air that has a P_iO_2 just lower than 0.21 atm, 0.20954 atm). Thus, regarding preconditioning, oxygen has the potential to have hormetic relationships in both the higher dose (i.e., hyperoxic) and lower dose (i.e., hypoxic) directions, and this has indeed been found to be the case.

4.3 Hypoxic preconditioning

For over 45 years, low oxygen has been one of the leading stressors known to confer protective preconditioning/hormetic effects [98]. These effects frequently relate to animals, both invertebrates and vertebrates, withstanding prolonged periods of anoxia or hypoxia. Such benefits of lower than normal oxygen are based on a hypothesis of "preparation for oxidative stress" (i.e., POS) [99], where, upon experiencing a decrease in oxygen levels, mitochondria prepare for the ensuing oxygen reperfusion by elevating cellular defenses, particularly oxidative stress defenses [100–102]. The need for antioxidant defenses with reperfusion of an ischemic wound results from the buildup of substances in the wound during the hypoxic or anoxic phase which, when the wound is reperfused with oxygen laden blood leads to the formation of reactive oxygen species with the potential to cause serious secondary injury [103].

An example of preconditioning at lower levels of oxygen than in room air entails a protective effect on the central nervous system. This was demonstrated through vascular remodeling which took place *via* two separate pathways in mice after 7 days of continuous hypoxic preconditioning with an oxygen concentration between 21 and 8% [104]. When breathing 13% oxygen, endothelial hyperplasia was triggered and expanded the capillary network. When breathing 12% oxygen, endothelial hypertrophy was triggered leading to expansion of large vessels and arteriogenesis. Such hypoxic conditioning had biphasic dose-response relationships with the maximum response when the mice were breathing about 10% oxygen [104].

4.4 Hyperoxic preconditioning

Exposures to hyperoxic conditions have also been demonstrated to protect against reduced delivery of oxygen and glucose to various tissues.

- Huang et al. [105] investigated the effects of HBO_2 PC (i.e., HBO_2 preconditioning) against reduced delivery of oxygen and glucose (OGD: oxygen glucose deprivation) as stress to the spinal cord. Heat shock proteins (HSP) were found in *in vitro* spinal neuron culture after only one exposure to HBO_2. When OGD or H_2O_2 stresses with and without HSP inhibitors were compared, the peak effect was found to be at 12 hours post-preconditioning, but active immediately afterwards. It was determined that HBO_2-PC protects by upregulating HSP 32 expression.

- Duan et al. [106] investigated hyperoxic preconditioning for stroke. Several regimens of hyperbaric oxygen preconditioning including once every other day for five sessions (A), once every other day for three sessions (B), once every day for five sessions (C), and once every day for three sessions (D) caused infarct size to be significantly reduced following middle cerebral artery occlusion. The greatest difference was for the A group. Preconditioning patterns of once every day for two sessions (E), once every 12 hours for four sessions (F), once every 12 hours for two sessions (G), and a single session (H) produced results statistically similar to untreated controls. The benefits of the hyperoxic preconditioning appeared to be related to stimulation of angiogenesis.

- Tähepõld et al. [107] reported on heart protection against simulated stroke in rats and mice from prior preconditioning with hyperoxic gas (i.e., up to 95% oxygen) at normal barometric pressure (i.e., 1.0 atmospheres absolute). They found that the PPO_2 and duration of the preconditioning impacted on effectiveness and there were also species variations.

- Touleimat et al. [108] found hyperbaric oxygen therapy administered at 2.4 ATA for 90 minutes 5 days in a week produced a small but significant change in lung diffusing capacity. When Dr. Conoscenti was queried about this following the report, he noted that after the subsequent week of hyperbaric oxygen therapy for the group included in the study, the lung function changes that were found after 1 week had normalized. Thus, the initial hyperbaric oxygen exposures apparently produced accommodation to the reported changes [109][5]

Other supporting facts for the hormetic nature of the oxygen dose-response can be found among conditions that have been treated with clinical HBO_2. These mirror the results of research and practical experience with normal wounds. With very high doses of oxygen, HBO_2 has been found to be of no benefit or even counterproductive and sometimes lethal with animal subjects due to oxygen poisoning. With lower doses, positive outcomes and/or practical benefits have been achieved. Some examples of this come from the literature on the survival of ischemic skin flaps:

- Negative outcomes: Kernahan et al. [87]; Caffee and Gallagher [88].

- Positive outcomes: Champion et al. [85]; Tan et al. [83]; Perrins [110]; Jurell and Kaijser [111].

All in all, since beginning to evolve our model of oxygen dose-response in 1996, some 26-plus years ago, the authors have yet to encounter research or practical application that did not fit the concepts of the model we have established and described here.

4.5 Oxygen toxicity

That oxygen is a biological toxin is well established [82, 112–119]. In sufficiently high doses, it is believed that oxygen is detrimental to all living cells [120]. Such effects result from the formation of reactive oxygen species (ROS) which damage many molecules in cells including DNA, RNA, and amino acids in proteins [118, 119, 121]. ROS also inactivates enzymes by oxidizing co-factors [122]. Polyunsaturated fats in membrane phospholipids are particularly sensitive to oxidation by ROS causing increased membrane rigidity, decreased activity of membrane-bound enzymes, altered activity of membrane

[5] Peterson RE. Personal communication with Craig Conoscenti MD., 1996.

receptors, and altered membrane permeability [119]. These effects are on the plasma and mitochondrial membranes of cells as well as their endomembrane system [122]. In view of such broad molecular and physiological impact of relatively high doses of oxygen, it is a logical conclusion that such actions should ultimately produce a net negative impact on the healing of damaged/wounded tissue which is overexposed to oxygen. Several studies on the impact of reactive oxygen species on tissue healing confirm this. A study by Ŝenel et al. [123] showed that ROS can adversely affect healing in ischemic wounds. A study by Stewart, Moore, Bennett et al. [124] showed that ROS can adversely affect the healing of wounds treated with hyperbaric oxygenation.

- Ŝenel et al. [123] conducted studies to determine the effect of oxygen radicals on wound healing in ischemic tissue. For this, they assessed the bursting force and, as an indicator of collagen metabolism, hydroxyproline content of the healing cross-member of an "H" incision on the back of rats as previously described by Quirina and Viidik [23]. These assessments were done at 7- and 14-days post-surgery in each of four groups: Untreated control group; group treated with superoxide dismutase (SOD), an oxygen radical scavenger; group treated with allopurinol, a xanthine oxidase inhibitor; control group with a normal, non-ischemic incisional skin wound (i.e., not an "H" incision) and no post-surgical treatments Ŝenel et al. [123]. In addition, a histopathological evaluation was conducted to assess the amount and organization of collagen in the healing cross-members of the "H" incisions on the backs of the rats in each of the three groups that received these.

  In this study, Ŝenel and Associates [123] found that allopurinol administration increased the bursting force of the "H" cross-member in comparison with the control group by 52% at 7 days ($p < 0.002$) and by 109% at 14 days ($p < 0.001$). The SOD administration, on the other hand, increased the bursting force of the "H" cross-member by 69% in comparison to the control group at both 7 and 14 days ($p < 0.003$ and $p < 0.002$, respectively). With respect to the other assessed parameters, the allopurinol-treated group was found to have a 75% greater hydroxyproline content than the control group on Day 7 ($p < 0.03$); the SOD-treated group was found to have 113% greater hydroxyproline content than the control group on Day 7 ($p < 0.001$). From the histopathological evaluation, the amount and organization of collagen was more prominent in the allopurinol- and SOD-treated groups than in the ischemic controls. Based on these outcomes, Ŝenel and Associates [123] concluded that oxygen free radicals play an important role in the failure of ischemic wound healing, and that antioxidants partially improve the healing of ischemic skin wounds.

- Stewart et al. [124] conducted studies of random-pattern skin flap healing in rats to determine whether treatment with hyperbaric oxygen (i.e., 2.5 ATA for 90 minutes once per day) and administration of free-radical scavengers (i.e., either superoxide dismutase plus catalase, or α-tocopheral acetate) or a free-radical inhibitor (i.e., allopurinol) would result in increased survival over hyperbaric oxygen, alone. Flap survival was determined by fluorescein injection, and tissue damage was determined by the degree of lipid peroxidation.

  At 7 days post-flap creation, hyperbaric oxygen plus both free-radical scavengers significantly improved flap survival ($p < 0.05$) while hyperbaric oxygen alone, allopurinol alone, and allopurinol in combination with hyperbaric oxygen did not produce a significantly different outcome than no treatments, whatsoever. At the same point post-surgery, lipid peroxidation associated with the hyperbaric oxygen was prevented by the administration of both free-radical scavengers, but not by the free-radical inhibitor.

With respect to the effectiveness of the two different scavengers (i.e., superoxide dismutase (SOD) plus catalase, or α-tocopheral acetate), the α-tocopheral acetate was found to be slightly superior. In conclusion, the investigators determined that moderate doses of free-radical scavengers or antioxidants in combination with conservative hyperbaric oxygen can improve the survival of random pattern skin flaps [124] in comparison with no hyperoxic therapy, or hyperoxic therapy administered without such antioxidant defenses.

In addition, the 1990 study by Barth et al. [61] introduced previously in this report, demonstrates that the holes drilled in proximal and distal metaphyses of rat femurs filled in 3 weeks through primary ossification when HBO_2 was administered once a day, in 4 weeks through enchondral ossification without HBO_2, and in 5 weeks through enchondral ossification when HBO_2 was administered twice a day. In prior research conducted by Bassett and Herrmann [125], it was determined that *in vitro* connective tissue cells, cut free from a clot of such cells and exposed to modestly elevated levels of oxygen (i.e., 35% with 5% CO_2 and balance N_2) would compact and differentiate directly to osseous tissue (primary ossification). Connective tissue cells cut free from the larger mass and exposed to reduced levels of oxygen (i.e., 5% with 5% CO_2 and balance N_2) would compact and differentiate to cartilage (enchondral ossification). This suggests that while one treatment per day of HBO_2 produced the expected result with hyperoxic treatments in the Barth study, rapid filling of the hole through primary ossification, no HBO_2 treatments and two treatments per day both behaved as if exposed to *hypoxic* levels of oxygen and filled the holes through enchondral ossification. Thus, in the case of two HBO_2 treatments per day in the Barth study, the benefits of the first treatment were more than offset by the second so an outcome less than that of no HBO_2 treatments was achieved. Consequently, the logical explanation for the dose-response relationship shown in **Figure 4** and supported by the studies discussed above is that as the treatment dose increases, the impact of the toxic effects of oxygen progressively inhibits, interferes with, and eventually more than cancels out the beneficial effects of hyperoxic therapy for healing the wounded tissue.

In view of the above, the outcome of hyperoxic treatment can be seen as the net result of the various beneficial and adverse effects at the specific wound site, and here, we are referring to "wound" in the broadest sense, so this could be an ulcerating wound such as a Wagner Grade 5 diabetic foot or the mildest of delayed onset muscle soreness (DOMS). This provides for a continuum of results with hyperoxic treatments from non-existent to optimally beneficial to neutral to negative depending on the local balance between all factors involved.

Acknowledgments

By Russell E. Peterson, Ph.D: I would like to thank my mother, Pauline W. Peterson, whose interest in medicine and the medical sciences led to my career in diving and hyperbaric medicine and physiology. I would also like to acknowledge my graduate school mentor, Christian J. Lambertsen, M.D., whose guidance to believe in one's own observations rather than the beliefs of others was a critical element in the evolution of this publication.

By Michael W. Allen: I would like to thank my parents, Phyllis P. and William G. Allen, who blessed me with an inquisitive mind and a need for constant learning. I would also like to thank Philip B. James M.D., Ph.D, my early mentor and lifelong friend who fostered my interest in pressure physiology and the potential offered by the use of oxygen in medicine.

Funding statement

The entire literature review, development of concepts, and preparation of this report were funded by the authors. No outside funding was sought or received from any source.

Conflict of interest

The authors are the Founding Partners of Microbaric® Oxygen Systems, LLC, now known as NEMO Therapeutics, LLC, which was established to provide an organization through which research in applications of normobaric oxygen therapy, particularly autism spectrum disorders, could be investigated and, as possible and appropriate, made available as a mainstream medical therapy for autism and other neurological conditions for which there is currently no effective treatment. This organization has been funded in full by the Founding Partners. No outside funding or income has been received to support the research and writing of business-related activities or this review of oxygen dose response.

Data availability

All publications cited as journal or book references in this manuscript are available from the National Center for Biotechnology Information, U.S. National Library of Medicine: 8600 Rockville Pike, Bethesda MD, 20894. www.ncbi.nlm.nih.gov/pubmed and other scientific and university databases.

Author details

Russell E. Peterson* and Michael W. Allen
NEMO Therapeutics, LLC, Sarasota, Florida, USA

*Address all correspondence to: repeterson@nemotherapy.com

References

[1] Lundgren C, Sandberg N. Influence of hyperbaric oxygen on the tensile strength of healing wounds in rats. In: Ledingham IM, editor. Hyperbaric Oxygenation: Proceedings of the Second International Congress. London: ES Livingston Ltd; 1965. pp. 293-396

[2] Kulonen E, Niinikoski J, Penttinen R. Effect of the supply of oxygen on the tensile strength of healing skin wounds and granulation tissue. Acta Physiologica Scandinavica. 1967;**70**:112-115

[3] Niinikoski J. Effect of oxygen supply on wound healing and formation of experimental granulation tissue. Acta Physiologica Scandinavica. 1969;**334**(Suppl.):1-72

[4] Barr P-O, Perrins DJD. Prolonged use of hyperbaric oxygen (HBO) in indolent ulcers of the leg. In: Proceedings of the Eighth International Congress on Hyperbaric Medicine. Long Beach, California August 20-22. 1984. pp. 217-222

[5] Sadeghani K, Gottlieb SF, Van Meter K, Farris B. The effect of increased oxygen tensions on healing surgical wounds. In: Undersea and Hyperbaric Medical Society, Inc. Annual Scientific Meeting Held 6-11 June 1989. Honolulu, Hawaii, USA: Hawaiian Regent Hotel. Available from: http://archive.rubicon-foundation.org/6629

[6] Hill RK Jr. Is more better: A comparison of different clinical hyperbaric treatment pressures – A preliminary report. In: Undersea and Hyperbaric Medical Society, Inc. Annual Scientific Meeting Held July 7-10, 1993. Halifax, Nova Scotia, Canada: World Trade Centre; 1993

[7] Ehler WJ, Marx RE, Peleo MJ. Oxygen as a drug: A does response curve for radiation necrosis. SPUMS Journal. 1995;**25**(2):86-87

[8] Fife CE, Smith L, Warriner RA, Sheffield PJ, Schmitz G, Ramos J, Swaby K, Otto G. Is there an Ideal Treatment Pressure? Treatment at 2.0 VS 2.4 ATA: The Effect of Treatment Pressure on Transcutaneous Oximetry (TCOM) Abstract Undersea and Hyperbaric Medical Society, Inc. 2004. Available from: http://archive.rubicon-foundation.org/1592

[9] Efrati S, Ben-Jacob E. How and why hyperbaric oxygen therapy can bring new hope for children suffering from cerebral palsy – An editorial perspective. Undersea & Hyperbaric Medicine. 2014;**41**(2):71-76

[10] Efrati S, Ben-Jacob E. Reflections on the neurotherapeutic effects of hyperbaric oxygen. Expert Review of Neurotherapeutics. 2014;**14**(3):233-236. DOI: 10.1586/14737175.2014.884928

[11] Deng Z, Chen W, Jin J, Zhao J, Xu H. The neuroprotection effect of oxygen therapy: A systematic review and meta-analysis. Nigerian Journal of Clinical Practice. 2018;**21**:401-416

[12] Krajčovičová Z, Meluš V, Zigo R, Matišáková I, Večeřa J, Králová E. Hyperbaric oxygen therapy in treatment of sudden sensorineural hearing loss: Finding for the maximal therapeutic benefit of different applied pressures. Undersea & Hyperbaric Medicine. 2019;**46**(5):665-672

[13] Margolis GS, Roth RN, Hardy KR. The pressure is on. JEMS: A Journal of Emergency Medical Services. 2000;**25**(5):76-87

[14] Mehm WJ, Pimsler M, Becker RL, Lissner CR. Effect of oxygen on in vitro fibroblast cell proliferation and collagen biosynthesis. Journal of Hyperbaric Medicine. 1988;**3**(4):227234

[15] Anderson LH, Mehm WJ. Effect of oxygen tension on macrophage migration in a complement C5a gradient. Undersea & Hyperbaric Medicine. 1994;**21**(Suppl.):56

[16] Niinikoski J, Hunt T. Oxygen tensions in healing bone. Surgery, Gynecology & Obstetrics. 1972;**134**:746-750

[17] Abbot NC, Swanson-Beck J, Carnochan FMT, Gibbs JH, Harrison DKJ, PB, Lowe JG. Effect of hyperoxia on 1 and 2 ATA on hypoxia and hypercapnia in human skin during experimental inflammation. Journal of Applied Physiology. 1994;**77**(2):767-773

[18] Sheffield PJ. Tissue oxygen measurements. In: Davis JC, Hunt TK, editors. Problem Wounds: The Role of Oxygen. New York: Elsevier Science Publishing Company; 1988. pp. 17-51

[19] Hunt TK, Zederfeldt B, Goldstick TK. Oxygen and healing. American Journal of Surgery. 1969;**118**:521-525

[20] Yablon IG, Cruess RL. The effect of hyperbaric oxygen on fracture healing in the rat. The Journal of Trauma. 1968;**8**:186-202

[21] Hunt TK, Niinikoski J, Zederfeldt BH, Silver IA. Oxygen in wound healing enhancement: Cellular effects of oxygen. In: Davis JC, Hunt TK, editors. Hyperbaric Oxygen Therapy. Bethesda: Undersea Medical Society; 1977. pp. 111-122

[22] Kindwall EP, Gottlieb LJ, Larson DL. Hyperbaric oxygen in plastic surgery: A review article. Plastic and Reconstructive Surgery. 1991;**88**(5):898-908

[23] Quirinia A, Viidik A. The effect of hyperbaric oxygen on different phases of healing of ischaemic flap wounds and incisional wounds in skin. British Journal of Plastic Surgery. 1995;**48**(8):583-589

[24] Tiidus PM. Alternative treatments for muscle injury: Massage, cryotherapy, and hyperbaric oxygen. Current Reviews in Musculoskeletal Medicine. 2015;**8**:162-167. DOI: 10.1007/s12178-015-9261-3

[25] James PB, Scott B, Allen MW. Hyperbaric oxygen therapy in sports injuries. Physiotherapy. 1993;**79**(8):571-572

[26] Fisher B, Seville C, Young M, Baracos V. A comparison of hyperbaric oxygen therapy and a nonsteroidal anti-inflammatory in the treatment of acute muscle injury in rats: A controlled study. Canadian Journal of Respiratory Therapy. 2000;**36**(4):31-36

[27] Mekjavic IB, Exner J, Tesch PA, Eiken O. Recovery of exercise-induced loss of muscle strength and muscle soreness is unaffected by HBO therapy. In: Marroni A, Oriani G, Wattel F, editors. Proceedings of the International Joint Meeting on Hyperbaric and Underwater Medicine. XXII Annual Meeting of the EUBS, XII International Congress on Hyperbaric Medicine, III Consensus Conference of the ECHM 1996 Sept 4-8, Milano, Italy. Bologna: Grafica Victoria; 1996. pp. 557-560

[28] Mekjavic IB, Exner JA, Tesch PA, Eiken O. Hyperbaric oxygen therapy does not affect recovery from delayed onset muscle soreness. Medicine and Science in Sports and Exercise. 2000;**32**(3):558-563

[29] Ehler WJ, Stefko RM, Colleton C. Effect of hyperbaric oxygenation (HBO) on autogenic long bone grafts in

the canine. Undersea & Hyperbaric Medicine. 1997;**24**(Suppl.)

[30] Soolsma SJ. The effect of intermittent hyperbaric oxygen on short-term recovery from grade II medial collateral ligament injuries [dissertation]. Vancouver: University of British Columbia. 1996. Available from: https://circle.ubc.ca/bitstream/id/15769/ubc_1996-0490.pdf

[31] Yagishita K, Enomoto M, Takazawa Y, et al. Effects of hyperbaric oxygen therapy on recovery acceleration in Japanese professional or semi-professional rugby players with grade 2 medial collateral ligament injury of the knee: A comparative non-randomized study. Undersea & Hyperbaric Medicine. 2019;**46**(5):647-654

[32] Abbadi SM, Elrefai JM. The role of hyperbaric oxygen in managing ankle sprain. JRMS. 2004;**11**(1):21-23

[33] Webster DA, Horn P, Amin HM, Weissbrich O, Mascia MF, Werner FW. Effect of hyperbaric oxygen on ligament healing in a rat model. Undersea Hyperbaric Medicine. 1996;**23**(Suppl.):13

[34] Horn PC, Webster DA, Amin HM, Mascia MF, Werner FW, Fortino MD. The effect of hyperbaric oxygen on medial collateral ligament healing in a rat model. Clinical Orthopaedics and Related Research. 1999;**360**:238-242

[35] Ishii Y, Miyanaga Y, Shimojo H, Ushida T, Tateishi T. Effects of hyperbaric oxygen on procollagen synthesis with the healing of rat tendon laceration. Tissue Engineering. 1999;**5**(3):279-286

[36] Ishii Y, Ushida T, Tateishi T, Shimojo H, Miyanaga Y. Effects of different exposures of hyperbaric oxygen on ligament healing in rats. Journal of Orthopaedic Research. 2002;**20**(2):353-356

[37] Mashitori H, Sakai H, Koibuchi N, Ohtake H, Tashiro T, Tamai K, et al. Effect of hyperbaric oxygen on the ligament healing process in rats. Clinical Orthopaedics and Related Research. 2004;**423**:268-274

[38] Yeh W-L, Lin S-S, Yuan L-J, Lee K-F, Lee MY, Ueng SWN. Effects of hyperbaric oxygen treatment on tendon graft and tendon-bone integration in bone tunnel: Biochemical and histological analysis in rabbits. Journal of Orthopaedic Research. 2007;**25**(5):636-645

[39] Alogogiannis K, Marshall KW. Early hyperbaric oxygen therapy ameliorates muscle after blunt trauma [abstract]. In: 32nd Annual Meeting of the Canadian Orthopedic Research Society, Ottawa, Canada, June 20-23, 1998

[40] Oyaizu T, Enomoto M, Yamamota N, et al. Hyperbaric oxygen reduces inflammation, oxygenates injured muscle, and regenerates skeletal muscle via macrophage and satellite cell activation. Scientific Reports. 2018;**8**(1):1288. DOI: 10.1038/s41598-018-19670-x

[41] Ishii Y, Miyanaga Y, Asano K, Shimojo H, Shiraki H. Metabolic effects of hyperbaric oxygen on muscle tear in the hind limb of rats. Advances in Exercise and Sports Physiology. 1998;**4**(1):11-15

[42] Best TM, Loitz-Ramage B, Corr DT, Vanderby R. Hyperbaric oxygen in the treatment of acute muscle stretch injuries. Results in an animal model. The American Journal of Sports Medicine. 1998;**26**(3):367-372

[43] Gregorevic P, Lynch GS, Williams DA. Hyperbaric oxygen improves contractile function of regenerating rat skeletal muscle after

myotoxic injury. Journal of Applied Physiology. 2000;**89**:1477-1482

[44] Gregorevic P, Williams DA, Lynch GS. Hyperbaric oxygen increases the contractile function of regenerating rat slow muscles. Medicine and Science in Sports and Exercise. 2002;**34**(4):630-636

[45] Horie M, Enomoto M, Shimoda M, Okawa A, Miyakawa S, Yagishita K. Enhancement of satellite cell differentiation and functional recovery in injured skeletal muscle by hyperbaric oxygen treatment. Journal of Applied Physiology. 2014;**116**:149-155

[46] Yagishita K, Yamami N, Togawa S, Nakayama T, Mano Y. The effects of hyperbaric oxygen therapy on patients with muscle injury. Undersea & Hyperbaric Medicine. 2007;**34**(4 Suppl.) Abstracts from the 2007 Annual Scientific Meeting:B2

[47] Chen YC, Chou WY, Ko JY, Mel SL, Wu RW. Early recovery of exercise-related muscular injury by HBOT. BioMed Research International. 2019;**2019**: 6289380, 10 p. DOI: 10.1155/2019/6289380

[48] Uhl E, Sirsjo A, Haapaniemi T, Nilsson G, Nylander G. Hyperbaric oxygen improves wound healing in normal and ischemic skin tissue. Plastic and Reconstructive Surgery. 1994;**93**:835-841

[49] Rud'ko VF, Volozhin AI, Chichua ZD, Karapetian IS. The use of hyperbaric oxygenation for the prevention of complications in local plastic operations on the face and neck. Stomatologiia (Mosk). 1989;**68**(2):33-34

[50] Johnsson K, Hansson A, Granström G, Jacobsson M, Turesson I. The effects of hyperbaric oxygenation on bone-titanium implant interface strength with and without preceding irradiation. The International Journal of Oral & Maxillofacial Implants. 1993;**8**(4):415-419

[51] Potkin RT, Wigington K, Lee R, Comer M. Effect of hyperbaric oxygen on wound healing in patients undergoing laser skin resurfacing – A preliminary study. Undersea & Hyperbaric Medicine. 1997;**24**(Suppl.):37

[52] Fulton JE. The use of hyperbaric oxygen (HBO) to accelerate wound healing. Dermatologic Surgery. 2000;**26**(12):1170-1172

[53] Llorente EN, Wicker RR. Hyperbaric oxygen therapy in the treatment of controlled laser induced thermal burns. Hyperbaric Medicine Today. 2001;**1**(5):12-14

[54] Butler J, Foex B. Best evidence topic report. Hyperbaric oxygen therapy in acute fracture management. Emergency Medicine Journal. 2006;**23**(7):571-572

[55] Bennett MH, Stanford R, Turner R. Hyperbaric oxygen therapy for promoting fracture healing and treating fracture non-union. Cochrane Database of Systematic Reviews. 2005;**1**:CD004712

[56] Bennett MH, Stanford RE, Turner R. Hyperbaric oxygen therapy for promoting fracture healing and treating fracture non-union. Cochrane Database of Systematic Reviews. 2012;**11**:CD004712. DOI: 10.1002/14651858.CD004712.pub4

[57] Coulson DB, Ferguson AB, Diehl RC. Effect of hyperbaric oxygen on the healing femur of the rat. Surgical Forum. 1966;**17**:449-450

[58] Natiella JR, Green GW, Gage AA. The effect of hyperbaric oxygenation on

bone healing after cryogenic injury. In: Trapp WG, Bannister EW, Davidson AJ, et al., editors. Proceedings of the Fifth International Conference on Hyperbaric Medicine. BC, Canada: Simon Fraser University; 1974. pp. 270-279

[59] Wilcox JW, Kolodny SC. Acceleration of healing of maxillary and mandibular osteotomies by use of hyperbaric oxygen. Oral Surgery. 1976;**41**(4):423-429

[60] Karapetian IS, Volozhin AI, Oleĭnik NN, Druzhinina RA. Treatment of mandibular fractures using hyperbaric oxygenation. Stomato logiia (Mosk). 1985;**64**(3):35-38. Russian

[61] Barth E, Sullivan T, Berg E. Animal model for evaluating bone repair with and without adjunctive hyperbaric oxygen therapy (HBO): Comparing dose schedules. Journal of Investigative Surgery. 1990;**3**:387-392

[62] Kitakoji T, Takahashi S, Ono Y, Hattori T, Takahashi H, Iwata H. Effect of hyperbaric oxygenation treatment on lengthened callus. Undersea & Hyperbaric Medicine. 1999;**26**(3):165-168

[63] Kawada S, Wada E, Matsuda R, Ishii N. Hyperbaric hyperoxia accelerates fracture healing in mice. PLoS One. 2013;**8**(8):e72603. DOI: 10.1371/journal.pone.0072603

[64] Ishii Y, Miyanaga Y, Shimojo H, Shiraki H. The experience of hyperbaric oxygen therapy for soft tissue injuries of sports athletes. Japanese Journal of Orthopaedic Sports Medicine. 1997;**17**(7):7-14

[65] Todorovic BS. Sports injuries and hyperbaric oxygen. In: Marroni A, Oriani G, Wattel F, editors. Proceedings of the International Joint Meeting on Hyperbaric and Underwater Medicine. XXII Annual Meeting of the EUBS, XII International Congress on Hyperbaric Medicine, III Consensus Conference of the ECHM, 1996 Sep 4-8, Milano, Italy. Bologna: Grafica Victoria; 1996. pp. 561-564

[66] Strauss MB, Borer RC, Winant DM. Cosmetic surgical applications of hyperbaric oxygen. Undersea & Hyperbaric Medicine. 1998;**25**(Suppl.):16

[67] Hodgson M. Hyperbaric experience with sports injuries. In: Hyperbaric Technicians and Nurses Association, 8th Annual Scientific Meeting on Diving and Hyperbaric Medicine. The Mercure Hotel - Brisbane, Australia, 7-9 September 2000

[68] Dolezal V. Hyperbaric oxygen therapy in the management of sports injuries. Casopís Lékařů Českých. 2002;**141**(10):304-306

[69] Peterson RE, Allen MW. The adjunctive use of hyperbaric oxygen therapy for the treatment of sports injuries. Hyperbaric Medicine Today. 2003a;**2**(1):22-24

[70] Peterson RE, Allen MW. The adjunctive use of hyperbaric oxygen therapy for the treatment of sports injuries, part 2. Hyperbaric Medicine Today. 2003b;**2**(2):54-57

[71] Kulonen E, Niinikoski J. Effect of hyperbaric oxygenation on wound healing and experimental granuloma. Acta Physiologica Scandinavica. 1968;**73**:383

[72] Wray JB, Rogers LS. Effect of hyperbaric oxygenation upon fracture healing in the rat. The Journal of Surgical Research. 1968;**8**(8):373-378

[73] Penttinen R, Niinikoski KE. Hyperbaric oxygenation and fracture

healing. Acta Chirurgica Scandinavica. 1972;**138**:3944

[74] Davis JC, Hunt TK, editors. Hyperbaric Oxygen Therapy. Bethesda MD: Undersea Medical Society; 1977

[75] Niinikoski J, Penttinen R, Kulonen E. Effect of oxygen supply on the tensile strength of healing wound and of granulation tissue. Acta Physiologica Scandinavica. 1966;**277**(Suppl.):146

[76] Niinikoski J, Juva K, Kulonen E. Effect of the supply of oxygen on the healing skin wound and experimental granulation. Scandinavian Journal of Clinical and Laboratory Investigation. 1967;**95**(Suppl.):1-87

[77] Niinikoski J, Penttinen R, Kulonen E. Effect of oxygen supply on the tensile strength of healing wound and of granulation tissue. Acta Physiologica Scandinavica. 1968;**68**(Suppl. 277):1-146

[78] Penttinen R, Niinikoski RJ, Kulonen E. Effects of hyperbaric oxygenation and reduced barometric pressure on the nucleic acid contents of healing fractures. Acta Chirurgica Scandinavica. 1972;**138**:269-274

[79] Meltzer T, Myers B. The effect of hyperbaric oxygen on the bursting strength and rate of vascularization of skin wounds in the rat. The American Surgeon. 1986;**56**(12):659-662

[80] Peterson RE, Allen MW. Dose dependence of hyperbaric oxygen therapy. Review of the scientific literature and oxygen uptake considerations and implications. In: Undersea and Hyperbaric Medical Society, Gulf Coast Chapter Annual Scientific Meeting Conjoint with UHMS Associates and Baromedical Nurses Association, Yesterday, Today, and Tomorrow. San Antonio Texas, October 12-14, 2000; Abstract 6

[81] Peterson RE, Allen MW. Dose dependence of hyperbaric oxygen therapy: A review of the scientific literature and oxygen uptake considerations; implications. In: UHMS Associates BNA Conjoint Annual Scientific Meeting, Orlando, Florida, June 22-24, 2006

[82] Clark JM, Lambertsen CJ, Gelfand R, Flores ND, Pisarello JB, Rossman MD, et al. Effects of prolonged oxygen exposure at 1.5, 2.0, or 2.5 ATA on pulmonary function in men (predictive studies V). Journal of Applied Physiology. 1999;**86**(1):243-259

[83] Tan CM, Im MJ, Myers RAM, Hoopes JE. Effects of hyperbaric oxygen and hyperbaric air on the survival of island skin flaps. Plastic and Reconstructive Surgery. 1984;**73**(1):27-30

[84] Yagishita K. Enhancement of satellite cell differentiation and functional recovery in injured skeletal muscle by hyperbaric oxygen treatment. Journal of Applied Physiology. 2014;**116**:149-155

[85] Champion WM, McSherry CK, Goulian D. Effect of hyperbaric oxygen on the survival of pedicle skin flaps. The Journal of Surgical Research. 1967;7:583-586

[86] Suleiman M, Abbadi MD, Elrefai JM. Journal of the Royal Medical Services. 2004;**11**(1):21-23

[87] Kernahan DA, Zingg W, Kay CW. The effect of hyperbaric oxygen on the survival of experimental skin flaps. Plastic and Reconstructive Surgery. 1965;**36**:19-25

[88] Caffee HH, Gallagher TJ. Experiments on the effects of hyperbaric oxygen on flap survival in the pig. Plastic and Reconstructive Surgery. 1988;**81**:751-754

[89] Peterson RE. Tracking of cumulative oxygen dose in decompression and therapy. In: Lambertsen CJ, editor. Symposium on Decompression Sickness and its Therapy. Allentown, PA: Air Products and Chemicals, Inc.; 1979. pp. 125-141

[90] Snedecor GW, Cochran WG. Statistical Methods. Ames, IA: Iowa State University Press; 1989. pp. 83-106

[91] Table of critical values of t: One-tailed significance level. Available from: https://users.sussex.ac.uk › ~grahamh.RM1web

[92] Calabrese EJ. Hormesis and medicine. British Journal of Clinical Pharmacology. 2008;**66**(5):594-617

[93] Calabrese EJ, Dhawan G, Kapoor R, Kozumbo WJ. Radiotherapy treatment of human inflammatory diseases and conditions: Optimal dose. Human & Experimental Toxicology. 2019;**38**(8):888-898. DOI: 10.1177/0960327119846925

[94] Berry R, Lopez-Martinez G. A dose of experimental hormesis: When mild stress protects and improves animal performance. Comparative Biochemistry and Physiology Part A: Molecular & Integrative Physiology. 2020;**242**:110658

[95] Schirrmacher V. Less can Be more: The Hormesis theory of stress adaptation in the global biosphere and its implications. Biomedicine. 2021;**9**:293. DOI: 10.3390/biomedicines9030293

[96] Wikipedia Contributors. Hormesis. Wikipedia, The Free Encyclopedia. Available from: https://en.wikipedia.org/wiki/Hormesis [Accessed: 02 November 2022]

[97] Calabrese EJ. Preconditioning is hormesis part I: Documentation, dose-response features and mechanistic foundations. Pharmacological Research. 2016;**110**:242-264

[98] Robinson AS. Influence of anoxia during gamma irradiation on the fertility and competitiveness of the adult male codling moth, Laspeyresia pomonella (L.). Radiation Research. 1975;**61**:526-534. DOI: 10.2307/3574127

[99] Giraud-Billoud M, Rivera-Ingraham GA, Moreira DC, Burmester T, Castro-Vazquez A, Carvajalino-Fernández JM, et al. Twenty years of the 'preparation for oxidative stress' (POS) theory: Ecophysiological advantages and molecular strategies. Comparative Biochemistry and Physiology A. 2019;**234**:36-49. DOI: 10.1016/j.cbpa.2019.04.004

[100] Hermes-Lima M, Storey JM, Storey KB. Antioxidant defenses and metabolic depression. The hypothesis of preparation for oxidative stress in land snails. Comparative Biochemistry and Physiology Part B: Biochemistry and Molecular Biology. 1998;**120**(3):437-448. DOI: 10.1016/S0305-0491(98)10053-6

[101] Hermes-Lima M, Storey JM, Storey KB. Antioxidant defenses and animal adaptation to oxygen availability during environmental stress. In: Storey KB, Storey JM, editors. Cell and Molecular Responses to Stress 2001, Protein Adaptations and Signal Transduction. Vol. 2. Amsterdam: Elsevier Press; pp. 263-287

[102] Hermes-Lima M, Zenteno-Savin T. Animal response to drastic changes in oxygen availability and physiological oxidative stress. Comparative Biochemistry and Physiology Part C: Toxicology and Pharmacology. 2002;**133**(4):537-556

[103] Wu MY, Yiang GT, Liao WT, Tsai APY, Cheng YL, Cheng PW, et al.

Current mechanistic concepts in ischemia and reperfusion injury. Cellular Physiology and Biochemistry. 2018;**46**:1650-1667

[104] Boroujerdi A, Milner R. Defining the critical hypoxic threshold that promotes vascular remodeling in the brain. Experimental Neurology. 2015;**263**:132-140. DOI: 10.1016/j.expneurol.2014.10.007

[105] Huang G, Xu J, Xu L, Wang S, Li R, et al. Hyperbaric oxygen preconditioning induces tolerance against oxidative injury and oxygen-glucose deprivation by up-regulating heat shock protein 32 in rat spinal neurons. PLoS One. 2014;**9**(1):e85967. DOI: 10.1371/journal.pone.0085967

[106] Duan S, Shao G, Yu L, Ren C. Angiogenesis contributes to the neuroprotection induced by hyperbaric oxygen preconditioning against focal cerebral ischemia in rats. International Journal of Neuroscience. 2015;**125**(8):625-634. DOI: 10.3109/00207454.2014.956101

[107] Tähepõld P, Ruusalepp A, Lia G, Vaageb J, Starkopf J, Valena G. Cardioprotection by breathing hyperoxic gas—Relation to oxygen concentration and exposure time in rats and mice. European Journal of Cardio-Thoracic Surgery. 2002;**21**:987-994

[108] Touleimat B, Conoscenti C, Chen LC, Selmont D, Fine J. Effects of multiple hyperbaric oxygen treatments on pulmonary function. Undersea & Hyperbaric Medicine. 1995;**22**(Suppl. 1): 46-46

[109] Bean JW. Effects of oxygen at increased pressure. Physiological Reviews. 1945;**25**(1):1-147

[110] Perrins DJD. Hyperbaric oxygenation of ischemic skin flaps and pedicles. In: Brown IW Jr, Cox BG, editors. Proceedings of the Third International Conference on Hyperbaric Medicine. Washington, DC: National Academy of Science – National Research Council; 1966. pp. 613-620

[111] Jurell G, Kaijser L. The influence of varying pressure and duration of treatment with hyperbaric oxygen on the survival of skin flaps. Scandinavian Journal of Plastic and Reconstructive Surgery. 1973;**7**(1):25-28

[112] Bert P. La pression barometrique. In: Recherches de physiologie experimentale. Paris: Masson; 1878 (Translated by Hitchcock MA, Hitchcock FA, Barometric Pressure. Researches in Experimental Physiology. Originally published by College Book Co, Columbus Ohio, 1943: Republished by Undersea Medical Society, Bethesda MD, 1978)

[113] Lorrain-Smith J. The Pathological Effects Due to Increase of Oxygen Tension in the Air Breathed. Queen's College, Belfast: From the Pathological Laboratory; 1899. pp. 19-35

[114] Comroe JH, Dripps RD, Dumke PR, Deming M. Oxygen toxicity – The effect of inhalation of high concentrations of oxygen for twenty-four hours on normal men at sea level and at a simulated altitude of 18,000 feet. JAMA. 1945;**128**(10):710-717

[115] Clark JM, Lambertsen CJ. Pulmonary oxygen toxicity: A review. Pharmacological Reviews. 1971;**22**(2):38-133

[116] Deneke SM, Fanburg BL. Normobaric oxygen toxicity of the lung. NEJM. 1980;**303**(2):76-86

[117] Davis WB, Rennard SI, Bitterman PB, Crystal RG. Early reversible changes in human alveolar structures induced by hyperoxia. NEJM. 1983;**309**(15):878-883

[118] Thompson L, Paton J. Oxygen toxicity. Paediatric Respiratory Reviews. 2014;**15**:120-123

[119] Phaniendra A, Jestadi DB, Periyasamy L. Free radicals: Properties, sources, targets and their implication in various diseases. Indian Journal of Clinical Biochemistry. 2015;**30**(1):11-26. DOI: 10.1007/s12291-014-0446-0

[120] Lambertsen CJ. Effects of oxygen at high partial pressure. In: Fenn WO, Hahn H, editors. Handbook of Physiology, Section 3 Respiration. Vol. 2. Washington DC: American Physiological Society; 1965. pp. 1027-1046

[121] Jamieson D. Oxygen toxicity and reactive oxygen metabolites in mammals. Free Radical Biology and Medicine. 1989;7:87-108

[122] Nita M, Grzybowski A. The role of the reactive oxygen species and oxidative stress in the pathomechanism of the age-related ocular diseases and other pathologies of the anterior and posterior eye segments in adults. Oxidative Medicine and Cellular Longevity. 2016; Art. ID 3164734:1-23. DOI: 10.1155/2016/3164734

[123] Ŝenel O, Cetinkale O, Özbay G, Ahçioğlu F, Bulan R. Oxygen free radicals impair wound healing in ischemic rat skin. Annals of Plastic Surgery. 1997;**39**:516-523

[124] Stewart RJ, Moore T, Bennett B, Easton M, Newton GW, Yamaguchi KT. Effect of free-radical scavengers and hyperbaric oxygen on random-pattern skin flaps. Archives of Surgery. 1994;**129**:982-988

[125] Basset CAL, Herrmann I. Influence of oxygen concentration and mechanical factors on differentiation of connective tissues in vitro. Nature. 1961;**190**:460-461

Chapter 2

Dose-Response Relationship of Therapeutic Oxygen: More Is Not Necessarily Better and May Be Inferior to No Supplemental Oxygen – Part 2: Implications and Consequences

Russell E. Peterson and Michael W. Allen

Abstract

In the late 1980s to mid-1990s, the authors had consistently positive experience in the treatment of typical sports injuries and cosmetic surgical wounds with hyperbaric oxygen. The treatments in these cases generally consisted of oxygen at 2.0 atmospheres absolute (ATA) for 60 minutes. We were thus surprised to find that experts in the field of hyperbaric medicine did not believe this modality to be effective for such *normal wounds*. Consequently, we asked Eric Kindwall, M.D., a professional acquaintance and published proponent of this prevalent view, what the bases for his beliefs on this matter were. Starting with references provided by Dr. Kindwall, we began an extensive literature review to try to reconcile our practical successes with the prevailing hyperbaric medical dogma. The finding that the outcomes of oxygen therapy have a *hormetic* dose-response relationship explains the mistaken conclusions drawn concerning the treatment of uncompromised or *normal* wounds. Further, consideration of this and related facts provides insights which can assist in a more accurate understanding of published findings relating to hyperoxic therapy and in optimizing clinical treatments conducted with hyperoxic gases at both normobaric and hyperbaric pressures.

Keywords: dose, dose response, hormesis, hormetic, hyperbaric, hyperoxia, hypoxia, normobaric, oxygen, oxygenation, supplementation, therapy

1. Introduction

This chapter is the second part of a publication discussing the aspects of therapeutic oxygen dose-response. Part 1 presents verification for the existence of oxygen dose-response and its nature which is hormetic. Part 2 below presents characteristics of the oxygen dose-response; the implications these have for the conduct of oxygen therapy at both normobaric and hyperbaric pressures; several beneficial applications of knowledge about oxygen dose-response.

2. Characteristics of oxygen dose-response

2.1 Oxygen dose-response is not static

In considering oxygen dose-response from the standpoint of wound healing, the perspectives of critical importance are the characteristics of the tissue of particular interest over time as suggested by Barr and Perrins [1]. Thus, though the dose of oxygen for a hyperoxic treatment may typically be thought of and prescribed as the partial pressure of inspired oxygen, the duration of the treatments, the frequency of the treatments, and the total number of treatments, these factors do not necessarily relate to the tissue of interest insofar as the outcome of the treatment is concerned (**Figure 1**). Rather, there must be a body of experience that the prescribing physician is familiar with and/or confident in that enables him to judge that the oxygen treatment dose parameters will provide the desired outcome for the specific wound he wishes to address. The oxygen pressure in the arterial blood will be factored at the wound site by any compromise of blood flow to that site because of capillary and/or other vascular damage, by any compromise of oxygen diffusion from the capillaries resulting from edema and material such as fibrin in the interstitial spaces local to that wound site, and by the degree of infection and inflammation in the wounded tissue which can greatly influence the amount of oxygen needed to effectively support healing. This view dictates that:

1. Uncompromised wounds to a particular tissue will be treated optimally with lower doses of oxygen than wounds to the same tissue where oxygen delivery has been compromised by such things as circulatory disruption, edema, and inflammation (**Figure 2**). This is because at a given partial pressure of oxygen, the amount of oxygen delivered to a wound site is inversely proportional to the degree of compromise to the circulation, diffusion, and inflammation at that site.

2. As events such as angiogenesis and the reduction of edema and/or inflammation occur during treatment at a wound site, relative local oxygen delivery will increase, and the optimal inspired oxygen level for therapy will decline correspondingly [2, 3]. This produces a leftward shift in the optimal dose-response relationship as shown in **Figure 2**.

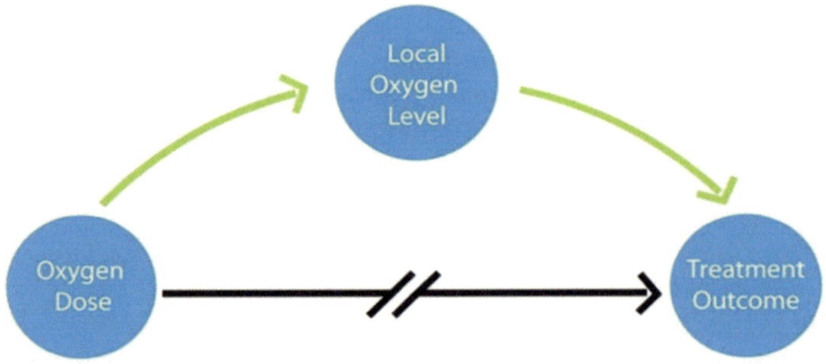

Figure 1.
Relationship between inspired oxygen dose and the actual local dose of oxygen at the wound site of concern.

DOI: http://dx.doi.org/10.5772/intechopen.1003699

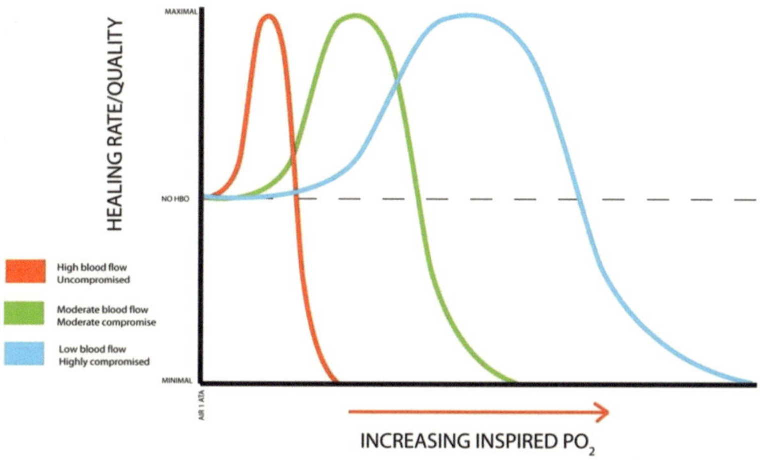

Figure 2.
Shift in oxygen dose-response relationship resulting from differences in local tissue oxygen delivery (circa 2006 by the authors). In the three cases illustrated, the left-most curve represents the tissue with the greatest perfusion rate or a particular tissue with the least compromise of oxygen delivery. The middle curve represents the tissue with the middle perfusion rate of the three or the particular tissue with the intermediate compromise of oxygen delivery. The right-hand curve represents the tissue with the lowest perfusion rate of the three or the particular tissue with the greatest degree of compromise to oxygen delivery of the three cases.

3. Where tissues have inherently different perfusion rates and, therefore, oxygen deliveries, the tissue with the higher natural delivery of oxygen, independent of compromise (i.e., high perfusion dose-response in **Figure 2**), will most often be optimally treated with lower doses of oxygen than tissues with lower natural delivery of oxygen (i.e., **Figure 2**). As an example, Neubauer [4] determined that appropriate oxygen treatment pressures for a central nervous system (i.e., CNS) condition such as multiple sclerosis (MS) was 1.5–2.0 ATA. HBO_2 for other tissues and organs with inherently lower oxygen deliveries than the brain is invariably conducted between 2.0 and 3.0 ATA.

Point 1 above is implicit in our derivation of the oxygen dose-response relationship. In research, it has been demonstrated by Karapetian et al. [5] in their study of the healing of mandibular fractures in rats with adjunctive HBO_2. With uncompromised fractures, HBO_2 administered at 2.0 atm improved healing while HBO_2 delivered at 2.5 atm hindered it [5]. If the fractures were compromised by inflammation, however, Karapetian and associates suggest that HBO_2 delivered at 2.5 atm would be more effective, thus predicting a rightward shift in the dose-response relationship with greater initial compromise to oxygen delivery.

Point 2 follows logically and predicts a leftward shift in the oxygen dose-response relationship as healing occurs (Figure 7, Part 1). Such a shift has been demonstrated in research conducted by Quirinia and Viidik [6] and Sadeghani et al. [7] using the healing of ischemic flaps and incisional wounds in rats, respectively. Hyperbaric oxygen treatments conducted once a day at 2.4 ATA for 90 minutes over 3 days produced benefits in almost all force parameters of healing ischemic flaps in comparison to the untreated control animals [6]. After 9 days of HBO_2 with the hyperoxic treatment parameters as described previously, however, the force parameters of the HBO_2-treated wounds fell below those of the controls [6]. Thus, as healing progressed, it seems that the effective dose-response curve shifted to the left. Sadeghani and associates, on the other hand, created 2.5 cm incisions on the backs of rats with the surrounding skin dissected from the subcutaneous tissue. At 8 days post-wounding, the bursting strengths of the wounds treated with 1.0 atm of O_2 and 2.5 atm of O_2 were very close. At 14 days post-wounding, however, the wounds healed with the 1.0 atm O_2 treatments were significantly stronger than those healed with the 2.5 atm O_2 treatments [7] indicating a shift in the oxygen dose response to the left. With healing in progress in both of these studies, it is only logical that the dose-response shift be to the left so that continued hyperbaric oxygen treatments using the higher treatment parameters produced adverse outcomes rather than beneficial ones.

Point 3 above also suggests a set of dose-response curves like those shown in **Figure 2**. In this case, however, the curves represent different uncompromised tissues where the leftmost curve is for the tissue with the greatest perfusion rate, and the rightmost curve is for the tissue with the lowest perfusion rate. Local oxygen consumption will of course be an important factor and could impose shifts in the curves for specific tissues. This does not change the basic nature of the relationships, however.

This latter aspect of our dose-response model has been demonstrated practically. Based on the research of Holbach and associates [8–10], Pierce and Jacobson [11] concluded that lower pressures were advisable for the treatment of brain edema and recommended a range of 1.5–2.0 ATA. A similar range of hyperbaric oxygen therapy has commonly been utilized for several cerebral neurological applications including stroke [12] and multiple sclerosis [4]. In the latter study, 1.5 ATA was found to be a more effective treatment pressure than 2.0 ATA. Highly relevant to this situation, we believe, is the fact that the brain typically receives 15–20% of the total cardiac output in humans though its mass makes up only 2.5% of the total body mass, on average. Normal clinical pressures for the treatment of systemic conditions with hyperbaric oxygen therapy such as those endorsed by the Undersea and Hyperbaric Medical Society (UHMS) commonly range from 2.0 to 2.8 ATA (UHMS Committee Report HBO Indications 14th Edition [13]).

2.2 Increased pressure is not essential with hyperoxic PO2's $\leq$ 1 ATA

Between 2005 and 2011, studies utilizing *mild hyperbaric oxygen therapy* ($mHBO_2$) in inflatable, zip-up "chambers" (**Figure 3**) were conducted for autism [14–18]. These *chambers* are typically flushed with enriched air having approximately 24% oxygen at 1.3 ATA, giving an inspired partial pressure of oxygen of 0.312 atm. The results of such studies, except for the two conducted by the Center for Autism and Related Disorders (CARD) whose business is to provide psychosocial treatments for autism based on the principals of applied behavior analysis (ABA) [17, 18], have not been appreciably different than those of HBO_2 at greater pressures. This was one of the bases upon which we decided to try hyperoxic therapy at normal barometric pressure for ASD [19, 20].

Research has also been conducted for other neurological conditions with hyperbaric oxygen therapy having sham controls at increased pressure. These control subjects have typically breathed air in standard clinical chambers with a partial pressure of oxygen greater than 0.21 atm (e.g., air at 1.3 ATA for a P_iO_2 of 0.272 atm). The research on autism using $mHBO_2$ and the controls for other neurological studies conducted with air at an increased pressure, though never exceeding an inspired oxygen pressure of air at 1.5 ATA (i.e., ≈0.314 atm) that we are aware of, have shown that such *treatments* may be beneficial for addressing at least some brain disorders. These include autism [21], mild traumatic brain injury [22] and persistent post-concussion symptoms in military personnel [23], chronic stroke [24], and cerebral palsy (CP)[1] (**Table 1**) [25, 26].

[1] Peterson RE. Personal communication with Pierre Marois MD. July 2008.

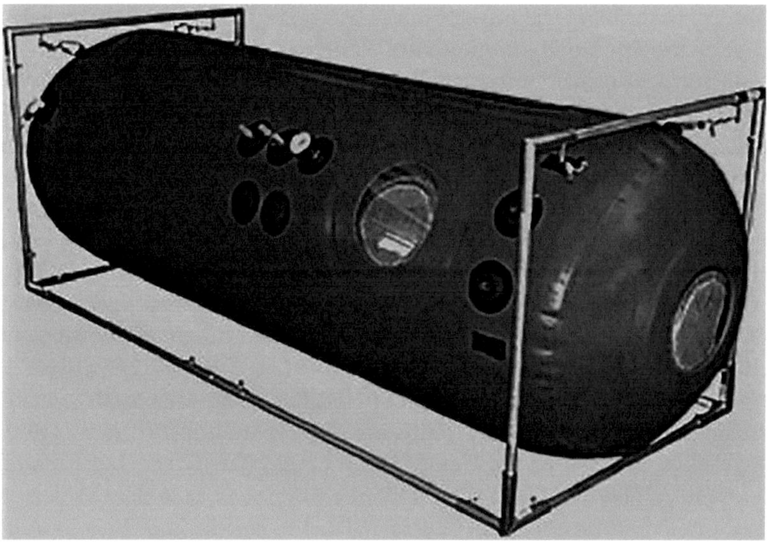

Figure 3.
"Mild" hyperbaric oxygen chamber (courtesy of Atlanta Hyperbaric Center, Smyrna, GA, USA).

	Ref.	Condition	Control		Test HBO_2		Best result
			P (ATA)	P_iO_2 (ATM)	P (ATA)	P_iO_2 (ATM)	
Sampanthavivat et al. [21]	[25]	ASD	1.15	0.241	1.50	1.50	NO DIFF
Wolf et al. [22]	[26]	Mild TBI	1.30	0.272	2.40	2.40	CONTROL
Miller et al. [23]	[27]	Post-Concussion	1.20	0.251	1.50	1.50	HBO_2
Anderson et al. [24]	[28]	Chronic Stroke	1.50	0.314	1.50	1.50	CONTROL
Collet et al. [25]	[29]	Cerebral Palsy	1.30	0.272	1.75	1.75	NO DIFF

Table 1.
Studies conducted for neurological conditions with blinded sham controls treated with air at elevated pressures in a whole-body chamber. It is important to note that in all these studies, both the hyperbaric sham air and test oxygen treatments produced notable benefits in comparison to no treatments at all. Further, there was no statistically important difference between the outcomes of the test and sham treatments.

It is most interesting that in these studies, the control and hyperbaric oxygen test conditions provided benefits not appreciably different from each other, and both were clearly better than no treatments at all. Invariably, however, the principal investigators considering only their own study's outcome each concluded that since the test hyperbaric oxygen treatments were not significantly better than the presumed hyperbaric hyperoxic placebo treatments, neither the control nor test treatments were of benefit. The explanations given for these outcomes were *Hawthorne effects* [22]; *placebo effects* [23]; *participation effects* [25]; an incomplete study, though the results obtained weighed heavily in favor of the control-treated stroke patients having the best result [24]; and the parents of autistic children overrating their child's improvement because they were extremely anxious for them to make progress [21].
Thus, neither the hyperoxic hyperbaric control nor test treatments were given any credit, whatsoever, for improving the symptoms of the afflicted subjects. Taken as a

group, however, we believe the impact made by the hyperoxic control treatments on the variety of cases studied is too much for coincidence. Further, in our own experience, the parents of one child with autism treated with our normobaric hyperoxic therapy were quite conscious of their desire for their child to improve so were very careful not to overrate his progress. Rather, they underrated it until the evidence of change overwhelmed their doubts.

A critical issue for the practical application of low-dose hyperoxia (i.e., a P_iO_2 less than or equal to 1.0 atm of oxygen) was whether or not increased pressures as provided by whole-body hyperbaric chambers in HBO_2 and $mHBO_2$ are necessary to achieve the desired outcomes. We believed increased ambient pressure would not be essential for conditions other than gas embolism and decompression sickness and determined to test this hypothesis [19].

Following a number of pilot studies of normobaric hyperoxia for autism [19, 20], cosmetic surgery (**Figures 4** and **5**)[2] [28], and hair transplant surgery (**Figure 6**)[3] [29], some of which produced remarkable outcomes, it appears that for such cases, no matter how much below 1.0 atm the dose of oxygen is, it is the oxygen pressure, alone, and not hydrostatic pressure that is critical to producing these outcomes (**Figure 6**).

To date, properly controlled studies have not yet been carried out to establish the validity of such claims to current scientific standards. In the meantime, however, a 2019 publication by Ding and colleagues [27] has provided independent support for the potential offered by normobaric hyperoxic therapy administered at 1.0 ATA (i.e., NBO_2) for treating acute stroke and the associated ischemic penumbra as well as short-term symptoms and long-term outcomes for other conditions produced by chronic circulation insufficiency (CCCI). Other research by Van Allen et al. [28] indicates that normobaric oxygen therapy benefits bladder dysfunction in cases with multiple sclerosis.

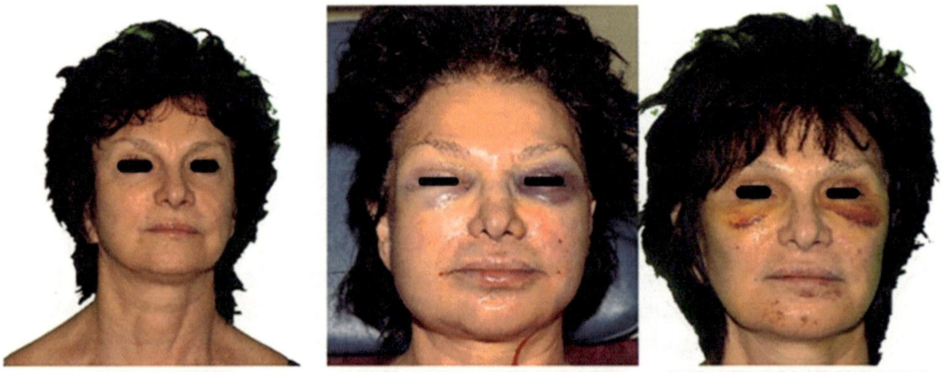

Figure 4.
A typical recovery following cosmetic sculpting of the face with autologous fat injection without adjunctive normobaric oxygen therapy being administered. Note bruising under eyes at one-week post-surgery. Source: Courtesy of James Goodnight, M.D., Everlasting Beauty, Ridgewood, N.J.

[2] Goodnight JW, Peterson RE, Allen MW. Unpublished data.

[3] Ballon J, Peterson RE, Allen MW. Unpublished data.

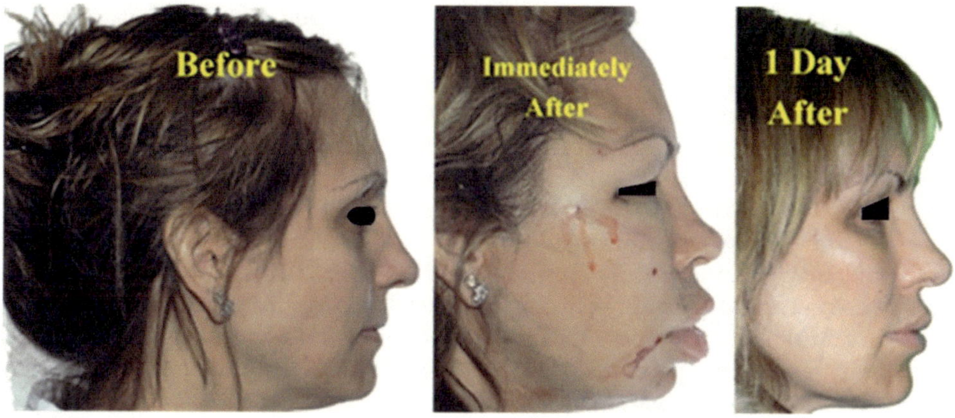

Figure 5.
One patient's transformation over the course of a single day: Times indicated are relative to the surgical procedure. This case illustrates the absence of bruising and rapid reduction in swelling following cosmetic sculpturing of the face with autologous fat injection and normobaric oxygen therapy being administered. The final picture is at 1 day post-surgery, not 1 week (courtesy of James Goodnight, M.D., Everlasting Beauty, Ridgewood, N.J.).

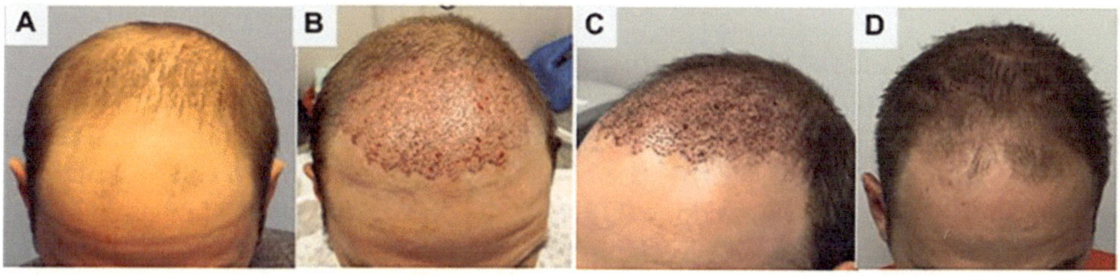

Figure 6.
Application of normobaric oxygen therapy following follicular unit extraction (FUE) hair transplant surgery: A. Immediately prior to the surgery. B. Immediately post-surgery. C. One day post-surgery. D. Eleven weeks post-surgery. At eleven weeks post-surgery, the hair transplant surgeon found it incredible that the patient was thrilled with the results so quickly and considered his appearance to be already "acceptable," to the point that he no longer felt it necessary to wear a hat. The patient also said that for the first time in the last 16 years (i.e., since he was 22-years old), he "could actually spike his hair up" (courtesy of Jon Ballon, M.D., Esthetics Hair Restoration, Alpharetta, GA).

3. Applications of knowledge of oxygen dose response

3.1 Treating wounds at normobaric pressure before they become intractable

In view of Kulonen and associates' [29] research demonstrating the capacity of improved healing of normal wounds with hyperoxia at 1 ATA (i.e., 35 and 70% oxygen in comparison to 21% oxygen as in air), there could be capacity for P_iO_2s up to 1 atm to improve wound healing when there is some degree of compromise to oxygen delivery. Thus, it may be possible to head off problem wounds (i.e., non-healing wounds) with hyperoxic therapy administered at 1 ATA before such wounds progress to a point where routine care must give way to hyperbaric oxygen therapy (e.g., Wagner Grade 3 and Grade 4 diabetic ulcers). With the great difference in cost, convenience, and risk between normobaric oxygen and hyperbaric oxygen [19], the possibility of heading off intractable wounds before they require hyperbaric oxygen therapy would seem to present considerable opportunity to reduce overall healthcare costs and risk to patients as well as improve the patients' ongoing quality of life. Confirmation of this possibility has been reported by Moon et al. [30], who have concluded that normobaric oxygen therapy significantly augments tissue oxygen pressure in the feet of human diabetic patients and may reinforce wound healing potential via impact on multiple healing processes.

Regarding pathological brain conditions, as shown with our autism spectrum disorder (ASD) pilot studies with normobaric oxygen therapy and almost 11 years of follow-up without regression at the time of this publication [19, 20], normobaric oxygen therapy may provide an opportunity to decrease costs and risk, and to improve convenience in treating certain neurological disorders. Conditions such as mild traumatic brain injury [22] and persistent post-concussion symptoms [23], chronic stroke [24], and cerebral palsy (CP)[1] [25, 26] have research findings with HBO_2 that parallel those of ASD. Further, in view of the sensitivity of the brain to changes in oxygen and the authors' results with ASD [19, 20], it is likely that a course of hyperbaric oxygen therapy at any increased atmospheric pressure may ultimately provide too great a partial pressure of oxygen (i.e., greater than 1.0 atm) to carry therapies of such conditions to their optimal conclusions [27, 31].

3.2 More accurate interpretation of research

One incident stands out as illustrating the importance of understanding the general nature of oxygen dose response to more accurately interpret the results of research relating to clinical HBO_2. In late 2004, Djillali Annane and associates in France published the results of a randomized, prospective, double-blind study of hyperbaric oxygen therapy of osteoradionecrosis of the mandible (ORN) in the Journal of Clinical Oncology [32]. The study protocol included two 90-minute oxygen treatments at 2.4 ATA per day to minimize patient inconvenience and expenses related to the overall length of time to administer the requisite number of treatments for the established Marx therapy protocol [33] on a once-a-day basis.

When the results of the study were revealed and examined at an interim point as originally planned, however, it was discovered that the HBO_2-treated group was doing less well (i.e., only 19% success) than the untreated control group (i.e., 32% success) [32]. Though this relatively large difference was not statistically significant, the test cases were clearly doing no better than the controls. Thus, the study was terminated for ethical reasons [32].

After the study was published, Blue Cross/Blue Shield in several U.S. states announced that they would stop or actually did stop reimbursing for the treatment of osteoradionecrosis of the mandible with hyperbaric oxygen therapy. This was despite the facts that:

- A randomized, prospective clinical study established the effectiveness of the protocol developed by Marx for the treatment of ORN based on aggressive surgical principles and sequential HBO_2 *once a day* [34].

- ORN was one of the relatively limited number of conditions for which HBO_2 was recognized by CMS and reimbursed for by Medicare, Medicaid, and other third-party health insurers in the U.S.

- ORN was one of the several most common conditions for which HBO_2 was prescribed, and its treatment with HBO_2 in the U.S. had been successfully conducted for many years.

In their attempts to explain Annane's results in a positive light on behalf of the hyperbaric medical community in the U.S., several prominent members of the Undersea and Hyperbaric Medical Society (i.e., Richard E. Moon, M.D., a former president of the of the Society, together with two university-associated oral and maxillofacial surgeons; and John J. Feldmeier, D.O., who was to become president of the Society some years later) pointed out in separate communications to the editor of the UHMS's journal, Undersea & Hyperbaric Medicine, that the general standard of care of Annane's patients was below the existing level in the United States [35, 36]. In doing this, they made a strong case that a missing element in the study approach was aggressive debridement of the wounds, which had been shown by Marx to be essential for the effectiveness of HBO_2 in the treatment of osteonecrosis of the mandible [33]. On this basis, it would seem Marx's and other positive research conducted in the U.S., as well as the long history of successful treatment of osteoradionecrosis with HBO_2, prevailed, and this indication continues to be recognized and reimbursed by health care insurers in the U.S. including Blue Cross and Blue Shield.

In another letter to the editor re Annane's study [37], however, as well as in Feldmeier's mentioned above [35], attention was drawn to the administration of two treatments a day in the study while Marx's protocol calls for one treatment per day for twice the number of days. Feldmeier, though, seemed to excuse this deviation, pointing out that at least one well-known hyperbaric medical center in the U.S. routinely treats patients twice a day for the same reason as Annane did [32, 35]. Regardless, Annane responded to these queries about the use of two treatments per day in print saying that "there is no evidence from both experimental and clinical studies to suggest that one HBO_2 session per day is superior to two sessions per day" [38]. Obviously, this reply by Annane would seem to be in ignorance of and contrary to the outcome of the study of Barth et al. [39] and other publications concerning HBO_2 and bone healing, but it was never formally rebutted by any party we are aware of. In addition, angiogenesis, the promotion of which is the objective of the Marx treatment protocol for ORN, like any physiological process, requires time to occur. Thus, unless the rate of angiogenesis were doubled by two treatments per day, which seems highly unlikely, the ultimate outcome of HBO_2 administered twice a day would not seem comparable to administration once a day per Marx's established protocol.

As a final point on this matter, there is the issue of Annane's study producing substantially poorer results, though not statistically significantly so, for the HBO_2-treated cases of ORN [32]. Annane and his associates never addressed this matter, and as Marx's explanation for the benefits provided by HBO_2 for the treatment of osteoradionecrosis was alteration of the existing hypoxia, hypocellularity, and hypovascularity [33], it is difficult to accept that even without adequate debridement, the HBO_2-treated cases would do less well than the placebo control cases rather than at least as well. Feldmeier [35] seems to have had the same thought, though he expressed it in opposite terms, noting that Annane and associates [32] offered no explanation for why the placebo arm of their study had a notably higher though not statistically significant rate of recovery from ORN. Based on the biphasic nature of the oxygen dose-response for the clinical use of oxygen established in this report and the two treatments per day administered in the Annane study, too much oxygen would certainly seem the logical explanation for why the HBO_2-treated patients in that study did not do as well as the untreated controls.

As this situation now stands, and in view of the evidence assembled in this report relating to oxygen dose-response, it seems there are still unanswered questions concerning the efficacy of HBO_2 for osteoradionecrosis of the mandible related to two treatments per day. Research comparing the outcomes of one and two HBO_2 treatments per day for ORN with the appropriate standards of care, and other conditions for which two treatments per day are used but not validated through controlled clinical research, would seem appropriate to conduct to clarify the uncertainties about such therapeutic practices currently in use or that are being considered to be put into practice.

3.3 Treatment of sports injuries

We trust the lengthy discussion at the beginning of Part 1 of this publication has made the point that normal wounds, such as sports injuries, can be effectively treated with hyperoxia at an appropriate dose. There is one "injury" that has been frequently used as representative of sports injuries. This is delayed onset muscle soreness (DOMS). For the purpose of rounding out the discussion of *normal* sports injuries in this report, further comment on the treatment of this condition is warranted.

3.3.1 Delayed onset muscle soreness

DOMS is a mild muscle over-use or unaccustomed-use injury that is convenient to design research around for either human or animal subjects. Thus, when the authors' efforts in the mid-1990s began to recruit professional sports teams in the United Kingdom and North America to utilize hyperbaric oxygen therapy to treat their injured athletes, a number of DOMS studies were initiated[4] [40–49]. For the most part, the conclusions of these studies were that HBO_2 was not an effective treatment for DOMS, and a review from the standpoint of evidence-based medicine by Bennett and associates in 2005 [50] found that the studies they included in their analyses provided an insufficient basis upon which to draw conclusions.

When examining these DOMS-based studies [43–49, 51–53] from the standpoint of oxygen dose-response, however, it is clear that these were primarily cases of overdosing very minor injuries with hyperoxia, in some cases utilizing full clinical doses for human subjects (i.e., 2.4 ATA oxygen for 120 minutes [44]; 2.5 ATA oxygen for 100 minute [46, 49].

Toward the lower end of the oxygen doses utilized to treat DOMS in human research relating to sports injuries [42, 45, 48], 2.0 atm oxygen for 60 minutes once a day has been an effective dose for a variety of serious but uncompromised sports injuries including severe muscle contusions and strains, as well as ligament and tendon injuries[5,6] [52, 54]. Thus, even these relatively low doses of hyperbaric oxygen used in research would seem to be too high for DOMS. In view of this, perhaps normobaric oxygen or even a lower concentration of oxygen would prove to be an effective regimen for the treatment of DOMS. The Uchimaru study[4] would seem to establish a dose that under-treats DOMS, however. In that study, 28% oxygen at 1.3 ATA (effectively $mHBO_2$ with a P_iO_2 of 0.364) did not significantly improve recovery compared to normobaric air. This matter really has little relevance to sports injuries, however. In our substantial experience in this regard, DOMS is not, as it is described by Mekjavic et al. [41] or Delaney and Montgomery [53], an injury that professional athletes have

[4] Uchimaru J, Li S, Takamura H, Suzuki S, Sato T. Effect of hyperbaric oxygen treatment on the delayed onset muscle soreness after eccentric exercise (abstract). American College of Sports Medicine. 2010.

[5] James PB. Hyperbaric Oxygen in Soft Tissue Injury. Report to the Directors of Dundee United F.C. 1989.

[6] Peterson RE, Allen MW. The adjunctive use of hyperbaric therapy for the treatment of sports injuries. Hyperbaric Medicine, 1995, Columbia, South Carolina. 20-22 March 1995.

used hyperbaric oxygen therapy to treat or would likely do so, especially because such treatment has not proven to provide any enhancement of healing.

3.3.2 With mild hyperbaric oxygen therapy

Currently, some manufacturers of inflatable, mild HBO_2 "chambers," with 510(k) clearance as substantially equivalent to the Gamow bag for treatment of acute mountain sickness, if they in fact have any FDA clearance at all [50], have promoted these systems for the treatment of neurological disorders and athletic injuries. Such promotion has attracted the interest of elite athletes who have adopted these systems for home use.[7]

While some studies have used $mHBO_2$ systems to administer therapy for neurological conditions such as autism spectrum disorders [14–16], no results of studies on the use of such equipment for typical sports injuries have been published to our knowledge. Rather, the promotion of $mHBO_2$ systems for the treatment of sports injuries would seem to depend on the results published for research with conventional clinical HBO_2 chambers using appropriate doses of oxygen as discussed above [50].

With respect to physical trauma to soft tissue, connective tissue, and bone, the two forms of treatment are not at all comparable. Further, several studies of sports injuries with control data reasonably like $mHBO_2$ have shown that the results of $P_iO_2s \leq 1.0$ ATA are significantly inferior to HBO_2 treatments conducted at 2.0 and 2.5 ATA breathing 100% oxygen.

Abbadi and Elrefai [55] showed that treating recently occurring acute ankle sprains seven times for 90 minutes, each, over a five-day period produced significant pain relief, with HBO_2 administered at 2.0 ATA (80% pain relief) and 2.5 ATA (97% pain relief), and no pain relief attributable to the oxygen treatments given at 1.0 ATA. In comparison to this last treatment condition, however, typical $mHBO_2$ has less than one-third the P_iO_2. Thus, based on this study, $mHBO_2$ could not be expected to provide any benefits over and above no treatment administration.

Chen et al. [56] treated first-degree muscle strains in baseball players with HBO_2 at 2.5 ATA for 70 minutes per treatment twice a week for 10 weeks. Each treatment had two 5-minute air-breaks taken from the 70 minutes and two appended 15-minute periods, one at the start for compression to the treatment pressure, and the other at the end for decompression from the treatment pressure to surface pressure. These subjects were compared to blinded control subjects breathing air at 1.3 ATA on the same treatment schedule, though the control group breathed oxygen during the 15-minute decompression time to surface pressure. The P_iO_2 during the control treatment phase was 0.2724 atm, just slightly below the typical PiO2 of $mHBO_2$, 0.312 atm. At the end of this course of therapy, the HBO_2-treated subjects were significantly better than the control subjects in most assessment categories and inferior in none. Those assessment categories with superior outcomes were:

- Muscular enzymes including reduced serum levels of CK (creatine kinase), GOT (glutamic-oxaloacetic transaminase), and MB (myoglobin), which were positive indications of recovery from muscular injury.

- Subscales of the Brief Pain Inventory including improved general activity, mood, sleep, and enjoyment of life.

[7] Terrell Owens uses his "hyperbaric" chamber—Vitaeris 320. https://www.youtube.com/watch?v=8SrzFEnDal8

As with the Abbadi and Elrefai [55] research, Chen and associates' [56] control data failed to show results that would suggest benefits for $mHBO_2$ in the treatment of typical sports injuries.

Another study to include in this discussion was conducted by Horie et al. [57]. They investigated recovery with HBO_2 from injury to the tibialis anterior muscles of rats induced by injecting cardiotoxin (CTX) into them. The HBO_2 treatments consisted of 120 minutes of oxygen at 2.5 ATA once a day, 5 days per week for 2 weeks. As well as untreated controls, other post-injury management utilized air breathing at 2.5 ATA (having a P_iO_2 of about 0.524 atm) and oxygen breathing at 1.0 ATA, with the other treatment parameters like those for the HBO_2-treated subjects [57]. It should be noted that both the hyperbaric air and normobaric oxygen treatments had P_iO_2s substantially greater than those typical of $mHBO_2$. Assessments comparing the HBO_2-treated rats to untreated controls, normobaric oxygen-treated animals, and hyperbaric-air-treated animals included histological analyses and measurement of the maximum force producing capacity of the regenerating muscle fibers. The results showed that HBO_2 treatments, but not hyperbaric air or normobaric oxygen treatments, accelerated satellite cell proliferation and myofiber maturation in rat muscle that was injured by a CTX injection, particularly at the end of the 2-week course of treatments. Thus, again, there was no indication of benefits from oxygen breathing conditions somewhat greater than those of $mHBO_2$.

To this point, a primary focus of this report has been the significant over-treating of normal wounds with hyperoxia and, thus, giving a false impression that such therapy is not beneficial for uncompromised trauma. In the fourth study to be discussed below, however, we have a first case in which all the hyperoxic treatments administered to subjects would appear to have been under-treatments. In this particular study reported by Uchimaru and associates (2010), 28% oxygen at 1.3 ATA (effectively $mHBO_2$ with a PiO_2 of 0.364 atm) did not significantly improve recovery from DOMS compared to normobaric air. This strongly suggests, therefore, that $mHBO_2$, usually with a slightly lower PiO2 (i.e., 0.312 ATA), would be an under-treatment for typical, more serious (i.e., than DOMS) sports injuries. On this basis, it seems that $mHBO_2$ is not likely to benefit any athlete seeking to expedite recovery from an injury he has sustained through participation in sport that we would expect to be more severe than DOMS.

4. Conclusions

Through extensive review of the scientific and clinical literature examining the issue of whether or not hyperbaric oxygen therapy could be an effective treatment for normal wounds (i.e., wounds that heal normally [58], it became evident to the authors that for therapeutic applications, hyperoxia is dose dependent. It also became apparent that the dose-response relationship for the clinical use of oxygen is biphasic in character, with beneficial effects in the lower dose range and negative impact in the higher dose range (i.e., hormetic in nature) when starting with the breathing of room air at one atmosphere absolute. The descending limb at higher doses in the dose-response relationship ultimately produces outcomes inferior to no hyperoxic therapy being administered at all (**Figure 4**, Part 1). This result is caused by the toxic effects of oxygen, which, in relative overdose, can have negative impact on all cells [59].

Another aspect of the dose-response relationship of hyperoxic therapy is that medical applications have a continuum of doses beginning at just greater than the partial pressure of oxygen in air at one atmosphere (i.e., 0.20954 atm) and extending to 3.0 atm of oxygen, which is the highest partial pressure deemed safe for clinical use over a limited time period. With this model, it is our experience that hydrostatic pressure is only essential to raise the oxygen partial pressure to values greater than 1.0 atm to reach a PiO_2 sufficient to get a positive response from the tissue or tissues being addressed, except for the treatment of gas phase/embolic (i.e., bubble) disorders (i.e., arterial and venous gas embolism, and decompression sickness). In these latter cases, the physical size of the gas phase can be reduced by increased pressure in a whole body chamber to accomplish such things as clearing gas-phase obstructions and thereby improving oxygen delivery to tissues through the circulation, enhancing gas phase elimination by concentrating gas molecules in smaller bubble volumes, and reducing pain produced by the physical size of the gas phase.

Obviously, if it will positively impact a given condition, normobaric oxygen therapy is more convenient, less risky, and less costly to administer than hyperbaric oxygen therapy. As we have shown in our autism studies over the last 11+ years years (as of early 2024), with an appropriate breathing gas assembly, normobaric hyperoxic therapy prescribed by a physician is suitable and safe for use with children in their homes [19] and, thus, we contend, for adults in assisted living situations. The administration, per se, can be easily and properly done by nonprofessionals, including suitably trained parents of children who are receiving the therapy.

In considering conditions that may be effectively treated with hyperoxia at normobaric pressure, some neurological disorders including autism spectrum disorder [19], Alzheimer's and other dementia [60], traumatic brain injury [22], chronic stroke [24], post-traumatic stress disorder [23], and cerebral palsy [25, 26] have promise. Also, wounds that do not respond to routine care such as diabetic ulcers of the lower extremities might benefit from early intervention with normobaric hyperoxia before they progress to intractable Wagner Grade 3 and 4 wounds that require hyperbaric oxygen therapy for management, with this latter therapy increasing the cost of care and decreasing the quality of life of the patients involved.

In conclusion, understanding the nature of oxygen dose-response and that the healing of normal wounds can be enhanced with oxygen therapy in proper dose in either normobaric or hyperbaric conditions provides opportunities to expand the overall applications of hyperoxic therapy and improve outcomes for patients as well as reduce their overall cost of care. This could include improved treatment protocols for hyperbaric oxygen therapy resulting from the leftward shift of the relevant oxygen dose-response relationship over a course of therapy and the possibility of physicians being able to treat some conditions more effectively with normobaric oxygen therapy or even normobaric gases with less than 1.0 ATA of oxygen.

Acknowledgements

By Russell E. Peterson, Ph.D.: I would like to thank my mother, Pauline W. Peterson, whose interest in medicine and the medical sciences led to my career in diving and hyperbaric medicine and physiology. I would also like to acknowledge my graduate school mentor, Christian J. Lambertsen, M.D., whose guidance to believe in one's own observations rather than the beliefs of others was a critical element in the evolution of this publication.

By Michael W. Allen: I would like to thank my parents, Phyllis P. and William G. Allen, who blessed me with an inquisitive mind and a need for constant learning.

I would also like to thank Philip B. James M.D., Ph.D, my early mentor and lifelong friend who fostered my interest in pressure physiology and the potential offered by the use of oxygen in medicine.

Funding statement

The entire literature review, development of concepts, and preparation of this report were funded by the authors. No outside funding was sought or received from any source.

Conflict of interest

The authors are the Founding Partners of Microbaric® Oxygen Systems, LLC, now known as NEMO Therapeutics, LLC, which was established to provide an organization through which research in applications of normobaric oxygen therapy, particularly autism spectrum disorders, could be investigated and, as possible and appropriate, made available as a mainstream medical therapy for autism and other neurological conditions for which there is currently no effective treatment. This organization has been funded in full by the Founding Partners. No outside funding or income has been received to support the research and writing of this review of oxygen dose response.

Data availability

All publications cited as journal or book references in this manuscript are available from the National Center for Biotechnology Information, U.S. National Library of Medicine: 8600 Rockville Pike, Bethesda MD, 20894. www.ncbi.nlm.nih.gov/pubmed and other scientific and university databases.

Author details

Russell E. Peterson* and Michael W. Allen
NEMO Therapeutics, LLC, Sarasota, Florida, USA

*Address all correspondence to: repeterson@nemotherapy.com.

References

[1] Barr P-O, Perrins DJD. Prolonged use of hyperbaric oxygen (HBO) in indolent ulcers of the leg. In: Proceedings of the Eighth International Congress on Hyperbaric Medicine; August 20-22; Long Beach, California. CA, USA: Best Publishing Company; 1984. pp. 217-222

[2] Hunt TK, Zederfeldt B, Goldstick TK. Oxygen and healing. The American Journal of Surgery. 1969;**118**(4):521-525

[3] Sheffield PJ, Fitzpatrick EL, Hutching DJ. Long-term effect on PO2 of the healing wound (abstract). In: Reprints of 1979 Annual Scientific Meeting. Washington, D.C.: Aerospace Medical Association; 1979

[4] Neubauer RA. Exposure of multiple sclerosis patients to hyperbaric oxygen at 1.5-2 ATA. A preliminary report. Journal of Florida MA. 1980;**87**(5):498-504

[5] Karapetian IS, Volozhin AI, Oleĭnik NN, Druzhinina RA. Treatment of mandibular fractures using hyperbaric oxygenation. Stomato Logiia (Mosk). 1985;**64**(3):35-38. Russian

[6] Quirinia A, Viidik A. The effect of hyperbaric oxygen on different phases of healing of ischaemic flap wounds and incisional wounds in skin. British Journal of Plastic Surgery. 1995;**48**(8):583-589

[7] Sadeghani K, Gottlieb SF, Van Meter K, Farris B. The effect of increased oxygen tensions on healing surgical wounds. In: Undersea and Hyperbaric Medical Society, Inc. Annual Scientific Meeting; 6-11 June, 1989; Hawaiian Regent Hotel, Honolulu, Hawaii, USA. Available from: http://archive.rubicon-foundation.org/6629

[8] Holbach KH. Discussion of Miller and Ledingham paper. In: Wada J, Iwa T, editors. Proceedings of the Fourth International Congress on Hyperbaric Medicine. Baltimore: Williams and Wilkins; 1969. pp. 453-458

[9] Holbach KH, Gott U. Effect of hyperbaric oxygenation therapy (HOT) on neurosurgical patients. In: Wada J, Iwa T, editors. Proceedings of the Fourth International Congress on Hyperbaric Medicine. Tokyo: Igaku Shoin Ltd; 1970. pp. 441-447

[10] Holbach KH, Caroli A. Oxygen tolerance and the oxygenation state of the injured human brain. In: Trapp WG et al., editors. Fifth International Hyperbaric Congress Proceedings, 1973. Burnaby, B.C., Canada: Simon Fraser University; 1974. pp. 350-361.87

[11] Pierce EC, Jacobson JH. Cerebral edema. In: Davis JC, Hunt TK, editors. Hyperbaric Oxygen Therapy. Bethesda MD: Undersea Medical Society; 1977. pp. 267-301

[12] Neubauer RA, End E. Hyperbaric oxygenation as an adjunct therapy in strokes due to thrombosis. A review of 122 patients. Stroke. 1980;**11**(3):297-300

[13] Hyperbaric Oxygen Therapy Indications. 14th edition. Ed: RE Moon Pub: Undersea Hyperbaric Medical Society

[14] Rossignol DA, Rossignol LW, James SJ, Melnyk S, Mumper E. The effects of hyperbaric oxygen therapy on oxidative stress, inflammation, and symptoms in children with autism: An open-label pilot study. BMC Pediatrics. 2007;7:36-48

[15] Rossignol DA, Rossignol LW. Hyperbaric oxygen therapy may improve

symptoms in autistic children. Medical Hypothesis. 2006;**67**:216-228

[16] Rossignol DA, Rossignol LW, Smith S, Schneider C, Logerquist S, et al. Hyperbaric treatment for children with autism: A multicenter, randomized, double-blind, controlled trial. BMC Pediatrics. 2009;**9**:21-36

[17] Granpeesheh D, Tarbox J, Dixon DR. Randomized trial of hyperbaric oxygen therapy for children with autism. Research in Autism Spectrum Disorders. 2010;**4**:268-275

[18] Jepson B, Granpeesheh D, Tarbox J, Tarbox J, et al. Controlled evaluation of the effects of hyperbaric oxygen therapy on the behavior of 16 children with autism Spectrum disorders. Journal of Autism and Developmental Disorders. 2011;**41**:575-588

[19] Peterson RE, Allen MW. Evolution and preliminary testing of a hyperoxic therapy for autism spectrum disorders. Autism Open Access. 2018;**8**:233. DOI: 10.4172/2165-7890.1000233

[20] Peterson RE, Allen MW. Hypothesis for how hyperoxic therapy may facilitate effective biologic "correction" of autism spectrum disorders. Autism Open Access. 2020;**10**:250. DOI: 10.35248/2165-7890.20.10.250

[21] Sampanthavivat M, Singkhwa W, Chaiyakut T, Karoonyawanich S, Ajpru H, et al. Hyperbaric oxygen in the treatment of childhood autism: A randomised controlled trial. Diving Hyperbar Medicine. 2012;**42**:128-133

[22] Wolf EG, Cifu D, Baugh L, Carne W, Profenna L. The effect of hyperbaric oxygen on symptoms after mild traumatic brain injury. Journal of Neurotrauma. 2012;**29**:2606-2612

[23] Miller RS, Weaver LK, Bahraini N, Churchill S, Price RC, et al. Effects of hyperbaric oxygen on symptoms and quality of life among service members with persistent post-concussion symptoms: A randomized clinical trial. JAMA Internal Medicine. 2015;**175**(1):43-52. DOI: 10.1001/jamainternmed.2014.5479

[24] Anderson DC, Bottini AG, Jagiella WM, Westphal B, Ford S, et al. A pilot study of hyperbaric oxygen in the treatment of human stroke. Stroke. 1991;**22**:1137-1142

[25] Collet JP, Vanasse M, Marois P, Amar M, Goldberg J, et al. Hyperbaric oxygen for children with cerebral palsy: A randomised multicentre trial. Lancet. 2001;**347**:582-586

[26] Senechal C, Larivee S, Engelbert R, Marois P. Hyperbaric oxygenation therapy in the treatment of cerebral palsy: A review and comparison to currently accepted therapies. Journal of the American Physician Surgeons. 2007;**12**:109-113

[27] Ding J, Zhou D, Lui C, Pan L, Ya J, Ding Y, et al. Normobaric oxygen: A novel approach for treating chronic cerebral circulation insufficiency. Clinical Intervent Aging. 2019;**14**:564-570

[28] Van Allen HW, Anderson EL, Schroeter GA, Herman H. Efficacy of 100% 1 ATA (normalbaric) oxygen therapy on bladder dysfunction in patients with central nervous system inflammatory auto immune disease [chronic progressive and chronic stable multiple sclerosis patients] (abstract). Undersea Biomedical Research. 1985;**12**(1):29

[29] Kulonen E, Niinikoski J, Penttinen R. Effect of the supply of oxygen on the tensile strength of healing skin wounds

and granulation tissue. Acta Physio Scandinavia. 1967;**70**:112-115

[30] Moon KC, Han SK, Lee YN, Jeong SH, Dhong ES, Kim WK. Effect of normobaric hyperoxic therapy on tissue oxygenation in diabetic feet: A pilot study. Journal of Plastic Reconstruct Aesthetic Surgery. 2014;**67**:1580-1586

[31] Hunt TK, Niinikoski J, Zederfeldt BH, Silver IA. Oxygen in wound healing enhancement: Cellular effects of oxygen. In: Davis JC, Hunt TK, editors. Hyperbaric Oxygen Therapy. Bethesda, Maryland: Undersea Medical Society; 1977. pp. 111-122

[32] Annane D, Depondt J, Aubert P, Villart M, Gehanno P, Gaidos P, et al. Hyperbaric oxygen therapy for radionecrosis of the jaw: A randomized, placebo-controlled, double-blind trial from the ORN96 Study Group. Journal of Clinical Oncology. 2004;**22**:4893-4900

[33] Marx RE. A new concept in the treatment of osteoradionecrosis. Journal of Oral and Maxillofacial Surgery. 1983;**41**(6):351-358

[34] Marx RE, Johnson RP, Kline SN. Prevention of osteoradionecrosis: A randomized prospective clinical trial of hyperbaric oxygen versus penicillin. Journal of the American Dental Association. 1985;**111**(1):49-54

[35] Feldmeier JJ. In response to the negative randomized controlled hyperbaric trial by Annane et al. in the treatment of mandibular ORN. Undersea & Hyperbaric Medicine. 2005;**32**:141-143

[36] Moon RE, McGraw TA, Blakey G III. Hyperbaric oxygen therapy for radiation necrosis of the jaw: Comments on a randomized study. Undersea & Hyperbaric Medicine. 2005;**32**:145-147

[37] van Merkesteyn R, Bakker DJ. Comment on "Hyperbaric oxygen therapy for radionecrosis of the jaw: A randomized, placebo-controlled, double-blind trial from the ORN96 study group". Journal of Clinical Oncology. 2005;**23**(19):4465-4466

[38] Annane D, Chevret S. In reply. Journal of Clinical Oncology. 2005;**23**(19):4466-4468

[39] Barth E, Sullivan T, Berg E. Animal model for evaluating bone repair with and without adjunctive hyperbaric oxygen therapy (HBO): Comparing dose schedules. Journal of Investigative Surgery. 1990;**3**:387-392

[40] Mekjavic IB, Exner J, Tesch PA, Eiken O. Recovery of exercise-induced loss of muscle strength and muscle soreness is unaffected by HBO therapy. In: Marroni A, Oriani G, Wattel F, editors. Proceedings of the International Joint Meeting on Hyperbaric and Underwater Medicine. XXII Annual Meeting of the EUBS, XII International Congress on Hyperbaric Medicine, III Consensus Conference of the ECHM 1996 Sept 4-8, Milano, Italy. Bologna: Grafica Victoria; 1996. pp. 557-560

[41] Mekjavic IB, Exner JA, Tesch PA, Eiken O. Hyperbaric oxygen therapy does not affect recovery from delayed onset muscle soreness. Medicine and Science in Sports and Exercise. 2000;**32**(3):558-563

[42] Edwards D, Phillips G, Van Someren K. A Study Investigating the Effects of Hyperbaric Oxygen on Recovery from Exercise Induced Muscle Damage [Report]. London: St. Mary's University College; 1995

[43] Staples JR, Clement DB, McKenzie DC, et al. The effects of intermittent hyperbaric oxygen on biochemical muscle metabolites of

eccentrically exercised rats [abstract]. Canadian Journal of Applied Physiology. 1995;**20**(Suppl):49

[44] Byrnes WC, Robinson D, Stevens B, Kearney JT, Sade E, Davison WM, et al. The effect of hyperbaric oxygen on delayed onset of muscle soreness as quantified by magnetic resonance imaging. In: Genser M, editor. Collection of Manuscripts for the XXIV Annual Scientific Meeting of the European Underwater and Baromedical Society. Stockholm, Sweden; 1998. p. 131

[45] Staples JR, Clement DB, Taunton JE, McKenzie DC. Effects of hyperbaric oxygen on a human model of injury. The American Journal of Sports Medicine. 1999;**27**(5):600-605

[46] Harrison BC, Robinson D, Davison BJ, Foley B, Sada E, Byrnes WC. Treatment of exercise induced muscle injury via hyperbaric oxygen therapy. Medicine and Science in Sports and Exercise. 2001;**33**(1):36-42

[47] Webster AL, Syrotuik DG, Bell GJ, Jones RL, Hanstock CC. Effects of hyperbaric oxygen on recovery from exercise-induced muscle damage in humans. Clinical Journal of Sport Medicine. 2002;**12**(3):139-150

[48] Babul S, Rhodes EC, Taunton JE, Lepawsky M. Effects of intermittent exposure to hyperbaric oxygen for the treatment of an acute soft tissue injury. Clinical Journal of Sports Medicine. 2003;**134**(3):138-147

[49] Germain G, Delaney J, Moore G, Lee P, Lacroix V, Montgomery D. Effect of hyperbaric oxygen therapy on exercise-induced muscle soreness. Undersea & Hyperbaric Medicine. 2003;**30**(2):135-145

[50] Bennett MH, Stanford R, Turner R. Hyperbaric oxygen therapy for promoting fracture healing and treating fracture non-union. Cochrane Database of Systematic Reviews. 2005;(1):CD004712

[51] James PB, Scott B, Allen MW. Hyperbaric oxygen therapy in sports injuries. Physiotherapy 1993;**79**(8):571-572

[52] Ishii Y, Miyanaga Y, Shimojo H, Shiraki H. The experience of hyperbaric oxygen therapy for soft tissue injuries of sports athletes. Japan Journal of Orthopaedic Sports Medicine. 1997;**17**(7):7-14

[53] Delaney JS, Montgomery DL. How can hyperbaric oxygen contribute to treatment. Physician and Sports Medicine. 2001;**29**(3):77-84

[54] Feldmeier J, Shah J, Peters J, Fache E. When it's better to be under more pressure 'mild hyperbaric' facilities need to comply with standards or cease and desist until they can. Pressure, UHMS Member Newsletter 2023;First Quarter:6-8 & 10

[55] Abbadi SM, Elrefai JM. The role of hyperbaric oxygen in managing ankle sprain. JRMS. 2004;**11**(1):21-23

[56] Chen YC, Chou WY, Ko JY, Mel SL, Wu RW. Early recovery of exercise-related muscular injury by HBOT. BioMed Research International. 2019;**6289380**:10. DOI: 10.1155/2019/6289380

[57] Horie M, Enomoto M, Shimoda M, Okawa A, Miyakawa S, Yagishita K. Enhancement of satellite cell differentiation and functional recovery in injured skeletal muscle by hyperbaric oxygen treatment. Journal of Applied Physiology. 2014;**116**:149-155

[58] Margolis GS, Roth RN, Hardy KR. The pressure is on. JEMS: A Journal

of Emergency Medical Services. 2000;**25**(5):76-87

[59] Lambertsen CJ. Effects of oxygen at high partial pressure. In: Fenn WO, Hahn H, editors. Handbook of Physiology, Section 3 Respiration. Washington DC: American Physiological Society; 1965;2. pp. 1027-1046

[60] Harch PG, Fogarty EF. Hyperbaric oxygen therapy for Alzheimer's dementia with positron emission tomography imaging: A case report. Medical Gas Research. 2018;**8**(4):181-184

Chapter 3

Biochemical Alterations and Antioxidant Levels in Patients Living with HIV

Bhawna Bhimte, Ranjit Patil, Rakesh Jagat, Hemant Verma, Daniya Nawaz and Bubul Kalita

Abstract

Acquired Immunodeficiency Syndrome (AIDS), is a contagious disease of the immune system caused by Human Immunodeficiency Virus (HIV). Present study aimed to find out biochemical parameters and antioxidant status of people living with HIV with or without co-morbidities. Total 110 patients enrolled in the study, maximum had no co-morbidities 56%, while 30% had tuberculosis. Majority of the patients were unemployed (35.5%) while 21.8% were unskilled workers. Total serum bilirubin (0.95 ± 0.51), total protein (7.22 ± 1.07) and alkaline phosphatase levels (134.52 ± 64.38) were found to be increased while serum albumin level was found to be decreased slightly (4.17 ± 0.79). Total antioxidant level was found to be reduced with or without co-morbidities in HIV patients. The study concluded for regular monitoring of biochemical parameters and antioxidant levels for better management of peoples living with HIV.

Keywords: AIDS, total antioxidant capacity, liver function test, co-morbidities, retrovirus, CD4- T cells, oxidative stress

1. Introduction

HIV, as name suggests damages the immune system. As the lentivirus travels via the lymphatic system, it affects the CD4 T cells by replicating in them and ultimately destroying them [1]. Cellular CD4 immunodeficiency at an early stage is a hallmark of HIV infection. AIDS has evolved itself from a mysterious illness to a global pandemic [2]. Data suggests that in the year 2021, around 650,000 people died from HIV-related grounds while 1.5 million people acquired HIV [3]. Highly reactive antiretroviral therapy (HAART), have been choice for management of HIV positive patients. Infected T lymphocytes leads to immune compromised situation. The body is faced with a dilemma of promoting apoptosis to eliminate HIV, yet consequently lowering the body's resistance to HIV.

Due to compromised immune system and the long-term ART therapy, people living with HIV may be at a higher risk of attaining co-morbidities related to cardio-vascular disease, chronic kidney disease, metabolic syndromes, hepatobiliary diseases etc. [4]. Moreover, HIV infection is complicated by various opportunistic infections (OIs) such as tuberculosis (TB), Hepatitis, candidiasis, herpes zoster, *Pneumocystis jerovicii*, cytomegalovirus (CMV) etc.

The involvement of the hepatobiliary system is a major concern in patients with HIV infection. Liver being the master organ for all the metabolic processes, approximately one third of the deaths in patients with HIV infection are in some way, related to liver disease. Opportunistic infections also add to the liver's burden. To ensure that the liver maintains its physiological normality throughout both the chronic and acute management of HIV infection, it is extremely crucial that people with HIV take care of their liver health [5].

Oxidative stress (OS) induced by the production of reactive oxygen species may play a critical role in the stimulation of HIV replication and the development of immunodeficiency. OS may have a principal contribution to both the expression of HIV and the development of AIDS. Oxidative stress is closely linked to chronic human immunodeficiency virus (HIV) infection, both alone and in combination with highly active antiretroviral therapy (HAART). Level of oxidative stress therefore also becomes a matter of concern in HIV patients, as it increases with disease progression. Studies also suggest a role of antioxidants in inactivation of viral replication, thereby making them an important early biochemical marker [6].

2. Material and methods

2.1 Study place

Study was conducted in the Department of Biochemistry in collaboration with the Department of Medicine and ART Centre at a tertiary care hospital of central India.

2.2 Inclusion criteria

- Patients registered at ART Centre, willing to participate and giving consent.
- Irrespective of their treatment status.
- Patients having any deranged parameters will be included and categorized for further data analysis.

2.3 Exclusion criteria

- Patient on oral antioxidant or multivitamins
- Newly detected patients

2.4 Study procedure

The study was conducted after obtaining clearance from the regional NACO Center and Institutional Ethical Committee. An informed consent in bilingual language was given and obtained from the study participants.

2.4.1 Sample size

The study group consisted of 110 HIV positive individuals, above 18 years of either sex. (Sample size calculated by sample size formula using total registered patients at ART centre).

2.4.2 Sample processing

Overnight fasting, 5 ml blood samples were collected following the universal aseptic precautions. A sterile vial without any anti-coagulant was used to collect a sample. The serum was separated after centrifugation and if required stored at -15° in deep freezer.

2.4.3 Biochemistry investigations

Following biochemical investigations were performed using Bio Systems BA400 analyzer.

- Serum bilirubin (Total and Direct) was measured by 2,4- Dichlorphenyl Diazonium (2,4- DCPD) method [7, 8];
- Alkaline phosphatase (ALP), Aspartate transaminase (AST) and Alanine transaminase (ALT) by modified IFCC method [7, 8].
- Serum albumin was assessed by (BCG) method [7],
- Total protein by Biuret method [8, 9] and
- Serum Globulin was calculated using the formula: Total protein - serum albumin.

Total antioxidant capacity (TAC) was measured by Colorimetric D Koracevic method [10].

CD4 count was done by flow cytometry.

2.4.4 Data collection and statistical analysis

Data was collected using MS Excel sheet. All the data was analyzed using Epi-info software. All variables were expressed as mean +/− SD (Standard Deviation). P value <0.05 was considered statistically significant.

3. Results and discussion

Present cross-sectional study of HIV positive patients, total 110 patients fulfilling all the inclusion and exclusion criteria were enrolled. Demographic profile showed diversity in socio-demography and HIV associated variables (**Figure 1**). The mean age of the patients reported was found to be 41.20 ± 10.44 years, out of them 62 of the subjects were males while 48 were females. Most of the subjects reported were unemployed (35.5%) followed by unskilled workers (21.8%) (**Table 1**). Study conducted by Amandeep Singh et al., showed similar results with maximum number of patients

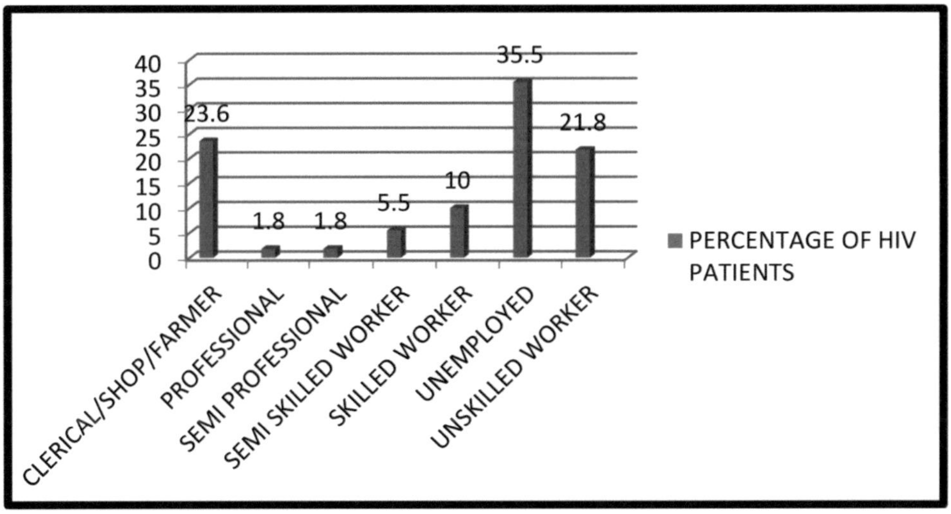

Figure 1.
Occupation wise distribution of study subjects. (classification of occupation is according to Kuppuswamy's classification).

Socio-demographic variables	HIV patients (Mean ± S.D.) (Percentage) n = 110
Age (in years)	41.20 ± 10.44
Male: Female Sex	62 (56.36%): 48 (43.64%)
Duration of HIV infection (in years)	6.43 ± 9.36

Table 1.
Age and sex distribution of HIV patients.

reported in their study that 73.8% patients belonged to the age group 41–60 years, 57.75% were males and 42.25% were females. They also reported predominance of patients from rural areas and from the lower middle and upper lower socio-economic classes [11].

Maximum number of HIV patients showed no co-morbidities (56%), while 30% had Tuberculosis. (**Figure 2**) This presents unique treatment challenges due to interactions between antitubercular and antiretroviral medications, overlapping drug toxicities, and the fact that HIV's immune-suppression delays the diagnosis of tuberculosis. In present study, 1% were infected with Hepatitis B, 5% with Hepatitis C and 2% with both hepatitis C and TB as co-infections. According to WHO guidelines co-infections are common among PLHIV, regardless of immune status. Some of those coinfections can be silent and do not cause significant impact on HIV disease nor are affected by it. In contrast, certain co-infections can affect the natural history of HIV infection and vice-versa, with implications in diagnosis, susceptibility, clinical presentation, and care, including timing and choice of drug regimens for treatment and prevention. WHO has developed specific guidance to manage some of these co-infections, focusing on the screening, prophylaxis, treatment and timing of ART for these conditions. The study by *A Treitinger*, et al., reported significant associations between hepatitis serological status and lipid profile [12].

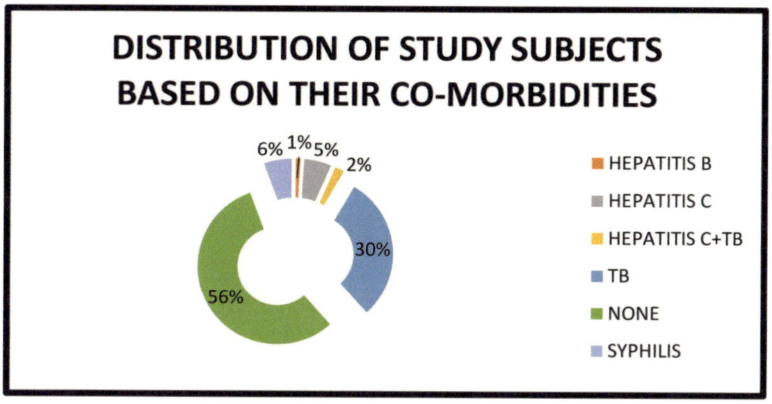

Figure 2.
Incidence of co-morbidities among HIV patients.

Table 2 shows levels of various biochemical parameters, levels of total bilirubin are significantly increased (0.95 ± 0.51) whereas levels of AST, ALT was deranged slightly. Total protein level was in normal range (7.22 ± 1.07) however serum albumin level was decreased (4.17 ± 0.79). According to Sunny Pathania et al., liver diseases account for almost 14–18% of all deaths in PLHA. They also reported hyperbilirubinemia (10.93%) and mild abnormalities in transaminases [13]. In a study by Sabir Kumar Dey et al., there was significant increase in total bilirubin levels of HIV positive patients as compared to normal [14].

Deranged parameters were also corelated on the basis of co-morbidities (**Table 3**), no strong association was found. This indicates that each co-morbidity has a different mechanism and it alters biochemical parameters in different ways. Hence there is need of assessment of each co-morbidity separately and the associated biochemical alterations.

Out of all co-morbidities, Tuberculosis (TB) had the highest percentage among the subjects. This presents unique treatment challenges due to interactions between antitubercular and antiretroviral medications, overlapping drug toxicities, and the

Biochemical parameters	Values (mean ± S.D.) n = 110
Liver function test	
Total bilirubin (mg/dl)	0.95 ± 0.51
AST (U/l)	35.13 ± 27.39
ALT (U/l)	30.94 ± 22.69
Serum albumin (g/dl)	4.17 ± 0.79
Total protein (g/dl)	7.22 ± 1.07
Serum globulin (g/dl)	3.05 ± 0.84
Alkaline phosphatase (IU/l)	134.52 ± 64.38

Table 2.
Mean values of common biochemical parameters in study subjects.

S.NO	Biochemical marker	Within range/ deranged	Comorbidities		Pearson Chi square	Df	P value
			Present	Absent			
1	Total bilirubin	Within range	33 (30%)	54 (49.09%)	3.911	1	0.041
		Deranged	14 (12.72%)	9 (8.18%)			
2	AST	Within range	40 (36.36%)	57 (51.81%)	0.745	1	0.284
		Deranged	7 (6.36%)	6 (5.45%)			
3	ALT	Within range	43 (39.09%)	60 (54.54%)	0.635	1	0.340
		Deranged	4 (3.63%)	3 (2.72%)			
4	Total protein	Within range	37 (33.63%)	50 (45.45%)	0.007	1	0.559
		Deranged	10 (9.09%)	13 (11.81%)			
5	Serum albumin	Within range	41 (37.27%)	55 (50%)	0.11	1	0.605
		Deranged	6 (5.45%)	8 (7.27%)			
6	Serum globulin	Within range	35 (31.81%)	45 (49.09%)	0.125	1	0.447
		Deranged	12 (10.9%)	18 (16.36%)			
7	Alkaline phosphatase	Within range	44 (40%)	50 (45.45%)	4.499	1	0.031
		Deranged	3 (2.72%)	13 (11.81%)			

Table 3.
Percentage of biochemical parameters in HIV patients with or without comorbidities.

fact that HIV's immune-suppression delays the diagnosis of tuberculosis. AST, ALT as well as ALP level was slightly elevated in patients with TB than without TB. Subir K et al., in their study of HIV patients with TB comorbidity reported elevated bilirubin, AST, ALT and ALP levels. But they reported low levels of albumin and globulin.

When oxidative stress was studied by measuring total antioxidant capacity of patients with co-morbidity, a clear correlation was seen (**Table 4**). It was seen that CD4 count was directly proportional to the total antioxidant capacity of patients. Similar study done by Suresh et al., reported strong association of oxidative stress with the level of CD4 count [15]. The discovery of HIV also led to a broadening of the view that ROS play a critical role in the expression of HIV and the development of AIDS. It has been reported that the virus induces OS by disturbing cellular anti-oxidant defense and initiating oxidative reactions. Advanced cases of HIV infection renders individuals susceptible to opportunistic infections, which take advantage of the progressive immunodeficiency caused by HIV [15]. Since cellular redox status is a normal physiological variable, any imbalance may elicit cellular response through proliferation, transcriptional activation, or apoptosis. For this reason, OS may be a principal mechanism in the progression of AIDS. Since OS can induce apoptosis, ROS may trigger apoptotic pathways responsible for the initial T-cell depletion upon HIV infection [15].

Biochemical parameter	Controls (mean ± S.D.)	HIV symptomatic patients (mean ± S.D.) N = 69	HIV asymptomatic patients (mean ± S.D.) N = 41	P value
Total antioxidant capacity (expressed in mmol/l)	1.08 ± 0.08	0.68 ± 0.14	0.75 ± 0.12	<0.02

Table 4.
Comparison of total antioxidant capacity with or without comorbidities.

4. Conclusion

It can be concluded from the present study that HIV causes either primary or treatment associated, liver function anomalies as well as OS. Majority of patients belonged to low socioeconomic status and productive age groups of their husband.

Due to the unique treatment challenges that TB + HIV co-infection poses and especially in a country like India who already suffers from a high TB load and a lack of resources, there's a need of careful monitoring of the interplay of anti-tubercular therapy with antiretroviral therapy, and that LFT and total antioxidant capacity are effective parameters that can be advised on a routine basis to assess any abnormalities. Total antioxidant capacity can be a novel early biomarker as it helps to assess the levels of oxidative stress in patients. Since present study has found direct correlation of OS with CD4 levels, the therapeutic effect of dietary anti-oxidant supplements and their role in delaying the progression of the disease comes into question. Further research will help to make ART regimens much better.

Author details

Bhawna Bhimte[1*], Ranjit Patil[2], Rakesh Jagat[1], Hemant Verma[3], Daniya Nawaz[1] and Bubul Kalita[1]

1 Gandhi Medical College, Bhopal, Madhya Pradesh, India

2 SSR Medical College, Mauritius

3 ART Plus Centre, Hamidia Hospital, Gandhi Medical College, Bhopal, Madhya Pradesh, India

*Address all correspondence to: bhawna_bhimte@yahoo.co.in

References

[1] Schacker T. The role of secondary lymphatic tissue in immune deficiency of HIV infection. AIDS. 2008;**22**(Suppl. 3):S13-S18

[2] Montagnier L. A history of HIV discovery. Science. 2002;**298**(5599):1727-1728

[3] World Health Organization. HIV/AIDS. World Health Organization. Available from: https://www.who.int/en/news-room/fact-sheets/detail/hiv-aids [Accessed: 26 December 2022]

[4] Goulet JL, Fultz SL, Rimland D, Butt A, Gibert C, Rodriguez-Barradas M, et al. Do patterns of comorbidity vary by HIV status, age, and HIV severity? Clinical infectious diseases. 2007;**45**(12):1593-1601

[5] Hernandez V. Liver function and HIV-1 infection. STEP Perspective. 1995 Summer;7(2):13-15

[6] Pandey M, Johri S, Talwar S.Role of Free Radicals during infection and the Advancement of Antioxidants to Improve the Treatment of Infectious Diseases. Antioxidant-Based Therapies for Disease Prevention and Management. 2021;(1):53-76

[7] Burtis CA, Ashwood ER, Bruns DE, WB Saunders Co. Tietz Textbook of clinical Chemistry and Molecular Diagnosis. 2005;**4**(1):1195-1197

[8] Friedman RB, Young DS. Effects of Disease on Clinical Laboratory Tests. AACC Press; 2002;**48**(4):682-683. DOI: 10.1093/clinchem/48.4.682a

[9] Gornall AG, Bardawill CS, David MM. Determination of serum proteins by means of biuret reaction. The Journal of Biological Chemistry. 1949;**177**:751-766

[10] Korvacevic D, Koracevic G, Djordjevic V, Andrejevic S, Cosic V. Method for measurement of antioxidant activity in human fluid. Journal of Clinical Pathology. 2001;**54**(5):356-361

[11] Singh A, Mahajan S, Singh T. Shyam sunder DeeptiSocio-demographic and clinical profile of HIV/AIDS patients attending the ART centre of Amritsar, Punjab. International Journal of Community Medicine and Public Health. 2018;**5**(5). DOI: 10.18203/2394-6040.ijcmph20181723

[12] Treitinger A, Spada C, da Silva LM, Hermes EM, Amaral JA, Abdalla DS. Lipid and acute-phase protein alterations in HIV-1 infected patients in the early stages of infection: Correlation with CD4+ lymphocytes. The Brazilian Journal of Infectious Diseases. 2001;**5**(4):192-199. DOI: 10.1590/s1413-86702001000400005

[13] Pathania S, Kaur N, Kumar S, Sashindran VK, Puri P. A cross-sectional study of liver function tests in HIV-infected persons in Western India. Medical Journal, Armed Forces India. 2017;**73**(1):23-28. DOI: 10.1016/j.mjafi.2016.12.004

[14] Dey SK, Ghosh I, Bhattacharjee D, Jha S, Dasgupta A, Dey SK. Liver function profile anomalies in HIV seropositive tuberculosis. Journal of Clinical and Diagnostic Research. 2013;7(6):1068-1072. DOI: 10.7860/JCDR/2013/5156.3047. Epub 2013 Jun 1

[15] Suresh DR, Annam V, Pratibha K, Prasad BV. Total antioxidant capacity--a novel early bio-chemical marker of oxidative stress in HIV infected individuals. Journal of Biomedical Science. 2009;**16**(1):61. DOI: 10.1186/1423-0127-16-61

Section 2

Hypoxia and Hemodynamics

Chapter 4

Relationship between Hypoxia and Pulmonary Microcirculation Hemorheology in Pediatric Patients with Patent Ductus Arteriosus Operated on at Moderate Altitude

Valeria Juárez García, Thalía Fernanda Camarillo González, Eunice Rut Rodríguez Cornejo and Pedro José Curi-Curi

Abstract

Hypobaric hypoxia due to altitude is a risk factor for patent ductus arteriosus (PDA). In order to explore a relationship between hypoxia and pulmonary microcirculation hemorheology in pediatric patients with surgically corrected PDA, a clinical case control study was carried out in a single medical center at a mean moderate altitude of 2240 meters above sea level (mASL). Patients were divided in two groups, with hypoxia (problems) and without hypoxia (controls), using conventional gasometric criteria. The problem group showed a higher hematocrit value. This suggests that an increase in blood viscosity due to the higher hematocrit level in response to altitude is a factor that promotes hypoxia in the pulmonary microcirculation. A pathophysiological explanation for this acute response in the problem group is provided.

Keywords: hypoxia, microcirculation, hemorheology, patent ductus arteriosus, altitude

1. Introduction

Patent ductus arteriosus (PDA) is one of the most frequent congenital heart diseases in countries located at an altitude above the sea level [1]. Ductus arteriosus is a fetal vascular structure that connects the left pulmonary artery with the descending thoracic aortic isthmus, and its function is to provide oxygen (O_2) as well as nutrients to the fetal lungs [2]. Its anatomic and functional closure occurs during the first hours after birth and is usually completed by up to the third month of extrauterine life. When the ductus arteriosis remains open from birth to the sixth week of extrauterine life and thereafter, it is considered as persistent [3]. Closure of PDA is due to the intake of oxygen in the first breath, the increase in blood oxygen partial pressure (PaO_2), and the decrease in the newborn prostaglandin E2 level [4–6]. Hypoxemia can lead to a delayed or non-closure of a PDA, however, developing changes in pulmonary microcirculation related to blood rheological properties [7].

Viscosity is the main rheological property of blood and depends on deformation and aggregation of erythrocytes, hematocrit, and plasma flow velocity in the pulmonary microcirculation. Pathological factors such as increases in leukocyte count and protein levels modify blood rheology [8, 9]. Since red blood cells (erythrocytes) are the most abundant blood components, their structure, function, and concentration are a main factor for blood rheology in the lungs. The function of red blood cells is to provide tissue oxygen *via* hemoglobin, which is a functional globular protein with high affinity for O_2 [10].

Altitude, considered as more than 1500 meters above the sea level (mASL), is a factor that affects interaction between hemoglobin and O_2 at the alveolar capillary level [11]. When ascending to high altitudes, the atmospheric pressure and the partial pressure of oxygen decrease. This leads to a reduction in the oxygen inspiratory fraction and less availability of this gas to be transported by hemoglobin. This condition is known as hypobaric hypoxia [12, 13]. The aim of this study is to analyze the relationship between hypoxia and hemorheology in the pulmonary microcirculation of pediatric patients with PDA operated on at a moderate altitude.

2. Methodology

A retrospective, observational, analytical, and cross-sectional case-control clinical trial was carried out. This included all pediatric patients with an echocardiographic diagnosis of PDA as the only cardiovascular pathology and who were operated on in a single-, high-, and specialized-level hospital located at a moderate altitude during a seven-year period of time. Exclusion criteria were patients without pre- and postsurgical laboratory data and those who were born at an altitude of less than 1500 mASL.

Patients were divided in two groups: Group 1 (problem: "WITH hypoxia") and Group 2 (control: "WITHOUT hypoxia"). Conventional gasometric criteria were used in order to include patients in the problem group: Alveolar oxygen pressure (PAO_2), arterial oxygen saturation (SAO_2), partial oxygen pressure/alveolar oxygen pressure (PaO_2/PAO_2), and PaO_2. Hypoxia was defined as the presence of one or more of the mentioned criteria (**Table 1**) [14–19].

Sociodemographic, clinical, echocardiographic, presurgical, postsurgical, and gasometric laboratory data were obtained from each patient's physical and electronic clinical record. According to the specific place of birth, the altitude and barometric pressure in millimeters of mercury (mmHg) corresponding to that geographical area was utilizrd to obtain PAO_2 and calculate the arterial-alveolar oxygen quotient.

A complete blood count was obtained as well as the blood gasometry of every patient, mainly within the first few days following their surgery. In neonates, gasometric samples were collected in heparinized capillary tubes. For infant patients, samples were taken in heparinized insulin syringes. Gasometric analysis was performed with the instrumentation Laboratory GEM 5000 premier system. Diagnosis of PDA was made by means of an echocardiogram, using GE Vivid S6 echocardiography equipment with neonatal and pediatric transducers.

Gasometric criteria	Reference values
Arterial SAO_2	Normal: 95–99% Acceptable: 90–95% Severe hypoxemia: <85%
PaO_2/PAO_2	Normal: >0.75 Hypoxemia: ≤0.75
Quotient PaO_2/FiO_2 adjusted ratio	Normal: >300 Mild hypoxia: ≤300 and >200 Moderate hypoxia: ≤200 and >100 Severe hypoxia: ≤100
PaO_2	Normal: 80–100 mmHg Acceptable: 60–80 mmHg Critical hypoxemia: 45–60 mmHg Severe hypoxemia: 45 mmHg

Abbreviations: SAO_2 = oxygen saturation, PaO_2 = partial oxygen pressure, PAO_2 = alveolar oxygen pressure, FiO_2 = oxygen inspired fraction, mmHg = millimeters of mercury.

Table 1.
Conventional gasometric criteria used to assess hypoxemia.

3. Statistical analysis

All the information was recorded in an electronic Excel spreadsheet and later processed with a SPSS v.21.0 statistical software. Continuous variables were expressed as mean ± standard deviation and categorical variables as absolute value and percentage in relation to the population at risk. Student's t-test was used to compare continuous variables and Fisher's exact test for categorical variables. A $p < 0.05$ was considered as statistically significant.

4. Results

A total of 18 patients (56.2%) were enrolled in the problem group and 14 (43.8%) in the control group. **Tables 2** and **3** show data results concerning the sociodemographic, clinical, and echocardiographic variables on both study groups. These are not significantly statistically different. The same is true for the data presented in **Tables 4** and 5. These include preoperative clinical variables, postsurgical follow-up details, hemodynamic stability parameters, gasometric criteria, and perioperative laboratory values. This means that both groups are fully comparable.

Although there are no statistically significant differences, it should be noted that in both study groups, infants made up the main population age group with the female gender predominating. Also, a higher percentage of patients with term birth live at an average altitude of 2683 mASL. Weight, height, and body mass index (BMI) showed low somatometric levels in the problem group according to child growth patterns established by the World Health Organization (WHO) [20]. According to the Center for Disease Control and Prevention (CDC) [21], however, both study groups had an adequate weight.

Most of the mothers of the problem group presented preeclampsia, and in the control group, the primary medications taken by the mothers during pregnancy were

Variables	WITHOUT hypoxia n (%)/mean ± SD (min-max)	WITH hypoxia n (%)/mean ± SD (min-max)	p
Age at surgery (years)	5.4 ± 3.70 (0.0–12.2)	4.0 ± 3.44 (0.1–11.9)	NS
Female	9 (64.2%)	14 (77.8%)	NS
Preterm	3 (21.4%)	6 (33.3%)	NS
Address (last 3 months)			
Mexico State	9 (64.28%)	16 (88.9%)	NS
Mexico City	4 (28.6%)	2 (11.1%)	NS
Hidalgo	1 (7.1%)	0 (0%)	NS
Somatometry			
Weight (kg)	26.6 ± 26.51 (1.1–109.0)	13.0 ± 7.78 (1.3–31.5)	NS
Size (cm)	113.9 ± 35.2 (36.0–163.0)	93.8 ± 22.68 (60.0–138.0)	NS
BMI (kg/m^2)	16.4 ± 7.54 (8.4–41.0)	13.6 ± 3.85 (2.3–20.4)	NS
Maternal morbidity	0 (0%)	6 (33.3%)	NS
Medication use in pregnancy	11 (78%)	14 (78%)	NS
Pregnancies			
Primigravida	4 (28.6%)	5 (27.8%)	NS
Multigesta	10 (71.4%)	13 (72.2%)	NS
Delivery way			
Vaginal	4 (28.6%)	9 (50.0%)	NS
Cesarean	10 (71.4%)	9 (50.0%)	NS
Type of pregnancy			
Single	13 (92.8%)	18 (100.0%)	NS
Multiple	1 (7.1%)	0 (0%)	NS
Fetal comorbidity	8 (57.1%)	7 (38.9%)	NS

Abbreviations: kg = kilograms, cm = centimeters, kg/m^2 = kilogram per squared meters, BMI = body mass index.

Table 2.
Comparison of sociodemographic and clinical variables between the studied groups.

multivitamins and betamethasone. Regarding fetal comorbidity, it should be noted that Down syndrome and congenital hypothyroidism predominated in the problem group. Regarding the preoperative clinical characteristics, the opportunity for surgery was elective in more than 80% of the patients. The primary operative technique used was extrapleural PDA section and suture. Very few patients required mechanical ventilation (18%) or the use of preoperative amines (5%) in either study groups.

It should be noted that 72% of the children in the problem group presented acute respiratory distress syndrome (ARDS) with different severity degrees and remained hypoxic, despite receiving an additional oxygen supply. This is corroborated by the significant increase in oxygen inspired fraction (FIO_2) and PAO_2 levels in this group. In contrast, patients in the control group did not require O_2 breathing since they were not determined to be hypoxic. **Table 6** shows the primary variables used to determine the relationship between hypobaric hypoxia and hematocrit in the pulmonary

Variables	**WITH hypoxia**	**WITHOUT hypoxia**	
	n (%)/mean ± SD (min-max)	**n (%)/mean ± SD (min-max)**	**p**
Smaller PDA mouth (mm)	6 ± 1.8 (3–10)	5.4 ± 1.9 (2–8)	NS
Smaller PDA mouth			
Pulmonary	10 (55.6%)	11 (78.6%)	NS
Aortic	6 (33.3%)	0 (0%)	NS
Same	2 (11.1%)	3 (21.4%)	NS
Aortic ring (mm)	11.2 ± 3.2 (7–17)	12.9 ± 3 (5–16)	NS
PDA/aortic ring ratio	0.6 ± 0.2 (0.3–1)	0.4 ± 0.1 (0.3–0.7)	NS
PDA size/Ao ring ratio			
Short	2 (11.1%)	4 (28.6%)	NS
Medium/large	13 (72.2%)	9 (64.3%)	NS
No data	3 (16.7%)	1 (7.1%)	NS
SPAP/SBP ratio	0.3 ± 0.1 (0.2–0.6)	0.3 ± 0.09 (0.2–0.5)	NS
PDA size/SPAP ratio			
Short	10 (55.6%)	9 (64.3%)	NS
Medium/large	1 (5.5%)	2 (14.3%)	NS
No data	7 (38.9%)	3 (21.4%)	NS
BP			
Systolic	99.6 ± 16.8 (67–134)	101.7 ± 20.4 (57–128)	NS
Dastolic	59.3 ± 15.8 (32–85)	59.5 ± 16.4 (38–89)	NS
Pulse pressure	40.3 ± 12.5 (21–70)	42.2 ± 13.8 (19–62)	NS
Mitral E/A ratio	1.5 ± 0.84 (0.7–2.5)	1.3 ± 0.7 (0.8–1.6)	NS

Abbreviations: Ao = aortic, Pu = pulmonary, PDA = patent ductus arteriosus, SPAP = systolic pulmonary artery pressure, SBP = systolic blood pressure, BP = blood pressure.

Table 3.
Comparison of echocardiographic variables between the studied groups.

microcirculation. A remarkable finding is the fact that the hematocrit values of the problem group were significantly higher than those of the control group. It can be seen that in addition to the already mentioned gasometric and hematocrit values, lactate also presents higher values in the problem group. Additionally, it can be observed that the echocardiographic diameter of the aorta at its interface with the heart had a statistical tendency to be greater in the problem group.

5. Discussion

Several reports show that healthy people who live at high altitudes have hypobaric hypoxia [22–24]. Since the closure of PDA is mainly related to O_2 concentrations, the presence of hypobaric hypoxia is an etiopathogenic risk factor for presenting this disease. The high prevalence of PDA in people living in hypoxic environments is associated with a delayed closure of PDA and postnatal pulmonary hypertension.

Variables	WITH hypoxia	WITHOUT hypoxia	
	n (%)/mean ± SD (min-max)	n (%)/mean ± SD (min-max)	p
Surgery opportunity			
Emergency	2 (11%)	2 (14%)	NS
Elective	16 (89%)	12 (86%)	NS
Surgical procedure			
Extrapleural SS	15 (83%)	13 (93%)	NS
Clip PDA closure	1 (5%)	1 (7%)	NS
Preoperative medications	15 (83%)	12 (86%)	NS
Invasive mechanical ventilation	2 (11%)	1 (7%)	NS
Preoperative vasopressor	1 (6%)	0 (0%)	NS
Preoperative (NYHA/Ross)			
I	4 (22%)	2 (14%)	NS
II	13 (72%)	12 (86%)	NS
III	1 (5%)	0 (0%)	NS
RACHS-1			
1	17 (94%)	13 (93%)	NS
2	1 (5%)	1 (7%)	NS
Postoperative (NYHA/Ross)			
I	18 (100%)	14 (100%)	NS
Surgical follow-up (months)	21.6 ± 16.4 (0–48)	10.9 ± 8.4 (2–25)	NS
Surgical morbidity/mortality	3 (17%)	2 (14%)	NS
Hemodynamic stability			
mPAP ≥25 mmHg	13 (72%)	10 (71%)	NS
Minor size PDA/Pu or Ao ring>1/3 (0.33)	11 (61%)	8 (57%)	NS
PDA minor diameter > 1.5 mm	1 (5%)	1 (7%)	NS
P pulse 25–30 mmHg	1 (5%)	0 (0%)	NS
PDA/Ao ring ratio > 0.5	1 (5%)	0 (0%)	NS
Mitral E/A ratio ≥ 1	1 (5%)	0 (0%)	NS
LV end-diastolic diameter with > +2	1 (5%)	1 (0%)	NS
AI/Ao > 1.3	1 (5%)	1 (0%)	NS

Abbreviations: NYHA = New York Heart Association, RACHS-1 = risk adjusted classification for congenital heart surgery-1, E/A = E wave/A wave ratio, LV = left ventricle, Ao = aorta.

Table 4.
Preoperative, follow-up, and hemodynamic stability clinical variables of the studied groups.

Variables	WITH hypoxia	WITHOUT hypoxia	p
	n (%)/mean ± SD (Min-Max)	**n (%)/mean ± SD (min-max)**	
Gasometry			
Preoperative	6 (33%)	11 (78%)	NS
Postoperative	11 (61%)	2 (14%)	NS
Unknown	1 (5%)	1 (7%)	NS
Arterial SaO_2			
Normal	13 (72.2%)	11 (78.6%)	NS
Hypoxemia	5 (27.8%)	0 (0%)	NS
Unknown	0 (0%)	3 (21.4%)	NS
PAO_2			
Hypoventilation	6 (33%)	0 (0%)	NS
Normal	7 (39%)	6 (43%)	NS
Unknown	5 (28%)	8 (57%)	NS
PaO_2/PAO_2			
Normal	8 (44%)	12 (86%)	NS
Hypoxia	5 (28%)	0 (0%)	NS
Unknown	5 (28%)	2 (14%)	NS
PaO_2/FIO_2			
Normal	1 (5%)	6 (43%)	NS
Mild	9 (50%)	0 (0%)	NS
Moderate	2 (11%)	0 (0%)	NS
Severe	2 (11%)	0 (0%)	NS
Unknown	4 (22%)	8 (57%)	NS
PaO_2			
Normal	5 (28%)	12 (86%)	NS
Acceptable	6 (33%)	0 (0%)	NS
Critical	2 (11%)	0 (0%)	NS
Unknown	5 (28%)	2 (14%)	NS
Hypoxia	18 (100%)	0 (0%)	NS
Preoperative laboratory			
Leukocytes	10 ± 3.8 (5.2–17.6)	7.9 ± 2.5 (4.6–12.9)	NS
Platelets	294.4 ± 71.2 (206–432)	245.9 ± 78.4 (92–356)	NS
Postoperative laboratory			
Hemoglobin	12.5 ± 1.7 (9.3–14.6)	12.9 ± 1.3 (9.6–14.7)	NS
Leukocytes	10.2 ± 4.3 (5.2–23.3)	9 ± 3 (5.9–14.9)	NS
Hematocrit	37.8 ± 4.9 (27.3–43.9)	39.2 ± 3.3 (31–43.1)	NS

Variables	WITH hypoxia	WITHOUT hypoxia	p
	n (%)/mean ± SD (Min-Max)	n (%)/mean ± SD (min-max)	
Platelets	290.9 ± 82.6 (171–435)	298 ± 122.4 (123–521)	NS

Abbreviations: SaO_2 = oxygen saturation, PAO_2 = oxygen alveolar pressure, PaO_2 = oxygen partial pressure, FIO_2 = oxygen inspired fraction.

Table 5.
Pre- and postoperative gasometric and laboratory variables of the studied groups.

The incidence of PDA therefore is higher in children who live at high altitudes in comparison to those who live at the sea level [25]. Under hypoxic conditions, juxtaglomerular cells of the kidney secrete erythropoietin (EPO), which stimulates bone marrow stem cells to produce red blood cells whose key component is hemoglobin. This increases O_2 transport to the different tissues as a hypoxia compensatory mechanism. Hematocrit levels, defined as the percentage fraction of erythrocytes contained in the blood, also increase in direct proportion to red cell count [26, 27].

Hematocrit is the main determinant of blood viscosity. Therefore, when there is a greater red blood cell count, blood viscosity increases [28]. To ensure a proper tissue oxygen and nutrient supply, it is necessary to maintain a normal blood flow rate, which depends on the length of blood vessels and the blood viscosity. Oxygen tissue supply depends on the arterial O_2 concentration and the blood flow through the vessels. Resistance is a factor that modifies blood flow velocity. This physiological relationship is stated mathematically by means of Poiseuille's Law, where the flow velocity of a fluid depends on the pressure and flow resistance. The flow resistance (R) is determined by the length of the blood vessel (L), the radius of the same vessel (r), and the viscosity of the fluid (η), in this case, blood [29, 30]. Any increase in blood viscosity and/or decrease in the diameter of blood vessels therefore leads to a decrease in the blood flow velocity [31].

The increase in blood viscosity causes a decrease in blood flow velocity in different organs such as the brain, heart, intestines, and lungs [32]. The slowdown in blood flow is a proven factor that promotes formation of microthrombi and alters the ventilation/perfusion ratio (V/Q) in the pulmonary microcirculation. This establishes a pattern in which there is ventilation without perfusion. The V/Q ratio in these circumstances tends to infinity. Such tissue is called physiological dead space and corresponds to areas of the lung that have adequate ventilation but not perfusion. Thus, they do not participate in gas exchange. The decreased oxygen concentration in blood leads to hypoxia and respiratory failure [33]. This is the reason why, despite the fact that the problem group has higher hematocrit values and therefore a greater oxygen transport capacity, hypoxia persists. Although it is true that the O_2 concentration is the same at different altitude levels, barometric pressure and therefore FiO_2 are lower as one ascends to higher altitudes. This value can also be modified if O_2 is supplied to the patient [34]. This is the case of the problem group, who, in addition to hypoxia, presented clinical data of respiratory failure for which additional oxygen was supplied. This increased the FiO_2 values in comparison to the control group and was therefore not an effect related to hypobaric hypoxia. Despite the fact that both groups presented similar altitude levels and barometric pressures, hypoxia and increased hematocrit values were only evidenced in the problem group.

The impact of blood viscosity in relation to hypoxia is a poorly studied parameter and is rarely considered in daily clinical practice. In this study, we showed that blood

Variables	WITH hypoxia n (%)/mean ± SD (min-max)	WITHOUT hypoxia n (%)/mean ± SD (min-max)	p
Demographics			
Altitude (mASL)	2258.1 ± 47.3 (2200–2400)	2301.9 ± 119.7 (2235.0–2667.0)	NS
Altitude ≥2300 (mASL)	2 (11.11%)	3 (21.43%)	0.432
Barometric pressure (mmHg)	581.6 ± 2.9 (572–584)	579.1 ± 7.5 (556–583)	NS
Echocardiographic			
Max gradient (mmHg)	57.2 ± 13.9 (25–80)	49.9 ± 20.4 (20–82)	NS
PDA length (mm)	9.8 ± 4 (5–24)	9.3 ± 3 (4–17)	NS
Aortic mouth (mm)	7.1 ± 1.6 (5–10)	9.1 ± 4.1 (4–17)	NS
Pulmonary mouth (mm)	6.9 ± 3.2 (3–17)	5.4 ± 1.9 (2–8)	NS
SPAP (mmHg)	29.5 ± 8.3 (20–50)	33.3 ± 11.2 (20–50)	NS
mPAP(mmHg)	32.1 ± 8.3 (22.6–52.6)	35.9 ± 11.3 (22.6–52.6)	NS
Preoperative laboratory			
Hemoglobin	13.3 ± 1.5 (10.9–17.3)	13.2 ± 2 (9.3–17.1)	NS
Hematocrit	40 ± 4.3 (34–53.2)	39.2 ± 5.5 (30–50.6)	NS
Gasometry			
pH	7.3 ± 0.2 (6.8–7.6)	7.4 ± 0.1 (7.2–7.6)	0.098
PaO_2	100.6 ± 82 (23–305)	155.8 ± 114.3 (38–397)	NS
$PaCO_2$	35 ± 8.4 (22–53)	31.7 ± 6.9 (20–46)	NS
SaO_2	91 ± 10.3 (64–100)	97 ± 2.4 (92–100)	0.042
HCO_3	20.1 ± 3.6 (14.9–28.3)	19.5 ± 3.4 (14.3–25)	NS
BE	−4.4 ± 8.4 (−25.2–10.5)	−3.9 ± 5.8 (−11.7–9.2)	NS
Lactate	1.4 ± 1 (0.5–4.3)	1 ± 0.4 (0.4–1.8)	NS
Hematocrit	33 ± 1.4 (31–34)	30.5 ± 4.9 (27–34)	0.047
FiO_2%	35.2 ± 19.2 (21–72)	21 ± 0 (21–21)	0.01
PAO_2	137.4 ± 101.8 (59.3–322.1)	74.8 ± 8.6 (64.7–86.1)	0.03
PaO_2/PAO_2	1 ± 0.7 (0.4–3.2)	1.9 ± 1.5 (1–5.1)	0.04
PaO_2/FiO_2	278.9 ± 144.9 (131.7–726.9)	520.1 ± 445 (313.5–1427.8)	0.03

Abbreviations: mASL = meters above sea level, mmHg = millimeters of mercury, mm = millimeters, SPAP = systolic pulmonary arterial pressure, mPAP = mean pulmonary arterial pressure, PaO_2 = oxygen arterial pressure, $PaCO_2$ = arterial carbon dioxide pressure, SaO_2 = oxygen saturation, HCO_3 = bicarbonate, BE = baseline excess, FIO_2 = oxygen inspired fraction, PAO_2 = oxygen alveolar pressure.

Table 6.
Demographic, echocardiographic, laboratory, and blood gas variables used to determine the relationship between pulmonary microcirculation and hemorheology.

viscosity is a factor that significantly influences the pulmonary microcirculation, favoring hypoxia. It seems that the increase in erythrocyte number and hematocrit level develops in order to improve hypoxia. This apparent compensatory mechanism, however, actually tends to perpetuate hypoxia rather than relieve it. The change in hemodynamics associated with increased viscosity promotes microthrombi as blood stasis is one of the factors that is part of Virchow's triad and is the main mechanism associated with thrombus genesis. Increased blood viscosity causes endothelial injury and affects blood flow turbulence, factors that contribute to platelet aggregation [35]. Pulmonary microcirculation is altered by the presence of microthrombi, which act as perpetuators of abnormal blood flow and therefore thrombosis promoters. Blood hyperviscosity, thrombosis and decreased pulmonary microcirculation, as well as endothelial injury and inflammation trigger the process of remodeling and interstitial fibrosis in the alveoli capillary unit in a medium- to long-term period of time. In hemodynamic terms, this factor produces a progressive increase in pulmonary vascular resistance and the consequent development of chronic thromboembolic disease as well as secondary pulmonary arterial hypertension [36].

On the other hand, it was additionally determined that in both of our study groups, most of the patients had a medium or large PDA diameter. Individuals who live permanently at moderate altitudes had increased pulmonary pressure and a larger diameter of PDA. This caused overload of pulmonary and left ventricular blood flow. A moderate or large PDA tends to be associated with moderate and severe pulmonary hypertension, respectively. More than 70% of the patients in both groups in our study had a mean pulmonary artery pressure > 25 mmHg, suggesting pulmonary hypertension. Thus, our study corroborates the literature [35, 36] that living at a moderate altitude predisposes to a greater diameter of the ductus arteriosus and therefore a greater probability of developing pulmonary hypertension. The diameter of the PDA, however, was not the most important factor associated with the presence of hypoxia in our problem group.

Finally, it is important to mention that our study has certain limitations such as the sample size and the retrospective nature of its design. Despite this, the trend of our results show a clear relationship between hypoxia and hemorheology in the pulmonary microcirculation produced by the increase in blood viscosity due to hematocrit level. If we increased the size of our sample, this tendency would likely be reinforced. In any case, it is highly recommended that future research should be carried out in this field in order to reliably confirm the tendencies identified in this study.

6. Conclusion

Though not statistically significant, the results of this study show a clear relationship between hypoxia and higher hematocrit values. This suggests that the increase in blood viscosity due to a higher hematocrit level in response to altitude, instead of controlling its hypobaric effects and being a compensatory mechanism, is a factor that promotes hypoxia in the pulmonary microcirculation. More clinical trials are needed to confirm this finding with statistical significance.

Conflict of interest

The authors declare no conflict of interest.

Appendices and nomenclature

PDA	patent ductus arteriosus
O_2	oxygen

PaO_2	oxygen partial pressure
mASL	meters above the sea level
PAO_2	alveolar oxygen pressure
SAO_2	arterial oxygen saturation
PaO_2/PAO_2	partial oxygen pressure/alveolar oxygen pressure
mmHg	millimeters of mercury
BMI	body mass index
WHO	World Health Organization
CDC	Center for Disease Control and Prevention
ARDS	acute respiratory distress syndrome
FIO_2	oxygen inspired fraction
EPO	Erythropoietin
R	resistance
L	length
r	radius
η	viscosity
V/Q	ventilation/perfusion
kg	kilograms
cm	centimeters
kg/m^2	kilogram per squared meters
Ao	aorta
Pu	pulmonary
SPAP	systolic pulmonary artery pressure
SBP	systolic blood pressure
BP	blood pressure
NYHA	New York Heart Association
RACHS-1	risk adjusted classification for congenital heart surgery-1
E/A	E wave/A wave ratio
LV	left ventricle
mm	millimeters
mPAP	mean pulmonary arterial pressure
$PaCO_2$	arterial carbon dioxide pressure
HCO_3	bicarbonate
BE	baseline excess

Author details

Valeria Juárez García[1,2], Thalía Fernanda Camarillo González[1,2],
Eunice Rut Rodríguez Cornejo[2,3] and Pedro José Curi-Curi[2*]

1 Facultad de Estudios Superiores, Universidad Nacional Autónoma de México, Mexico

2 Dirección de Planeación, Enseñanza e Investigación, Hospital Regional de Alta Especialidad de Ixtapaluca, Mexico

3 Escuela Superior de Medicina, Instituto Politécnico Nacional, Mexico

*Address all correspondence to: pcuricuri001@gmail.com

References

[1] Morales-Quispe JA, Espinola-Zavaleta N, Caballero-Caballero R, Merino-Pasaye LE, Solano-Gutierrez A, Rodríguez-Ortega F. Evolución posquirúgica de la hipertensión arterial pulmonar asociada a conducto arterioso permeable a una altitud de 2680 metros sobre el nivel del mar. Archivos de Cardiología de México. 2012;**82**(4):290-296

[2] Bunney PE, Zink AN, Holm AA, Billington CJ, Kotz CM. Diagnosis and management of ductus patent. Physiology & Behavior. 2017;**176**(1):139-148

[3] Lin TY, Yeh JL, Hsu JH. Role of extracellular matrix in pathophysiology of patent ductus arteriosus: Emphasis on vascular remodeling. International Journal of Molecular Sciences. 2020;**21**(13):1-17

[4] Liu C, Zhu X, Li D, Shi Y. Related factors of patent ductus arteriosus in preterm infants: A systematic review and meta-analysis. Frontiers in Pediatrics. 2021;**8**(January):1-13

[5] Martínez-Roque AM, Valle Leal J, Martínez Limón AJ, Álvarez-Bastidas L. Hemodynamic repercussions in neonates with patent ductus arteriosus: Associated factors. Archivos de Cardiología de México. 2017;**87**(3):248-251

[6] Gillam-Krakauer M, Reese J. Diagnosis and management of patent ductus arteriosus. NeoReviews. 2018;**19**(7):e394-e402

[7] Epçaçan S, Bulut MO, Kaya Y, Yücel İK, Çakır Ç, Şişli E, et al. Characteristics and transcatheter closure of patent ductus arteriosus in patients living at moderate to high altitude in eastern Anatolia. Turk Kardiyoloji Dernegi Arsivi. 2019;**47**(6):431-439

[8] Moggi L. Hemorreología y microcirculación. Revista Argentina de Anestesiología. 2011;**69**:61-84

[9] Saldanha C. Hemorheology, microcirculation and macrocirculation. Revista Portuguesa de Cardiologia. 2020;**39**(1):25-26

[10] Cross SJ, Linker KE, Leslie FM. Red blood cells: The forgotten player in hemostasis and thrombosis. Physiology & Behavior. 2016;**176**(1):100-106

[11] Herberg U, Knies R, Müller N, Breuer J. Altitude exposure in pediatric pulmonary hypertension-are we ready for (flight) recommendations? Cardiovascular Diagnosis and Therapy. 2021;**11**(4):1122-1136

[12] Moore LG. Measuring high-altitude adaptation. Journal of Applied Physiology. 2017;**123**(5):1371-1385

[13] Du X, Zhang R, Ye S, Liu F, Jiang P, Yu X, et al. Alterations of human plasma proteome profile on adaptation to high-altitude hypobaric hypoxia. Journal of Proteome Research. 2019;**18**(5):2021-2031

[14] Carrillo ÁA. Monitorización de la ventilación mecánica: gasometría y equilibrio acidobásico. Anales de Pediatría (English Edition). 2003;**59**(3):252-259

[15] Morales AA. Cociente PaO2/FiO2 o índice de Kirby: determinación y uso en población pediátrica. El Residente. 2015;**10**(2):88-92

[16] Donoso A, Arriagada D, Contreras D, Ulloa D, Neumann M. Monitorización respiratoria del paciente pediátrico en la Unidad de Cuidados Intensivos. Boletín

Médico del Hospital Infantil de México. 2016;**73**(3):149-165

[17] Román-Vistraín G, Mireya Muñoz-Ramírez C, Márquez-González H, Luis Álvarez-Valencia J, Zárate-Castañón P. Valoración respiratoria durante la guardia. El Residente. 2015;**10**(2):63-68

[18] Oliver P. Estudio de la oxigenación e interpretación de la gasometría arterial. Documentos de la SEQC. 2014;**2015**:31-47

[19] Garcia JCV, Padilla RP. Valores gasometricos estimados para las principales poblaciones y sitios a mayor altitud en Mexico. Revista del Instituto Nacional de Enfermedades Respiratorias. 2000;**13**(1):6-13

[20] Szkutnik M, Delgadillo M, Enrique P, Jacek B. Transcatheter closure of patent ductus arteriosus among native high-altitude habitants. Pediatric Cardiology. 2008;**29**:624-627

[21] Glowacki J, Zabal C, Bermúdez-Cañete R. Patent ductus arteriosus at low and high altitudes: Anatomical and haemodynamic features and their implications for transcatheter closure. Kardiologia Polska. 2011;**69**(5):431-436

[22] Getu A. Ethiopian native highlander' s adaptation to chronic high-altitude hypoxia. BioMed Research International. 2022;**2022**:1-5

[23] Zheng JY, Qiu YG, Li DT, He JC, Chen Y, Cao Y, et al. Prevalence and composition of CHD at different altitudes in Tibet: A cross-sectional study. Cardiology in the Young. 2017;**27**(8):1497-1503

[24] Suresh S, Rajvanshi PK, Noguchi CT. The many facets of erythropoietin physiologic and metabolic response. Frontiers in Physiology. 2020;**10**:1-20

[25] Ge RL, Witkowski S, Zhang Y, Alfrey C, Sivieri M, Karlsen T, et al. Determinants of erythropoietin release in response to short-term hypobaric hypoxia. Journal of Applied Physiology. 2002;**92**(6):2361-2367

[26] Pérez AG. Síndrome de hiperviscosidad. Características Fisiopatológicas y Clínicas. 2020;**59**(278):1-5

[27] Nader E, Skinner S, Romana M, Fort R, Lemonne N, Guillot N, et al. Blood rheology: Key parameters, impact on blood flow, role in sickle cell disease and effects of exercise. Frontiers in Physiology. 2019;**10**:1-14

[28] Secomb TW. Hemodynamics. Comprehensive Physiology. 2016;**6**(2):975-1003

[29] Cabrales P, Govender K, Williams AT. What determines blood viscosity at the highest city in the world? The Journal of Physiology. 2020;**598**(18):4121-4130

[30] Cakmak G, Alkan FA, Korkmaz K, Saglam ZA, Karis D, Yenigun M, et al. Blood viscosity as a forgotten factor and its effect on pulmonary flow. Translational Respiratory Medicine. 2013;**1**(1):1-5

[31] Fernández FR. Pathophysiology of gas exchange in ARDS. Medicina Intensiva. 2006;**30**(8):374-378

[32] Çınar T, Hayıroğlu Mİ, Selçuk M, Çiçek V, Doğan S, Kılıç Ş, et al. Association of whole blood viscosity with thrombus presence in patients undergoing transoesophageal echocardiography. The International Journal of Cardiovascular Imaging. 2022;**38**(3):601-607

[33] Patiño-Aldana AF, Sternberg ÁMR, Rondón ÁMP, Molano-Gonzalez N, Lima DRR. Interaction effect between hemoglobin and hypoxemia on COVID-19 mortality: An observational study from Bogotá, Colombia. International Journal of General Medicine. 2022;**15**:6965-6976

[34] Dhawan RT, Gopalan D, Howard L, Vicente A, Park M, Manalan K, et al. Beyond the clot: Perfusion imaging of the pulmonary vasculature after COVID-19. The Lancet Respiratory Medicine. 2021;**9**(1):107-116

[35] Białkowski J, Głowacki J, Zabal C, Garcia-Montes A, Bermudez-Canete R, Flores-Arizmendi R, et al. Patent ductus arteriosus at low and high altitudes: Anatomical and haemodynamic features and their implications for transcatheter closure. Kardiologia Polska. 2011;**69**(5):431-436

[36] Chinawa JM, BFCATC and COD. The effects of ductal size on the severity of pulmonary hypertension in children with patent ductus arteriosus (PDA): A multi-center study. BMC Pulmonary Medicine. 2021;**21**(79):1-8

Chapter 5

A Severe Clinical Example of Hypoxia: Sickle Cell Anemia

Büşra Tuğçe Akman

Abstract

Sickle cell anemia is a disease in which the erythrocyte changes shape due to a mutation in the beta chain of hemoglobin causing vascular occlusion (vaso-occlusion) and clinical symptoms. In sickle cell patients, intermittent vascular occlusion leads to reperfusion injury associated with granulocyte accumulation and increased production of reactive oxygen species. Sickle cells adhere to endothelial cells and other blood cells more than normal erythrocytes in the microvascular circulation. The increase in thrombin and fibrin decreases the procoagulant activity of tissue factor, which triggers hypercoagulation. Where NO accumulates, oxidative stress reactions occur with vaso-occlusion. This results in decreased NO bioavailability and increased vascular dysfunction. Tissue damage due to vaso-occlusion causes the release of inflammatory mediators that trigger pain. Cytokines are released into the circulation by platelets, white blood cells, and endothelial cells. Patients with this condition are taken to the hospital with various syndromes such as occlusive crisis, acute chest syndrome, infection, multiple organ failure, and acute stroke. Sickle cell anemia effectively illustrates the severity of clinical manifestations caused by hypoxia.

Keywords: hemolysis, hypoxia, oxidative stress, sickle cell disease, vaso-occlusion

1. Introduction

Sickle cell disease (SCD) is the most common monogenic disorder [1]. With the "malaria hypothesis" formulated by Haldane in 1949 and Allison in 1954, the sickle cell trait is thought to protect against severe malaria [2]. The prevalence of the disease is high in large areas of sub-Saharan Africa, the Mediterranean basin, the Middle East, and India due to its natural protection against malaria [3]. In our country, Turkey, which is a Mediterranean country, the total number of patients with SCD is around 1200, and the frequency of the mutant Hb (HbS) of SCD is 0.03% [4]. Because of population movements, the distribution of sickle cell disease is widespread. According to estimates in the United States, about 100,000 people are thought to have the disease [5]. Every year, it is predicted that 300,000 babies are born with sickle cell anemia [6]. The vast majority of these births occur in three countries: Nigeria, the Democratic Republic of the Congo, and India. Sickle cell disease rates are expected to increase in the coming years. Over the last 40 years, survival rates have increased significantly in high-income countries with early screening, immunization, and use of antibiotics and hydroxyurea. In these countries, childhood deaths with sickle cell anemia are now close to deaths in the general population with a median survival of more than 60 years [7]. In Africa, where newborn screening and routine childhood vaccinations are absent and malaria, malnutrition, and poverty remain major problems, the mortality rate among children under 5 years of age with SCD can be up to 90% [8].

SCD occurs as a result of a point mutation in the β-globin chain of hemoglobin (replacement of glutamic acid at position 6 by valine). This mutant hemoglobin is called HbS. Conversion of hydrophilic glutamate to hydrophobic valine leads to polymerization of Hb and sickle erythrocytes (RBC) when deoxygenated [9–11]. While normal erythrocyte lifespan is 120 days, the lifespan of these deformed and hard sickled erythrocytes is shortened to 10–20 days. Because of their lack of flexibility, these erythrocytes cannot pass through microcapillaries resulting in extravascular and intravascular hemolysis, vaso-occlusion, abnormal erythrocyte-endothelial interactions, and ischemia-reperfusion injury. Persistent vaso-occlusion triggers further acute tissue hypoxia and chronic organ damage resulting in cycling that contributes to the progression of SCD. Hypoxia is a critical element in this cycle. Various physiological and pathological processes such as angiogenesis and inflammation have been shown to be regulated by hypoxia through a family of transcription factors known as hypoxia-inducible factors (HIFs), specifically HIF-la [12, 13]. Their effects include vaso-occlusion, increased production of free hemoglobin by lysis of erythrocytes, increased inflammation, platelet activation, increased erythrocyte adhesion to the vascular endothelium, and abnormal nitric oxide metabolism. Tissue damage increases with the interaction of sequestered neutrophils with the endothelium. These abnormalities lead to multisystem dysfunction with chronic inflammation, vascular damage, and anemia [14].

2. Pathophysiology of sickle cell disease

Hemoglobin consists of 2 alpha and 2 beta chains. HbS is the result of a specific point mutation in the HBB gene that encodes hemoglobin beta chains. It occurs with the replacement of glutamic acid in the seventh amino acid with valine. SCD is inherited autosomal recessively. It occurs when HbS is in a homozygous state (HbSS) or with some other HBB variants (Hb C, D or E) or when compound heterozygosity is present with beta thalassemia. The sections below describe the changes in the pathway from HbS development to SCD formation.

2.1 HbS polymerization and change of erythrocyte morphology

HbS polymerization is the initiating event from which all other pathophysiological changes occur [15]. Normal HbS is soluble in the cytoplasm of the RBC. Oxygen-free HbS polymerizes and precipitates inside the cell as a solid crystal. The sickle fibers that make up the polymerization of HbS initiate a series of events including damage to the RBC membrane, cellular dehydration, sickle-shaped cell transformation, and hemolysis. The formation of hemoglobin polymerization is an unstable event. Conditions such as hypoxia, 2,3-diphosphoglycerate (2,3-DPG) concentration, pH, temperature, and dehydration enhance the formation of intracellular polymerization [16, 17]. There are three important pathways that affect the dehydration of erythrocytes. These are KCl transport, the Gardos channel, and the Na-K pump system. It is reported in studies that the most important of these pathways is the Gardos channel.

Even a minimal Gardos channel activation can lead to a potent and almost irreversible dehydration effect that promotes the sickling process [18]. The HbS polymer may cause reversible alterations to the RBC membrane. After repeated cycles, however, the red blood cell membrane becomes irreversibly damaged and sickle-shaped [19]. Sickle cells seen in peripheral smear are changed irreversibly [20]. Mature RBCs and reticulocytes can accumulate polymerized hemoglobin and transform into sickle cells. Immature, nucleated RBC progenitor cells do not sickle [21]. In sickle cells, abnormal globin chains cluster along the cell membrane and cause changes in cytoskeletal proteins such as band-3, ankyrin, and spectrin. Band-3 is an important integral membrane protein of erythrocytes and is required for the organization of the cytoskeleton, anion transport across the membrane, regulation of erythrocyte volume, and CO_2 transport. Band-3 damage in SCD contributes to the sickling processes. Aggregation of globin chain clusters along the cytoskeletal membrane promotes IgG aggregation and triggers monocyte chemotaxis. This leads to the removal of aged erythrocytes from the circulation [22, 23].

2.2 Adhesion of sickle cells

The expression of typically underexpressed proteins such as phosphatidylserine (PS), basal cell adhesion molecule (B-CAM), integrin-associated protein (IAP), and intercellular adhesion molecule-4 (ICAM-4) increases when sickle erythrocytes' membrane structure is damaged [24–26]. This situation facilitates the adhesion of erythrocytes to both endothelium and other blood cells and contributes to the pathogenesis of vaso-occlusive crises. According to research, the expression of adhesion molecules such as α4β1 (VLA-4) and CD36 is increased in the membrane of reticulocytes in SCD patients. This may play a role in the pathogenesis of cell adhesion and vascular occlusion [26]. As a result of the adhesion of the cells to the vascular endothelium, the transcription factor NF-KB is activated; oxygen radicals are released; and gene regulation and endothelial expression of adhesion molecules such as activated NF-κB, E-selectin, VCM-1, and ICAM-1 are increased [27].

2.3 Hemolysis and oxidative stress

In sickle cell disease, erythrocytes are exposed to intravascular and extravascular hemolysis and hemoglobin levels are 6–11 g/dl. While the rate of erythrocyte hemolysis is constant in patients with SCD during the stationary period, it increases during crisis. This increase varies according to the patient's genotype (HbSS, HbSB, HbSC) and HbF level. In patients with high erythrocyte hemolysis and low Hb levels in the normal period, organ dysfunction in the form of vascular damage, endothelial dysfunction, and pulmonary hypertension associated with high pulse pressure, diastolic left heart disease, and renal dysfunction may develop in the future. In SCD patients, intravascular hemolysis releases free hemoglobin and heme; the plasma proteins haptoglobulin and hemopexin bind with these compounds, respectively, and remove them from the circulation. These protective mechanisms become dysfunctional in many pathological conditions, however, and hemopexin becomes completely depleted. Due to the absence of hemopexin, extremely high quantities of free heme accumulate in the blood. As a result, reactive oxygen molecules (ROS) are formed, which cause oxidative stress and cell damage [28]. In addition, free heme is lipophilic and can join with the lipid membranes of the vascular endothelium. As a result of the adhesion of activated endothelial cells with leukocytes, an inflammatory response is initiated that damages the endothelium and increases vascular permeability. Oxy-Hb released during hemolysis reacts with nitric oxide (NO) and lowers the plasma NO level. This condition causes endothelial dysfunction and has been associated with end-organ vasculopathy including leg ulcers, nephropathy, priapism, pulmonary hypertension, and death [28–30]. Erythrocytes release free hemoglobin and ADP, which stimulate platelet activation and contribute to vascular thrombosis and pulmonary hypertension by activating coagulation pathways [31, 32]. They also activate TLR4 and inflammasome signaling pathways as well as innate immune pathways [33]. RBC life is the greatest indicator for hemolysis and is substantially correlated with reticulocyte percentage and HbF level. Hb and hematocrit are not associated with RBC survival, however [34].

2.4 Inflammation and hypoxia

Erythrocyte injury-related molecules (eDAMP) released by hemolysis contribute to ischemia-reperfusion injury by supporting the formation and progression of inflammation. Heme and its oxidized form, hemin, are potent TLR4 agonists that contribute to the proinflammatory and procoagulant state in SCD patients. It has been reported that this condition is associated with activation of leukocytes, platelets, and endothelial cells, tissue factor release, cytokine storm, NO depletion, and ROS formation [35–37]. In addition, heme has also been shown to increase ADP- and epinephrine-dependent platelet aggregation [38]. Recent studies have shown that heme affects the migration and phagocytosis functions of monocytes, macrophages, and neutrophils leading to impaired bacterial clearance. Also, the G-protein-coupled receptor (GPBR) signaling pathway causes neutrophil migration, neutrophil extracellular trap (NET) production, oxidative damage, IL-8 production, and increased neutrophil survival [39, 40]. NETs are released from neutrophils under various inflammatory conditions and induce tissue damage by promoting the activation of innate immune responses. Repeated atherosclerosis and reperfusion attacks cause ischemia-reperfusion injury by promoting transient hypoxia, ROS generation, microvascular dysfunction, activation of innate and adaptive immune responses, and cell death [41–43]. This results in the activation of cell death programs such as ROS-induced damage to cellular proteins, lipids, DNA, and ribonucleic acids, apoptosis, necrosis, autophagy, and NETosis (the release of NETs by neutrophils). This in turn causes the release of various tissue and cell-derived DAMPs [43]. HIF1a, released after hypoxia in tissues, mediates adenosine release. Adenosine plays a central role in regulating the physiological response to hypoxia. It has long been known to mediate vasodilation, reduce inflammation, and mediate cell protection during ischemia-reperfusion injury in many organs. It was also revealed that adenosine stimulates RBCs to produce more 2,3-BPG, resulting in increased oxygen release from Hb. Although this contributes to the reduction of hypoxia in healthy individuals, it worsens the situation in SCD patients. This effect of adenosine is mediated by the G-protein-coupled adenosine receptor ADORA2B on the erythrocyte. The effect of adenosine on the ADORA2A receptor on invariant natural killer T (iNKT) cells has been shown to reduce pulmonary inflammation [44].

3. Clinical findings and management of sickle cell disease

The clinical manifestations of SCD may differ between major genotypes and even between patients with the same genotype. As a general rule, individuals with both

SCD (homozygous HbS) and sickle-beta^0 thalassemia have more severe symptoms than those with HbSC disease or sickle-beta$^+$thalassemia, alone [1]. An exception is retinopathy, the most common complication in individuals with HbSC disease. Climate, meteorological changes, air quality, and infections are other environmental factors that affect the severity of the disease [45]. Acute and chronic complications are seen in sickle cell anemia. Painful crisis is the most common acute complication. Hemolytic crisis, splenic and hepatic sequestration crisis, acute chest syndrome, stroke, and priapism are other acute complications. Chronic complications are usually described in adults. Pulmonary hypertension, hepatopathy, kidney disease, splenomegaly, bone and joint deformities, retinopathy, iron deposition, and leg ulcers are its chronic complications. In addition, SCD patients have an increased susceptibility to infection. The life expectancy of patients with SCD has been shortened by at least 20 years, and the quality of life has decreased [14, 46]. Common complications and their management will be discussed below.

3.1 Acute and chronic pain

The most typical complication of SCD is severe intermittent acute pain (vaso-occlusive crisis), which is responsible for more than 70% of acute hospital visits in SCD patients [47]. Chronic daily pain increases with advanced age and occurs in 30–40% of adolescents and adults with SCD [48, 49]. Acute pain is largely associated with ischemia-reperfusion injury, tissue infarction, and vaso-occlusion of sickle red blood cells and occurs in an isolated anatomical site (e.g., arm, leg, back) or in multiple locations. Chronic pain may result from sensitization of the central and/or peripheral nervous system and is often accompanied by features of neuropathic pain [50, 51]. Disease complications such as avascular necrosis (hip, shoulder) and leg ulcers also cause chronic pain [52]. The aim of the intervention in acute pain is to relieve the patient's pain or reduce it to an acceptable level to restore daily functions. Oral or intravenous (IV) opioids and IV hydration are first-line therapies for acute pain. Analgesics should be initiated within 30–60 minutes of triage [53]. Ketamine, a non-opioid analgesic, can be given as adjuvant therapy in acute pain resistant to opioids. Non-steroidal anti-inflammatory drugs (NSAIDs) are routinely used as adjuvant therapy for the management of acute pain [53, 54]. Red cell transfusion is indicated to rapidly reduce HbS levels or correct acute anemia (if splenic sequestration, hemolytic, or aplastic crisis are present). In patients with chronic pain, opioids can be given after the cost-benefit ratio has been calculated. In long-term use at increasing doses, the possibility of side effects including myocardial infarction, bone fracture, increased risk of motor vehicle impact, sexual dysfunction, and mortality should be considered. Trifluoperazine, an antipsychotic drug, serotonin, and norepinephrine reuptake inhibitors (SNRIs), gabapentinoids, and tricyclic antidepressants (TCAs) can be used for chronic pain [53, 55]. Acupuncture can also be tried [56].

3.2 Cardiopulmonary disease

Cardiopulmonary disease is associated with increased morbidity and mortality in individuals with SCD. Pulmonary arterial hypertension (PAH) is present in up to 10% of adults with SCD [57]. Pulmonary hypertension is defined as the measurement of mean pulmonary artery pressure (PAP) $\geq$25 mmHg at rest with right heart catheterization. In addition, the tricuspid regurgitation velocity (TRV) is measured as >2.5 m/s (s) by transthoracic echocardiography. Chronic intravascular hemolysis is the greatest risk factor for the development of PAH and leads to pulmonary arteriolar vasoconstriction and smooth muscle proliferation. Obstructive lung disease, restrictive lung disease, obstructive sleep apnea, or nocturnal hypoxemia are pulmonary disorders that may be present [58–61]. Patients with SCD who have symptoms of cardiovascular illness, such as increased dyspnea, hypoxemia, or impaired exercise tolerance, should have a diagnostic ECHO and SFT. If there is snoring, witnessed apnea, breathing pauses, or hypoxia during sleep, daytime tiredness, or nocturnal enuresis, a sleep study should be performed in a diagnostic setting. Hydroxyurea or monthly red blood cell transfusions should be considered in the treatment of pulmonary hypertension. Endothelial receptor antagonists and prostanoids can be used in the selected patients. About 28% of children with SCD have asthma, associated with acute chest syndrome and higher mortality, as well as increased episodes of pain that may result from impaired oxygenation leading to sickling and vaso-occlusion [62–64]. First-line treatments include standard beta-adrenergic bronchodilators and oxygen as needed. When corticosteroids are indicated, they should be tapered off over a few days taking into account the risk of rebound SCD pain that may result from abrupt discontinuation of courses.

Patients with acute chest syndrome (AGS) usually present with a pneumonia-like clinical picture. It occurs due to vaso-occlusion in pulmonary vessels and manifests as hypoxia, fever, and new infiltration on chest X-ray. Since radiological findings may occur late, patients without infiltration should also be carefully evaluated with follow-up films. Although laboratory findings are not indicative, the hemoglobin concentration may drop suddenly. Although the most common etiological factor is infection, AGS can also occur from bone marrow embolism, intrapulmonary aggregates of communal cells, atelectasis, or pulmonary edema. It can very quickly lead to respiratory failure or death. It therefore requires urgent hospitalization. Treatment is antibiotics, oxygen support, and exchange transfusion in patients with respiratory failure. The risk of acute chest syndrome can be reduced with incentive spirometry and preoperative transfusions during hospitalization [14].

3.3 Central nervous system complications

Overt and silent cerebral infarctions cause significant morbidity in SCD patients. Eleven percent of patients by age 20 and 24% by age 45 will have had a detectable stroke [65]. Silent cerebral infarcts occur in 39% of adults at 18 years and > 50% at 30 years [66, 67]. Patients with both types of stroke have an increased risk of recurrent stroke [68]. Overt strokes occur in the great arteries, while silent cerebral infarcts occur in penetrating arteries. Overt strokes present as paresis, dysarthria or aphasia, seizures, sensory deficits, headaches, or altered consciousness. Silent infarctions are associated with cognitive deficits including low IQ and impaired academic performance. The diagnosis of overt stroke is made by evidence of acute infarction on brain MRI diffusion-weighted imaging and focal deficits on neurological examination. A silent cerebral infarction is defined by "fluid-attenuated inversion healing (FLAIR) MRI signal abnormality, at least 3 mm in one dimension and visible in 2 planes on T2-weighted images" and no defects on neurological examination [69]. Because silent cerebral infarcts are not clinically detectable, baseline brain MRI scanning is recommended in school-aged children with SCD [70]. Recent SCD clinical practice guidelines also recommend scanning the brain MRI in adults with SCD to facilitate rehabilitation services, patient, and family understanding of cognitive deficits, and further needs assessment [70]. Red blood cell exchange transfusion is the recommended treatment to rapidly reduce HbS below 30% in acute stroke [71]. A simple transfusion is usually given as an emergency measure when preparing for an exchange transfusion, however [70].

3.4 Renal disease

In SCD patients, glomerulopathy results from intravascular hemolysis and endothelial dysfunction in the renal cortex. Medullary hypoperfusion and ischemia also contribute to kidney disease in SCD causing hematuria, urinary concentration defects, and distal tubular dysfunction [72].

Glomerulopathy, characterized by hyperfiltration leading to albuminuria, is an early asymptomatic manifestation of SCD nephropathy. Hyperfiltration, defined as an absolute increase in the glomerular filtration rate, can be seen in 43% of children with SCD [73]. Albuminuria, defined by the presence of ≥30 mg/g urine albumin over 24 hours, was observed in 32% of adults with SCD [74]. About 20–40% of adults with SCD develop chronic kidney disease (CKD) and are at risk of developing end-stage renal disease (ESRD) [74]. Since microalbuminuria/proteinuria precedes CKD in SCD, annual urine microalbumin/protein screening is recommended starting at age 10 [46]. Kidney failure may be associated with the use of ketorolac in children with SCD hospitalized for pain. Although controlled clinical studies are lacking, hydroxyurea may be associated with improvements in glomerular hyperfiltration and urinary concentration ability in children with SCD [74, 75]. ACE-I or ARB therapy reduces microalbuminuria in patients with SCD [76]. ACE-I or ARB therapy has not been shown to improve kidney function or prevent CKD, however. Because of recent advances in renal graft survival and post-transplant mortality, renal transplantation should be considered in individuals with SCD and ESRD [77].

4. Modifying drugs used in treatment

Hydroxyurea, which is frequently used in SCD patients, is an antimetabolite that disrupts the DNA replication process. Stress induces fetal hemoglobin production through erythropoiesis, reduces inflammation, increases nitric oxide, and decreases cell adhesion. Other SCD-modifying drugs (i.e., L-glutamine, crizanlizumab, and voxelotor) were recently approved by the FDA. L-glutamine is required for the synthesis of nicotinamide adenine dinucleotide, glutathione, and arginine. This amino acid protects red blood cells against oxidative damage which is the basis for its proposed use in SCD. Crizanlizumab is a humanized monoclonal antibody that binds P-selectin and blocks the interaction of the adhesion molecule with its ligand (i.e., P-selectin glycoprotein ligand 1). P-selectin expression triggered by inflammation promotes adhesion of neutrophils, activated platelets, and sickle red blood cells to the endothelial surface and to each other thus promoting vaso-occlusion in SCD. Polymerization of the voxelotor Hb S in the deoxygenated state represents the first step in red blood cell sickling, which leads to reduced disfigurement of red blood cells and increased hemolysis. Voxelotor is the first allosteric modifier of HbS to increase oxygen affinity [78–80]. In addition to the modified drugs used in treatment, hematopoietic stem cell transplantation from HLA-matched sibling donors remains superior as the only curative treatment [81].

5. Conclusion

SCD, as a severe clinical example of hypoxia, progresses with complications including organ damage such as cardiopulmonary, cerebrovascular, and kidney disease resulting in increased morbidity and mortality. The survival of individuals with SCD is reduced compared to those without SCD, but the prognosis of SCD is steadily improving with neonatal screening, immunizations, antibiotics, hydroxyurea, and faster prevention and treatment. Where comprehensive care is available, the disease has evolved from a fatal pediatric illness to a chronic illness often associated with progressive deterioration in quality of life and organ function. Modifying drugs such as hydroxyurea L-glutamine, crizanlizumab, and voxelotor are frequently used for treatment. Fetal hemoglobin induction, sickle hemoglobin research on inhibition of polymerization, reduction of cell adhesion, and reduction of oxidative stress are continuing. Today, hematopoietic stem cell transplantation from HLA-matched sibling donors remains the only curative treatment.

Author details

Büşra Tuğçe Akman
Department of Hematology, Baskent Univercity, Ankara, Turkey

*Address all correspondence to: akmantugce@hotmail.com

References

[1] Rees DC, Williams TN, Gladwin MT. Sickle-cell disease. Lancet. 2010;**376**:2018-2031

[2] Elguero E, Délicat-Loembet LM, Rougeron V, et al. Malaria continues to select for sickle cell trait in Central Africa. Proceedings of the National Academy of Sciences of the United States of America. 2015;**112**:7051-7054

[3] Piel FB, Patil AP, Howes RE, et al. Global distribution of the sickle cell gene and geographical confirmation of the malaria hypothesis. Nature Communications. 2010;**1**:104

[4] Arcasoy A. Dünya'da ve Türkiye'de talasemi ve hemoglobinopatiler. In: Hemoglobinopati ve Talasemi Önlem Tanı Tedavi. Ulusal hemoglobinopati Konseyi Sağlık Bakanlığı. Baskı, Antalya; 2003. pp. 11-19

[5] Hassell KL. Population estimates of sickle cell disease in the U.S. American Journal of Preventive Medicine. 2010;**38**(Suppl):S512-S521

[6] Piel FB, Patil AP, Howes RE, et al. Global epidemiology of sickle haemoglobin in neonates: A contemporary geostatistical model-based map and population estimates. Lancet. 2013;**381**:142-151

[7] Gardner K, Douiri A, Drasar E, et al. Survival in adults with sickle cell disease in a high-income setting. Blood. 2016;**128**:1436-1438

[8] Grosse SD, Odame I, Atrash HK, Amendah DD, Piel FB, Williams TN. Sickle cell disease in Africa: A neglected cause of early childhood mortality. American Journal of Preventive Medicine. 2011;**41**(Suppl 4):S398-S405

[9] Ingram VM. A specific chemical difference between the globins of normal human and sickle-cell anaemia haemoglobin. Nature. 1956;**178**:792-794

[10] Chang JC, Kan YW. Antenatal diagnosis of sickle cell anaemia by direct analysis of the sickle mutation. Lancet. 1981;**2**:1127-1129

[11] Hebbel RP. Beyond hemoglobin polymerization: The red blood cell membrane and sickle disease pathophysiology. Blood. 1991;**77**:214-237

[12] Mucaj V, Shay JE, Simon MC. Effects of hypoxia and HIFs on cancer metabolism. International Journal of Hematology. 2012;**95**:464-470

[13] Eltzschig HK, Carmeliet P. Hypoxia and inflammation. The New England Journal of Medicine. 2011;**364**:656-665

[14] Kanter J, Kruse-Jarres R. Management of sickle cell disease from childhood through adulthood. Blood Reviews. 2013;**27**(6):279-287

[15] Sundd P, Gladwin MT, Novelli EM. Pathophysiology of sickle cell disease. Annual Review of Pathology. 2019;**14**:263

[16] Harmening DM. Hemoglobinopathies. Clinical Hematology and Fundamentals of Hemostasis. 3rd ed. Philadelphia. USA: FA Davis; 1997. pp. 173-192

[17] Brittenham GM, Schechter AN, Noguchi CT. Hemoglobin S polymerization: Primary determinant of the hemolytic and clinical severity of the sickling syndromes. Blood. 1985;**65**:183-189

[18] Brugnara c. Sickle cell dehydration: Pathophysiology and therapeutic

applications. Clinical Hemorheology and Microcirculation. 2018;**68**(2-3):187-204

[19] Serjeant GR, Petch MC, Serjeant BE. The in vivo sickle phenomenon: A reappraisal. The Journal of Laboratory and Clinical Medicine. 1973;**81**:850

[20] Ballas SK, Eckman JR. Chapter 20: Sickle cell pain: biology, etiology, and treatment. In: Steinberg MH, Forget BG, Higgs DR, Weatherall DJ, editors. Disorders of Hemoglobin. 2nd ed. Cambridge: Cambridge University Press; 2009. p. 564

[21] Grasso JA, Sullivan AL, Sullivan LW. Ultrastructural studies of the bone marrow in sickle cell anaemia. II. The morphology of erythropoietic cells and their response to deoxygenation in vitro. British Journal of Haematology. 1975;**31**:381

[22] Platt OS, Falcone JF. Membrane protein interactions in sickle red blood cells: Evidence of abnormal protein 3 function. Blood. 1995;**86**(5):1992-1998

[23] Bosman GJ. Erythrocyte aging in sickle cell disease. Cellular Molecular Biology (Noisy-le-grand). 2004;**50**(1):81-86

[24] Bunn HF. Pathogenesis and treatment of sickle cell disease. The New England Journal of Medicine. 1997;**337**:762-769

[25] Barabino GA, Platt MO, Kaul DK. Sickle cell biomechanics. Annual Review of Biomedical Engineering. 2010;**12**:345-367

[26] Smith RA, Mankelow TJ, Drizou D, et al. Large red cell-derived membrane particles are major contributors to hypercoagulability in sickle cell disease. Scientific Reports. 2021;**11**:11035

[27] Kaul DK, Finnegan E, Barabino GA. Sickle red cell-endothelium interactions. Microcirculation. 2009;**16**:97-111

[28] Rp R, Bell L, Hillmen P, Gladwin MT. The clinical sequelae of intravascular hemolysis and extracellular plasma hemoglobin: A novel mechanism of human disease. Journal of the American Medical Association. 2005;**293**:1653-1662

[29] Reiter CD, Wang X, Tanus-Santos JE, Hogg N, Cannon RO, et al. Cell-free hemoglobin limits nitric oxide bioavailability in sicklecell disease. Nature. 2002;**8**(12):1383-1389

[30] Hsu LL, Champion HC, Campbell-Lee SA, Bivalacqua TJ, Manci EA, et al. Hemolysis in sickle cell mice causes pulmonary hypertension due to global impairment in nitric oxide bioavailability. Blood. 2007;**109**:3088-3098

[31] Villagra J, Shiva S, Hunter LA, Machado RF, Gladwin MT, Kato GJ. 2007 platelet activation in patients with sickle disease, hemolysis-associated pulmonary hypertension, and nitric oxide scavenging by cell-free hemoglobin. Blood. 2007;**110**:2166-2172

[32] Kı A. Hypercoagulability and thrombotic complications in hemolytic anemias. Haematologica. 2009;**94**(11):1481-1484

[33] Gladwin MT, Ofori-Acquah SF. Erythroid DAMps drive inflammation in ScD. Blood. 2014;**123**:3689-3690

[34] Hebbel RP. Reconstructing sickle cell disease: A data-based analysis of the "hyperhemolysis paradigm" for pulmonary hypertension from the perspective of evidence-based medicine. American Journal of Hematology. 2011;**86**:123

[35] Serjeant GR, Serjeant BE, Milner PF. The irreversibly sickled cell; a determinant of haemolysis in sickle cell anaemia. British Journal of Haematology. 1969;**17**:527

[36] Allali S, Maciel TT, Hermine O, Montalembert M. Innate immune cells, major protagonists of sickle cell disease pathophysiology. Haematologica. 2020;**105**(2):273-283

[37] Dutra FF, Bozza MT. Heme on innate immunity and inflammation. Frontiers in Pharmacology. 2014;**5**:115

[38] Malik Z, Creter D, Cohen A, Djaldetti M. Haemin affects platelet aggregation and lymphocyte mitogenicity in whole blood incubations. Cytobios. 1983;**38**:33-38

[39] Kono M, Saigo K, Takagi Y, Takahashi T, Kawauchi S, et al. Heme-related molecules induce rapid production of neutrophil extracellular traps. Transfusion. 2014;**54**:2811-2819

[40] Graca-Souza A, Arruda MA, de Freitas MS, Barja-Fidalgo C, Oliveira PL. Neutrophil activation by heme: Implications for inflammatory processes. Blood. 2002;**99**:4160-4165

[41] Belcher JD, Bryant CJ, Nguyen J, Bowlin PR, Kielbik MC, et al. Transgenic sickle mice have vascular inflammation. Blood. 2003;**101**:3953-3959

[42] Kaul DK, Rp H. Hypoxia/reoxygenation causes inflammatory response in transgenic sickle mice but not in normal mice. Journal of Clinical Investment. 2000;**106**:411-420

[43] Eltzschig HK, Eckle T. Ischemia and reperfusion-from mechanism to translation. Nature. 2011;**17**:1391-1401

[44] Sun K, Xia Y. New insights into sickle cell disease: A disease of hypoxia. Current Opinion in Hematology. 2013;**20**(3):215-221

[45] Piel FB, Steinberg MH, Rees DC. Sickle cell disease. The New England Journal of Medicine. 2017;**376**(16):1561-1573

[46] Yawn BP, Buchanan GR, Afenyi-Annan AN, Ballas SK, Hassell KL, James AH, et al. Management of sickle cell disease: Summary of the 2014 evidence-based report by expert panel members. JAMA. 2014;**312**(10):1033-1048

[47] Brousseau DC, Owens PL, Mosso AL, Panepinto JA, Steiner CA. Acute care utilization and rehospitalizations for sickle cell disease. Journal of the American Medical Association. 2010;**303**(13):1288-1294

[48] Sil S, Cohen LL, Dampier C. Psychosocial and functional outcomes in youth with chronic sickle cell pain. The Clinical Journal of Pain. 2016;**32**(6):527-533

[49] Smith WR, Penberthy LT, Bovbjerg VE, McClish DK, Roberts JD, Dahman B, et al. Daily assessment of pain in adults with sickle cell disease. Annals of Internal Medicine. 2008;**148**(2):94-101

[50] Ballas SK, Darbari DS. Neuropathy, neuropathic pain, and sickle cell disease. American Journal of Hematology. 2013;**88**(11):927-929

[51] Sharma D, Brandow AM. Neuropathic pain in individuals with sickle cell disease. Neuroscience Letters. 2020;**714**:134445

[52] Dampier C, Palermo TM, Darbari DS, Hassell K, Smith W, Zempsky W. AAPT diagnostic criteria for chronic sickle

cell disease pain. The Journal of Pain. 2017;**18**(5):490-498

[53] Brandow AM, Carroll CP, Creary S, et al. American Society of Hematology 2020 guidelines for sickle cell disease: Management of acute and chronic pain. Blood Advances. 2020;**4**(12):2656-2701

[54] Lubega FA, DeSilva MS, Munube D, Nkwine R, Tumukunde J, Agaba PK, et al. Low dose ketamine versus morphine for acute severe vaso occlusive pain in children: A randomized controlled trial. Scandinavian Journal of Pain. 2018;**18**(1):19-27

[55] Molokie RE, Wilkie DJ, Wittert H, Suarez ML, Yao Y, Zhao Z, et al. Mechanism-driven phase I translational study of trifluoperazine in adults with sickle cell disease. European Journal of Pharmacology. 2014;**723**:419-424

[56] Mahmood LA, Reece-Stremtan S, Idiokitas R, Martin B, Margulies S, Hardy SJ, et al. Acupuncture for pain management in children with sickle cell disease. Complementary Therapies in Medicine. 2020;**49**:102287

[57] Mehari A, Alam S, Tian X, Cuttica MJ, Barnett CF, Miles G, et al. Hemodynamic predictors of mortality in adults with sickle cell disease. American Journal of Respiratory and Critical Care Medicine. 2013;**187**(8):840-847

[58] Cohen RT, Strunk RC, Rodeghier M, Rosen CL, Kirkham FJ, Kirkby J, et al. Pattern of lung function is not associated with prior or future morbidity in children with sickle cell anemia. Annals of the American Thoracic Society. 2016;**13**(8):1314-1323

[59] Kassim AA, Payne AB, Rodeghier M, Macklin EA, Strunk RC, DeBaun MR. Low forced expiratory volume is associated with earlier death in sickle cell anemia. Blood. 2015;**126**(13):1544-1550

[60] Sharma S, Efird JT, Knupp C, Kadali R, Liles D, Shiue K, et al. Sleep disorders in adult sickle cell patients. Journal of Clinical Sleep Medicine. 2015;**11**(3):219-223

[61] Rosen CL, Debaun MR, Strunk RC, Redline S, Seicean S, Craven DI, et al. Obstructive sleep apnea and sickle cell anemia. Pediatrics. 2014;**134**(2):273-281

[62] Knight-Madden JM, Barton-Gooden A, Weaver SR, Reid M, Greenough A. Mortality, asthma, smoking and acute chest syndrome in young adults with sickle cell disease. Lung. 2013;**191**(1):95-100

[63] Strunk RC, Cohen RT, Cooper BP, Rodeghier M, Kirkham FJ, Warner JO, et al. Wheezing symptoms and parental asthma are associated with a physician diagnosis of asthma in children with sickle cell anemia. The Journal of Pediatrics. 2014;**164**(4):821-771

[64] Takahashi T, Okubo Y, Handa A. Acute chest syndrome among children hospitalized with vaso-occlusive crisis: A nationwide study in the United States. Pediatric Blood & Cancer. 2018;**65**(3):e26885

[65] Ohene-Frempong K, Weiner SJ, Sleeper LA, Miller ST, Embury S, Moohr JW, et al. Cerebrovascular accidents in sickle cell disease: Rates and risk factors. Blood. 1998;**91**(1):288-294

[66] Bernaudin F, Verlhac S, Arnaud C, Kamdem A, Vasile M, Kasbi F, et al. Chronic and acute anemia and extracranial internal carotid stenosis are risk factors for silent cerebral infarcts in sickle cell anemia. Blood. 2015;**125**(10):1653-1661

[67] Kassim AA, Pruthi S, Day M, Rodeghier M, Gindville MC,

Brodsky MA, et al. Silent cerebral infarcts and cerebral aneurysms are prevalent in adults with sickle cell anemia. Blood. 2016;**127**(16):2038-2040

[68] Powars D, Wilson B, Imbus C, Pegelow C, Allen J. The natural history of stroke in sickle cell disease. The American Journal of Medicine. 1978;**65**(3):461-471

[69] DeBaun MR, Gordon M, McKinstry RC, Noetzel MJ, White DA, Sarnaik SA, et al. Controlled trial of transfusions for silent cerebral infarcts in sickle cell anemia. The New England Journal of Medicine. 2014;**371**(8):699-710

[70] DeBaun MR, Jordan LC, King AA, Schatz J, Vichinsky E, Fox CK, et al. American Society of Hematology 2020 guidelines for sickle cell disease: Prevention, diagnosis, and treatment of cerebrovascular disease in children and adults. Blood Advances. 2020;**4**(8):1554-1588

[71] Hulbert ML, Scothorn DJ, Panepinto JA, Scott JP, Buchanan GR, Sarnaik S, et al. Exchange blood transfusion compared with simple transfusion for first overt stroke is associated with a lower risk of subsequent stroke: A retrospective cohort study of 137 children with sickle cell anemia. The Journal of Pediatrics. 2006;**149**(5):710-712

[72] Cazenave M, Audard V, Bertocchio JP, Habibi A, Baron S, Prot-Bertoye C, et al. Tubular acidification defect in adults with sickle cell disease. Clinical Journal of the American Society of Nephrology. 2020;**15**(1):16-24

[73] Lebensburger JD, Aban I, Pernell B, Kasztan M, Feig DI, Hilliard LM, et al. Hyperfiltration during early childhood precedes albuminuria in pediatric sickle cell nephropathy. American Journal of Hematology. 2019;**94**(4):417-423

[74] Niss O, Lane A, Asnani MR, Yee ME, Raj A, Creary S, et al. Progression of albuminuria in patients with sickle cell anemia: A multicenter, longitudinal study. Blood Advances. 2020;**4**(7):1501-1511

[75] Zahr RS, Hankins JS, Kang G, Li C, Wang WC, Lebensburger J, et al. Hydroxyurea prevents onset and progression of albuminuria in children with sickle cell anemia. American Journal of Hematology. 2019;**94**(1):E27-E29

[76] Quinn CT, Saraf SL, Gordeuk VR, Fitzhugh CD, Creary SE, Bodas P, et al. Losartan for the nephropathy of sickle cell anemia: A phase-2, multicenter trial. American Journal of Hematology. 2017;**92**(9):E520-E528

[77] Gérardin C, Moktefi A, Couchoud C, Duquesne A, Ouali N, Gataut P, et al. Survival and specific outcome of sickle cell disease patients after renal transplantation. British Journal of Haematology. 2019;**187**(5):676-680

[78] Ataga KI, Kutlar A, Kanter J, Liles D, Cancado R, Friedrisch J, et al. Crizanlizumab for the prevention of pain crises in sickle cell disease. The New England Journal of Medicine. 2017;**376**(5):429-439

[79] Niihara Y, Miller ST, Kanter J, Lanzkron S, Smith WR, Hsu LL, et al. A phase 3 trial of L-glutamine in sickle cell disease. The New England Journal of Medicine. 2018;**379**(3):226-235

[80] Vichinsky E, Hoppe CC, Ataga KI, Ware RE, Nduba V, El-Beshlawy A, et al. A phase 3 randomized trial of voxelotor in sickle cell disease. The New England Journal of Medicine. 2019;**381**(6):509-519

[81] Gluckman E, Cappelli B, Bernaudin F, Labopin M, Volt F, Carreras J, et al. Sickle cell disease: An international survey of results of HLA-identical sibling hematopoietic stem cell transplantation. Blood. 2017;**129**(11):1548-1556

Section 3

Ischemia Reperfusion Injury

Chapter 6

Cellular and Molecular Effects of Ischemia on Brain Cells

Cláudio André Martins Roque

Abstract

The structural organization of the human body settles the central nervous system as responsible for the integration on information and the modulation of all other subsystems. A role that can only be played with mastery if inside of its walls, everything is working correctly. One of the major disruptive causes of this harmony is precisely the reduction of oxygen and nutrients supply to the cells during an ischemic stroke. Therefore, the scope of this chapter is precise to describe the several intracellular signaling pathways that are activated upon an ischemic period and summarize the way they interact with each other leading to cellular dysfunction of neurons, glial cells, and vascular cells. As well as to associate those mechanisms with the tissue injury that leads to systemic effects observed on patients and their consequent functional impairments. Not forgetting the impact that the knowledge of the cellular and molecular basis of this pathology may have on the development of integrative brain repair-based therapies that lead to the recovery of injured cells and, consequently, of the functions associated with those tissues.

Keywords: intracellular ischemic cascade, neurons, glial cells, ischemia-induced impairments

1. Introduction

The nervous system (NS) is considered the master controlling and communicating system of the human body and is organized into peripheral and central divisions [1]. While the peripheral nervous system (PNS) is associated with the transport of information to and from the central division [2]. The central nervous system (CNS) in the literature is classically considered as the most important part of NS because it is where the information is processed, integrated, and a response is produced; therefore, every thought, feeling, action, and emotion reflects its activity [1, 2].

This anatomical and functional organization ensures that the modulatory capacity over the visceral and somatic activity is especially associated with the CNS [1]. On the other hand, across the CNS territories, it is possible to identify areas specialized in specific functions, such as the primary motor area that controls voluntary movements, the primary visual area where vision begins to be decoded, the hypothalamus that modulates the physiological components, or for example the nuclei located in the brainstem that control breathing or heart rate, among others [1, 2].

However, as incredible as it may seem, only three types of cells contribute to all this complexity of actions, which are neurons, glial cells, and vascular cells, in what is called the neurovascular unit (NVU) [1]. Neurons are often referred to as the structural and functional unit of the CNS, and it is with this type of cell that major functions are associated [3]. Glial cells are classically considered as the support cells of the neuronal population and play a crucial role in neuronal homeostasis [1]. And finally, the vascular cells that form the blood vessels that irrigate the CNS, and whose function is fundamental to adequately supply this entire territory [1].

Naturally, something that interferes with any of these components, or with all of them at the same time, could thus lead to an imbalance in this system that could be reflected in the impairment of one or more areas of that territory, thus resulting in site-specific deficits [4]. In this sense, one of the major causes of CNS impairment are the injuries that result from ischemic periods, in what is called ischemic stroke (IS) [4].

By definition, IS is characterized by the reduction of blood flow to levels where it no longer meets the needs of brain tissues, thus leading to an ischemic injury [5, 6]. The first elements in this entire system to experience this reduction in blood flow are precisely the cells. From the moment there is no longer an adequate supply of oxygen and nutrients, various intracellular mechanisms that induce cell death are triggered (necrotic and apoptotic mechanisms) [4]. One of the major objectives of this work is precisely to describe all the mechanisms involved in what is the ischemic cascade and how this period affects different cell types differently, as well as to summarize the main deficits that are left.

The impact that this pathology has worldwide is elevated, with a high rate of associated mortality and morbidity [7, 8]. However, as incredible as it may seem and despite the countless efforts made in recent years, the only proven effective approach is in the acute phase, in the emergency department, in the sense of unclogging the affected blood vessel as quickly as possible [9]. For the subacute and chronic phases, the only approaches that exist are, above all, to reduce the associated deficits and not to recover the ischemic-injured tissues [9, 10]. In this sense, it is essential to continue exploring this field of medicine to identify integrative brain repair-based approaches that lead to the recovery of injured cells and, consequently, of the functions associated with those tissues [4], which will only be possible by deepening the existing knowledge about the cellular and molecular basis that is at the origin of this CNS disorder.

2. The central nervous system

The CNS is one of the most important components of the human body; this vital part of the organism works as a control tower that has the capacity to receive the information collected by the internal and external afferents and, based on that sensory input, develop an appropriate response to that specific situation, whether somatic and/or autonomous [1, 2]. This very important role of CNS is essentially due to its capacity to modulate the activity of all the other subsystems of the organism; therefore, something that disturbs its normal functioning could jeopardize the entire physiological system [1, 2].

Interestingly the CNS is also cloistered from all other subsystems in order to guarantee its protection in which the entry of molecules is a highly controlled process mediated by the blood–brain barrier and by the cerebrospinal fluid barrier [1]. Inside of their walls, there are basically three types of cells (neurons, glial cells, and vascular

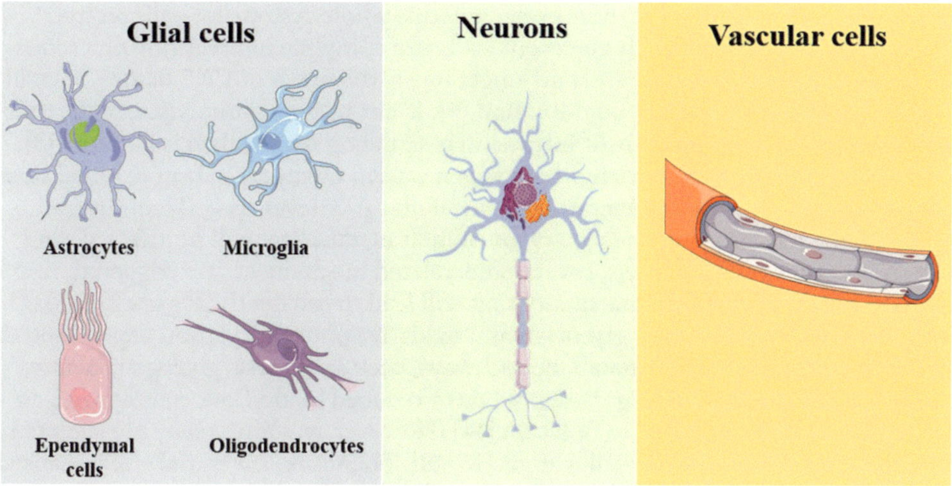

Figure 1.
Cell types present in central nervous system.

cells) in what is called the NVU (**Figure 1**) and from a biochemical point of view, the way they interact and cooperate is an extremely complex process, but at the same time exciting [1]. Neurons and Glial cells are the two major elements of this intricate communication system and establish complex interactions [2].

Historically, neurons are considered the most important cells of the CNS, and they are responsible for the input of sensory information, the integration of the brain and the output of information via their afferent division [2]. This is only possible due to their ability to communicate between themselves, which is done through action potentials and synaptic transmission [1]. To receive and send these action potentials is necessary to a shift in the membrane potential caused by the flow of ions through the neuronal membrane [1]. To maintain the ionic gradients, such mechanism requires large amounts of energy, therefore they need a constant supply of glucose and oxygen which associated to the fact that they do not have their own energy stores makes them the most sensitive cells of the human body to ischemia and any imbalance on this apport jeopardizes neuronal functions [3].

Glial cells of CNS, which include astrocytes, microglia, oligodendrocytes, and ependymal cells, are seen as the housekeeping cells of CNS, and their major function is to support neurons [1]. Associated with this type of cells, there are functions that in the literature have been described as secondary but which are fundamental for neuronal homeostasis, which include structural, metabolic, and trophic support to neurons, defense against pathogens, regulation of inflammatory responses, regulation of synaptic transmission, removal of metabolites, and the formation of the blood–brain-barrier the cerebrospinal fluid barrier [11–13].

3. The intracellular ischemic cascade

However, like every cell in the body, to properly perform their function, all those cells present inside of the CNS depend on one hand on a constant and adequate supply of energy, oxygen, nutrients, and water, and on the other hand, a correct removal of metabolites resulting from cellular metabolic processes (e.g., carbon dioxide, nitrogen, phosphates, and sulfates), for these exchanges this whole system depends on the bloodstream [14]. Therefore, if any event leads to a complete interruption or a reduction of blood flow to levels where it no longer meets the needs of CNS tissues, we will have the beginning of an ischemic situation [5]. If not reversed immediately, the cells begin to resent it, and a cascade of intracellular signaling mechanism is initiated [3].

The local depletion of nutrients and oxygen caused by the reduction of blood flow will progressively lead to a reduction in intracellular ATP levels [14]. Therefore, all energy-dependent processes necessary for cellular metabolism will be affected, and when ATP reaches critical levels, several interrelated mechanisms are triggered, resulting in damage to the cellular machinery that will lead to cell death (**Figure 2**) [15]. The synthesis of ATP mediated by glycolysis and oxidative phosphorylation depends on the available substrates for both metabolic pathways, such as glucose, glycogen, lactate, and fatty acids [16, 17]. During these periods of reduced blood flow, cells depend on these compounds to continue to function [14]. However, as soon as they are depleted, ATP production slows down until it stops [16–18]. Therefore, the initial effects caused by ischemia are dependent on the availability of alternative glycolytic and oxidative substrates and on the rate of ATP consumption by the cell [14, 15].

If there are alternative substrates for the metabolic pathways of ATP production in an initial phase, for oxygen, this does not happen [4]. Oxygen is an irreplaceable driver of mitochondrial respiration, the main source of cellular ATP [4]. Therefore, the deprivation of oxygen immediately and severely compromises ATP production, which results in a rapid decrease in their levels due to ongoing consumption [4]. This ischemia-induced interruption of oxidative phosphorylation also modifies ATP-synthase activity, which starts to consume ATP accelerating its loss as well as electron leak and the production of reactive oxygen species (ROS) [17].

Finally, after the inhibition of cellular respiration and with the cell trying to rapidly produce energy through glycolysis, the intracellular compartment begins to acidify due to the accumulation of several acidic compounds resulting from this

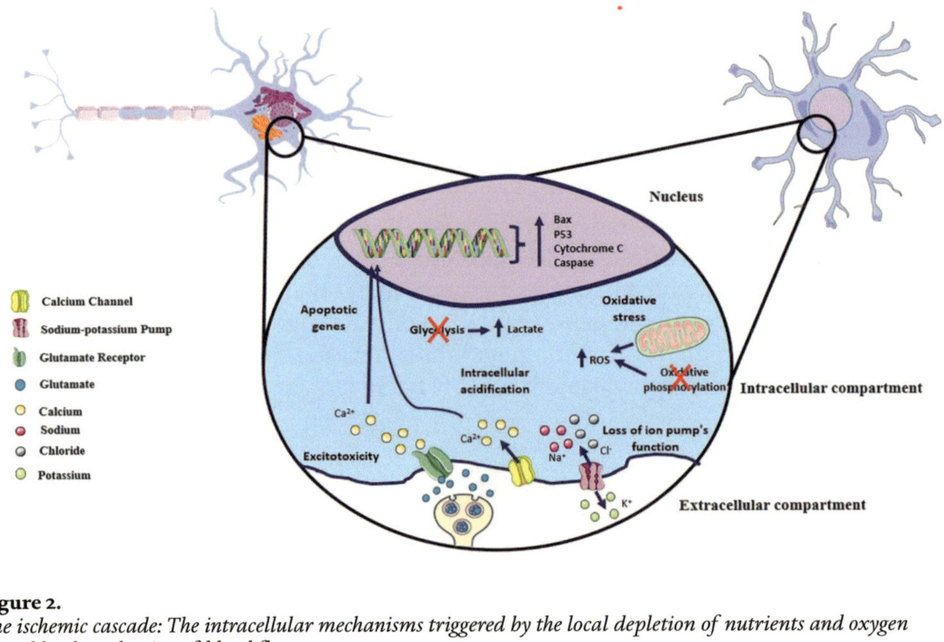

Figure 2.
The ischemic cascade: The intracellular mechanisms triggered by the local depletion of nutrients and oxygen caused by the reduction of blood flow.

metabolic process, such as protons and lactate [17]. This intracellular acidification and the above-mentioned reduction of cellular energy trigger several other secondary mechanisms that are associated with cell death, such as more production of ROS, the loss of ion pumps function and the release of excitatory neurotransmitters [4, 17].

The ischemia-induced increase of intracellular ROS levels drives the cell to oxidative stress, a well-known pro-apoptotic mechanism [4]. The radical species formed under ischemic conditions can react and damage almost all components of cellular machinery and extracellular structures, of which vascular endothelium is particularly relevant [15, 17]. This detrimental interaction impairs biochemical, functional, and metabolic processes, ultimately triggering apoptotic pathways [15, 17].

Ion pumps are crucial to maintaining neuronal homeostasis and for their ability to communicate with other neurons. These structures are responsible to establish an appropriate ionic gradient across the membrane [1]. However, in order to perform their work correctly, they require large amounts of ATP [19]. If the intracellular levels of this compound begin to decrease, the integrity of ion pumps is compromised, and the cell membrane potential will decrease, leading to the loss of ionic gradients [3]. This will lead to the efflux of potassium and influx of sodium, chloride, calcium, and water, which ultimately results in the swelling of cells and their lysis [19]. Associated with this cell death necrotic process is a release of the intracellular components that in turn promote the activation of inflammatory processes on nearby tissues [3].

The increase of intracellular calcium levels resulting from this influx of calcium due to the disturbance of ion pump function is also associated with the activation of several intracellular pro-apoptotic pathways as well as the release of excitatory neurotransmitters, such as glutamate [19]. The dissipation of the ionic gradient also leads to a dysfunction in the glutamate reuptake mechanisms [19]. The excessive accumulation of this neurotransmitter in the synaptic cleft results in the overactivation of glutamate receptors, namely N-methyl-D-aspartate receptors (NMDA-receptors), α-amino-3-hydroxy-5-methyl-4-isoxazolepropionic acid receptors, and kainite receptors, on a phenomenon called excitotoxicity [3]. Excitotoxicity itself is also associated with an imbalance in calcium homeostasis, oxidative stress caused by the synthesis of nitric oxide (NO) and by the production of ROS, as well as the activation of pro-apoptotic mechanisms [4].

The overall activation of the ischemic cascade results finally on the expression of pro-apoptotic genes (Bax and P53), followed by the release of pro-apoptotic molecules such as cytochrome c and apoptosis-inducing factor from mitochondria [4]. Consequently, the caspase pathway is activated, which also induces cell death [3]. However, not everything is bad; some studies indicate that during these detrimental mechanisms, some protective pathways could be activated as a defense against apoptotic and necrotic cell death (e.g., production of Bcl-2, heat shock protein 70, neurotrophin-3, or interleukin-10) [4].

4. The impact of ischemia on CNS cells

However, it is important to note that how different cell types respond to an ischemic period is variable and essentially depends on their metabolic needs and on their intrinsic characteristics, for example, the presence of energy stores or substrates to synthetize energy [4]. Therefore, cells that require more energy for their metabolic processes are more susceptible to ischemic periods [3, 4]. And this is precisely why neurons are extremely sensitive to ischemia; as mentioned before, neurons have a high metabolic rate to maintain their cellular processes and do not have their own energy stores [3, 4].

On the other hand, astrocytes, the most abundant glial cell type in the CNS, have intrinsic characteristics that make them less susceptible to ischemia [16]. Compared to neurons, this type of cell has a lower metabolic need, allowing them to maintain ATP levels for longer periods and delay severe ionic dysregulation [16]. Several factors underlie this well-known selective loss of neurons over astrocytes [13, 16]. Firstly, the majority of glycogen stores found in the CNS are precisely inside of astrocytes [13]. Secondly, astrocytes have a lower density of ionic channels, and consequently, less energy is required to maintain the ionic gradients [16]. And third, astrocytes express lower levels of ionotropic glutamate receptors than neurons and have better ionic buffering and antioxidant capacity [13].

Vascular cells and blood vessels are also affected by ischemia; under normal conditions, the BBB has powerful regulatory mechanisms that assure the perfusion of brain tissues according to its needs, blocking the passage of anything that might be harmful [20]. However, ischemia induces profound modifications in the mechanisms that control cerebral circulation, like the endothelial function, autoregulation, vascular reactivity to hypercapnia, and neurovascular coupling [20]. Being this associated with the impairment of endothelium-dependent regulation of vascular tone and basal receptor-mediated endothelium-dependent vasodilation [20]. The major cause of this detrimental ischemia-induced vascular alterations is the increase of ROS levels, which leads to oxidative stress, impairing the function of vascular cells [20]. Therefore, this dysregulation undermines the ability of the brain to maintain blood flow, aggravates the intensity of the ischemic insult, and leads to the BBB and the infiltration of leukocytes [20].

It is, therefore, clear that this entire ischemic cascade affects all cells present in CNS and results from a series of events that are in their genesis caused by the depletion of oxygen and nutrients, that at the same time induce the simultaneous activation of several intracellular signaling pathways which in turn have the ability to activate each other, resulting in cell death [4]. This is what happens in the brain parenchyma on the center of the cerebral tissue where ischemia occurs, the so-called ischemic core [21]. In this region of the injury, all cells are dead mostly by necrotic processes, and from a cell recovery point of view, there is not much to do [21]. However, around the core, there is an area in which we find cells that are not yet dead but that are also not properly working, in many of them pro-apoptotic mechanisms will soon be activated [4, 21]. This area is called the penumbra; hypothetically, these are the cells that can be rescued from their programmed death and thus reduce the size of the injury and, consequently, the impairments associated with an ischemic stroke (IS) [4].

5. Symptoms and impairments triggered by the ischemic injury

IS is a neurological disorder with sudden onset and characterized by neurological signs directly related to the brain regions that were deprived of oxygen and nutrients [5, 6]. There are several etiologies that can cause this catastrophic event for CNS, such as thrombosis, embolisms, systemic hypoperfusion, and venous thrombosis [3, 5]. Each indicating a different mechanism of blood vessel injury or of decreased blood flow [5]. The final infarct size depends on several factors like the duration and the severity of the ischemic period, the existence of collateral systems, and an adequate systemic blood pressure [22]. Being, the size and the site of the injury crucial to determine the potential neurological outcome that results from that specific injury [3].

The two most frequent signs and symptoms observed in hospitalized patients diagnosed with IS are paresis and sensorial deficits [23, 24]. Paresis on one side of the body is observed in approximately 87.6% of IS patients, most often in the arms (81.1%), legs (73.4%), and face (58.7%) [23, 24]. Whereas sensorial deficits are observed in approximately 49% of cases, most often in the arms (42.3%), legs (37.6%), and face (22.9%) [23, 24]. Apart from these, there are several other signs and symptoms that are often observed, such as aphasia (26.1%), severe headache (22.4%), diplopia and visual problems (15.4%), and gait disturbance (11.4%) [23, 24]. Less frequent are the cases in which patients present convulsions (3.2%) and vertigo (2.5%) [23, 24].

This pathology's impact on patients is high and is considered the leading cause of complex and serious long-term disability in developed countries [7, 8]. Dysfunctions have become chronic, with several functional and clinical problems persisting over the years; data indicate that approximately two-thirds of the patients have some form of neurological impairment and/or disability [7]. These impairments are closely related to the location, size, and severity of the injury and can be classified in physical, cognitive, and emotional and cause significant impact on life quality and restrictions to activities of daily life [7]. Half of the patients stay physically dependent, which translates also into a very large impact on those around them [8, 25].

The predominant cause of long-term disability is impairments left in motor control; a large number of patients who have suffered an IS have limitations in balance, coordination, and gait [7]. Physically, are also observed somatosensory and visual impairments [7]. Somatosensory deficits refer to the inability of patients to process and manipulate their environment and can range in severity from numbness or tingling in one part of the body to complete sensory neglect of a body part or one side of the body [7, 26]. Visual impairments can take the form of monocular vision loss, visual field loss on the left or the right side of the midline, or cortical blindness [7, 27]. Cognitively, the most common impairments are problems with concentration, attention, memory, orientation, visual–spatial perception, and apraxia [7, 28]. Additionally, and which may be more subtle, there are symptoms associated with the emotional state or with personality, like anxiety, frustration, anger, sadness, and a sense of loss [7, 29, 30]. Depression is the most common post-stroke mood disorder identified with a prevalence of approximately 40% [7, 29, 30].

6. Potential therapeutic strategies

Despite the numerous efforts made over the past decades by the scientific community, the therapeutic strategies are not yet fully effective [9]. In the acute phase in the medical emergency department, the concern of clinicians is to perfuse the injured area as soon as possible in order to minimize the neuronal loss triggered by ischemia [9]. In fact, cells in the penumbra are salvageable if reperfusion is established during the early hours after the ischemic event [31]. However, after this period and entering the subacute and chronic phases, most of the treatments (e.g., Physical therapy, speech therapy, occupational therapy) are focused on reducing the sequelae that ischemia has left or controlling modifiable risk factors (e.g., hypertension, diabetes, and coagulopathies) [9, 10].

In this sense, a strategy is needed that focuses on recovering the tissues that can still be recovered, the so-called brain repair-based therapies to post-stroke injured tissues [3]. The potential effectiveness of that type of therapy on the recovery of the penumbra area is high, and its major purpose is to reduce the infarct area and significantly attenuate the neurological dysfunctions of IS patients [31]. As mentioned, it is clear that the ischemia-induced cascade involves several cellular pathways and structures, and to recover the penumbra area should be used strategies that have an integrative approach by modulating several of the above-mentioned detrimental effects [3]. Several brain repair-based strategies are being studied that could lead to the recovery of these damaged areas, such as repetitive transcranial magnetic stimulation (rTMS), the modulation of inflammation, pleiotropic approaches, or the development of cerebrotectants.

In human trials, rTMS proved to be very effective in the improvement of neurological, motor, learning, memory, and cognitive ischemia-induced outcomes, as reviewed by Zong and colleagues [32]. Those effects are associated with the ability of rTMS after an ischemic event to prevent apoptosis, neurite rupture, and inflammation, as well as by increasing neuroprotection, neurogenesis, and synaptic plasticity as reported by studies performed in animals [32] and cellular models [33].

The modulation of the inflammatory process has been described as another important step to reduce the injury associated with the ischemic event [4]. It is known that several inflammatory responses are necessary for the protection of the injured areas due to their ability to induce cell migration, proliferation, matrix deposition, and tissue remodeling [34]. However, when this is exacerbated, it begins to be harmful to the tissues; it is documented that the reduction of innate immune responses effectively reduces acute brain damage [35]. Therefore, one of the potential strategies associated with this particular mechanism will effectively involve its modulation in order to enhance only the beneficial effects and inhibit the harmful ones, thus requiring further studies [34].

Additionally, researchers in this field of interest also have their attention focused on the development and application of other strategies to induce the recovery of the injured areas, such as cerebrotectants [36], ischemic conditioning [37], therapeutic hypothermia [38], activated protein C analogs [39], and pleiotropic approaches with the use of exosomes [40] and microRNAs [41].

Despite all these efforts, any approaches have yet passed the human trials and are being applied on a large scale, reinforcing the need to continue studying and developing brain repair-based therapies.

7. Conclusion

The knowledge of the molecular and cellular basis of the origin of diseases has always had great importance in understanding their phenomenon, symptoms, and therapy. However, with the revolution of science, and especially in the last 20 years, the data that have been collected point to an increasing preponderance when it comes to identifying new therapeutic approaches.

In the specific case of the ischemic cascade, the *in vivo* and *in vitro* models allowed to collect sufficiently robust data that help map the major signaling pathways that are activated and how they interact with each other. These data are especially relevant because, due to the pathophysiology of the ischemic injury, it is necessary to look at these mechanisms in order to develop integrative therapeutic approaches that focus on recovering the cells and tissues that can still be recovered, in order to obtain a functional improvement.

In an era of constant evolution both in therapeutic approaches and in the methodologies used in the study of pathologies. It seems clear that it is fundamental, on the one hand, to continue to explore the cellular and molecular mechanisms in order to increase our knowledge of the basis of the disease and, on the other hand, try to develop these same integrative approaches, which in the case of ischemic stroke could effectively involve the modulation of several pathways that are triggered by ischemia.

Acknowledgements

This work was developed within the scope of the CICS-UBI projects UIDB/00709/2020 and UIDP/00709/2020, financed by national funds through the Portuguese Foundation for Science and Technology/MCTES.

Author details

Cláudio André Martins Roque[1,2,3]

1 CICS-UBI–Health Sciences Research Centre, University of Beira Interior, Covilhã, Portugal

2 Faculty of Health Sciences, University of Beira Interior, Covilhã, Portugal

3 School of Health Sciences of the Polytechnic Institute of Guarda, Guarda, Portugal

*Address all correspondence to: claudio.am.roque@gmail.com

References

[1] Purves D, Augustine GJ, Fitzpatrick D, Katz LC, LaMantia A, McNamara JO, et al. Neuroscience. New York: Oxford University Press; 2018. pp. 1-29

[2] Waxman SG. Clinical Neuroanatomy. New York, USA: McGraw Hill; 2020

[3] Zhao Y, Zhang X, Chen X, Wei Y. Neuronal injuries in cerebral infarction and ischemic stroke: From mechanisms to treatment (review). International Journal of Molecular Medicine. 2022;**49**(2)

[4] Qin C, Yang S, Chu YH, Zhang H, Pang XW, Chen L, et al. Signaling pathways involved in ischemic stroke: Molecular mechanisms and therapeutic interventions. Signal Transduction and Targeted Therapy. 2022;7(1):215

[5] Caplan LR, Simon RP. In: Zigmond MJ, Rowland LP, Coyle JT, editors. Cerebrovascular Disease - Stroke. Neurobiology of Brain Disorders - Biological Basis of Neurological and Psychiatric Disorders. Cambridge, Massachusetts, USA: Academic Press; 2015. pp. 339-355

[6] Favate AS, Younger DS. Epidemiology of ischemic stroke. Neurologic Clinics. 2016;**34**(4):967-980

[7] Benjamin EJ, Virani SS, Callaway CW, Chamberlain AM, Chang AR, Cheng S, et al. Heart disease and stroke Statistics-2018 update: A report from the American Heart Association. Circulation. 2018;**137**(12):e67-e492

[8] Feigin VL, Krishnamurthi RV, Parmar P, Norrving B, Mensah GA, Bennett DA, et al. Update on the global burden of ischemic and hemorrhagic stroke in 1990-2013. Neuroepidemiology. 2015;**45**(3):161-176

[9] Powers WJ, Rabinstein AA, Ackerson T, Adeoye OM, Bambakidis NC, Becker K, et al. Guidelines for the early Management of Patients with Acute Ischemic Stroke. Stroke. 2018;**49**(3):e46-e110

[10] Cramer SC. Treatments to promote neural repair after stroke. Journal of Stroke. 2018;**20**(1):57-70

[11] Belanger M, Allaman I, Magistretti PJ. Brain energy metabolism: Focus on astrocyte-neuron metabolic cooperation. Cell Metabolism. 2011;**14**(6):724-738

[12] Harada K, Kamiya T, Tsuboi T. Gliotransmitter release from astrocytes: Functional, developmental, and pathological implications in the brain. Frontiers in Neuroscience. 2015;**9**:1-9

[13] Lee HG, Wheeler MA, Quintana FJ. Function and therapeutic value of astrocytes in neurological diseases. Nature Reviews. Drug Discovery. 2022;**21**(5):339-358

[14] Wang L, Xiong X, Zhang L, Shen J. Neurovascular unit: A critical role in ischemic stroke. CNS Neuroscience & Therapeutics. 2021;**27**(1):7-16

[15] Deb P, Sharma S, Hassan KM. Pathophysiologic mechanisms of acute ischemic stroke: An overview with emphasis on therapeutic significance beyond thrombolysis. Pathophysiology. 2010;**17**(3):197-218

[16] Rossi DJ, Brady JD, Mohr C. Astrocyte metabolism and signaling during brain ischemia. Nature Neuroscience. 2007;**10**(11):1377-1386

[17] Zhao Y, Wieman HL, Jacobs SR, Rathmell JC. In: Pyle AM, editor. Mechanisms and Methods in Glucose Metabolism and Cell Death. Methods in Enzymology. Vol. 442. 2008. pp. 439-457

[18] Gourdin M, Dubois P. Impact of ischemia on cellular metabolism. In: Aronow WS, editor. Artery Bypass. 2013

[19] Pivovarov AS, Calahorro F, Walker RJ. Na(+)/K(+)-pump and neurotransmitter membrane receptors. Invertebrate Neuroscience. 2018;**19**(1):1

[20] Hu X, De Silva TM, Chen J, Faraci FM. Cerebral vascular disease and neurovascular injury in ischemic stroke. Circulation Research. 2017;**120**(3):449-471

[21] Woodruff TM, Thundyil J, Tang SC, Sobey CG, Taylor SM, Arumugam TV. Pathophysiology, treatment, and animal and cellular models of human ischemic stroke. Molecular Neurodegeneration. 2011;**6**(11):1-19

[22] Sommer CJ. Ischemic stroke: Experimental models and reality. Acta Neuropathologica. 2017;**133**(2):245-261

[23] Ali M, van Os HJA, van der Weerd N, Schoones JW, Heymans MW, Kruyt ND, et al. Sex differences in presentation of stroke: A systematic review and meta-analysis. Stroke. 2022;**53**(2):345-354

[24] Rathore SS, Hinn AR, Cooper LS, Tyroler HA, Rosamond WD. Characterization of incident stroke signs and symptoms: Findings from the atherosclerosis risk in communities study. Stroke. 2002;**33**(11):2718-2721

[25] Cloud G, Hoffman A, Rudd A. National Sentinel Stroke Audit 1998-2011. Clinical Medicine. 2013;**13**(5):444-448

[26] Kessner SS, Bingel U, Thomalla G. Somatosensory deficits after stroke: A scoping review. Topics in Stroke Rehabilitation. 2016;**23**(2):136-146

[27] Pula JH, Yuen CA. Eyes and stroke: The visual aspects of cerebrovascular disease. Stroke and Vascular Neurology. 2017;**2**(4):210-220

[28] Sun JH, Tan L, Yu JT. Post-stroke cognitive impairment: Epidemiology, mechanisms and management. Annals of Translational Medicine. 2014;**2**(8):80-96

[29] Caeiro L, Ferro JM, Santos CO, Figueira ML. Depression in acute stroke. Journal of Psychiatry & Neuroscience. 2006;**31**(6):377-383

[30] Meng G, Ma X, Li L, Tan Y, Liu X, Liu X, et al. Predictors of early-onset post-ischemic stroke depression: A cross-sectional study. BMC Neurology. 2017;**17**(1):199

[31] Zhou Z, Lu J, Liu WW, Manaenko A, Hou X, Mei Q, et al. Advances in stroke pharmacology. Pharmacology & Therapeutics. 2018;**191**:23-42

[32] Zong X, Gu J, Geng D, Gao D. Repetitive transcranial magnetic stimulation (rTMS) for multiple neurological conditions in rodent animal models: A systematic review. Neurochemistry International. 2022;**157**:105356

[33] Roque C, Pinto N, Vaz Patto M, Baltazar G. Astrocytes contribute to the neuronal recovery promoted by high-frequency repetitive magnetic stimulation in in vitro models of ischemia. Journal of Neuroscience Research. 2021;**99**(5):1414-1432

[34] Boltze J, Aronowski JA, Badaut J, Buckwalter MS, Caleo M, Chopp M, et al. New mechanistic insights, novel

treatment paradigms, and clinical Progress in cerebrovascular diseases. Frontiers in Aging Neuroscience. 2021;**13**:623751

[35] Alawieh A, Langley EF, Tomlinson S. Targeted complement inhibition salvages stressed neurons and inhibits neuroinflammation after stroke in mice. Science Translational Medicine. 2018;**10**(441)

[36] Bosetti F, Koenig JI, Ayata C, Back SA, Becker K, Broderick JP, et al. Translational stroke research: Vision and opportunities. Stroke. 2017;**48**(9):2632-2637

[37] Landman TRJ, Schoon Y, Warlé MC, de Leeuw FE, Thijssen DHJ. Remote ischemic conditioning as an additional treatment for acute ischemic stroke. Stroke. 2019;**50**(7):1934-1939

[38] Wu C, Zhao W, An H, Wu L, Chen J, Hussain M, et al. Safety, feasibility, and potential efficacy of intraarterial selective cooling infusion for stroke patients treated with mechanical thrombectomy. Journal of Cerebral Blood Flow and Metabolism. 2018;**38**(12):2251-2260

[39] Lyden P, Pryor KE, Coffey CS, Cudkowicz M, Conwit R, Jadhav A, et al. Final results of the RHAPSODY trial: A multi-center, phase 2 trial using a continual reassessment method to determine the safety and tolerability of 3K3A-APC, a recombinant variant of human activated protein C, in combination with tissue plasminogen activator, mechanical Thrombectomy or both in moderate to severe acute ischemic stroke. Annals of Neurology. 2019;**85**(1):125-136

[40] Zhang ZG, Chopp M. Exosomes in stroke pathogenesis and therapy. The Journal of Clinical Investigation. 2016;**126**(4):1190-1197

[41] Sun P, Liu DZ, Jickling GC, Sharp FR, Yin K-J. MicroRNA-based therapeutics in central nervous system injuries. Journal of Cerebral Blood Flow and Metabolism: Official Journal of the International Society of Cerebral Blood Flow and Metabolism. 2018;**38**(7):1125-1148

Chapter 7

Advances in Ischemia Reperfusion Injury Prevention in Free Flaps and Vascularized Composite Allotransplantation

Nina Hadzimustafic, Andrew D'Elia, Cagdas Duru and Siba Haykal

Abstract

In Plastic and Reconstructive Surgery, ischemia reperfusion injury (IRI) prevention is of utmost importance in free flaps and vascularized composite allotransplantation (VCA) to continue increasing accessibility to these advanced reconstructive options. At present, free flaps and VCA undergo irreversible ischemic damage at 3 hours due to the highly metabolic nature of skeletal muscle, and static cold storage (SCS) can only extend this to 4–6 hours. It is important to understand that one of the major challenges with transplanting composite tissues is that each tissue has a unique tolerance and mechanism to ischemia-reperfusion. Research targeting attenuation of IRI can be subdivided into 3 time periods: the pre-ischemic, ischemic, and post-ischemic. In the pre-ischemic period, there are conditioning methods, the delay phenomenon, which is already used clinically, pharmacologic, and stem cell strategies. In the ischemic period, SCS is used clinically, whilst other preservation methods including cryopreservation, vitrification, machine perfusion, and pharmacologic strategies are being studied. Lastly, in the post-ischemic period, our greatest clinical tool is close post-operative monitoring, however conditioning methods, and pharmacologic strategies have been studied. This chapter covers IRI in tissues implicated in free flaps and VCA, and several prevention strategies either currently in use or in pre-clinical studies.

Keywords: reconstruction, free flaps, vascularized composite allotransplantation, ischemia reperfusion injury, static cold storage, pre-ischemic period, post-ischemic period, preservation strategies

1. Introduction

In Plastic and Reconstructive surgery, the focus of ischemia reperfusion injury (IRI) prevention research is in free flaps and vascularized composite allotransplantation (VCA). Free flaps and VCA are at the highest end of reconstructive complexity options available to patients with significant tissue defects. Both free flaps and VCA require the division of blood supply to transfer or transplant the tissue; survival is dependent on prompt revascularization at the recipient site to minimize total ischemia time. Clinically, we currently have limited options for targeting the pre-ischemic, ischemic, and post-ischemic periods to attenuate IRI. The delay phenomenon is the best described and most validated preconditioning method (see Section 3.1.2), static cold storage (SCS) remains the primary clinical intervention during the ischemic period (see Section 3.2.2), and the mainstay after microvascular anastomosis is close monitoring for microvascular complications (see Section 3.3.2). This chapter will describe several experimental methods and areas of advancement that are expected to be seen in clinical trials and use in coming years.

It is notable that the majority of cutting-edge research in the field is focused on the ischemic period, as simple SCS can no longer meet the demands of preserving tissue as the field advances. Solid organs can withstand varying times in SCS: lungs are considered acceptable for 6–8 hours [1], heart for 4–6 hours [2], kidneys for up to 24 hours but ideally less than 12 [3], and liver for 8–12 hours [4]. Similarly to cardiac muscle, free flaps and VCA include transplantation of highly metabolic tissues which limits ischemia time with no interventions to 3 hours before irreversible ischemic damage takes place. Permissible ischemia time can only be extended to 4–6 hours with the use of SCS which has historically been and continues to be the gold standard for storage. Due to the highly metabolic nature of the tissues, free flaps and VCA are particularly susceptible to IRI, and thus significant advancements in prevention of IRI are targeted at reducing ischemia through various preservation methods described in this chapter.

1.1 Fundamentals of flaps and VCA

A flap is a unit of tissue wherein the blood supply has been maintained. Flaps are transferred from donor to recipient sites, which may be close or distant in proximity [5]. Depending on the indication, flaps containing different tissue types, vascular configurations, or different conformations can be procured. Exploration of donor sites and vascular patterns have led to the categorization of flaps into various subtypes, which are classified based on circulation (blood supply), constituents (composition), contiguity (destination), construction (blood flow), conformation (geometry), and/or conditioning (preparation) of the tissue [6]. The term free flap is used to describe a unit of tissue whose blood supply has been temporarily detached at the pedicle. The free flap can then be anastomosed to a new blood supply at the recipient site to fill and/or cover defects [5]. Thus, free flap transfer is both subject to and limited by an obligatory ischemia time—with ischemic insult between division of the pedicle at the time of flap elevation and eventual microvascular anastomosis. Although heavily criticized at first, technical advances and perfection of this technique has rendered free flap transfer a highly reliable option for reconstructive surgery [7], with reported success rates of 93–98.8% [8]. Free flap transfer is successful when adequate blood supply has been re-established, ischemia time is minimized, and vascular complications such as thrombosis are thwarted [8]. As alluded to, flaps can have varying composition where constituents have different capacities to withstand ischemia.

Skin flaps which are composed of just skin, subcutaneous fat, and superficial fascia are often used to cover wound defects where skin edges cannot be approximated together tension-free, or where there is inadequate vascular supply for a skin graft to survive [9]. Muscle flaps are most often used to fill large oncologic or traumatic defects as they are well vascularized, and if used with overlying skin, a myocutaneous flap, may obliviate the need for an overlying skin graft [10]. Fascial flaps are often used when a vascular flap is required, but with minimal tissue bulk for good cosmetic outcome [11]. Fasciocutaneous flaps contain skin, subcutaneous fat, and deep fascia, are thin like fascial flaps, but remove need for overlying skin graft [12]. Bone and osteocutaneous flaps are most often used for reconstruction of large bony defects, such as in craniofacial reconstruction [13]. With each different composition, different considerations regarding IRI may play a role and affect viability of the tissue being transferred.

VCA is the most complex and most novel reconstructive option for people suffering from significant tissue loss which offers functional recovery. Unlike solid organ transplantation, VCA refers to the procurement and transplantation of multiple tissues as a functional unit, including skin, nerves, muscle, bone, tendons, ligaments, adipose tissue, and vasculature. Clinically, VCA applications include limb, face, larynx, penile, uterine, and abdominal wall transplants. Since the development of VCA in 1998, the most common form of VCA performed has been hand and upper extremity transplant with 148 total reported between 1998 and 2022 [14]. From 2005 to 2020, 48 face transplants have been described world-wide [15], and since 2005 5 penile transplants have been performed [16]. As well, 42 uterine transplants, commonly performed as male-to-female gender affirming surgery, have been performed with at least 12 live births [17]. Despite significant advances in the field, VCA failure rates continue to be high, and it is thus not a routinely pursued reconstructive option if other options are available. This highlights the need for continued research and innovation in the field [18, 19].

2. Mechanisms of ischemia reperfusion injury

In ischemia, the loss of oxygenated blood flow results in a mandatory shift from aerobic to anaerobic respiration in all tissue types [20]. At the mitochondrial level, oxygen is required to accept electrons in the electron transport chain (ETC), and in hypoxic conditions, the ability to produce ATP through the ETC is therefore lost [20]. Cells become reliant on glycolysis which can produce 2 ATP per glucose molecule [20, 21]. Glycolysis is dependent on the presence of the coenzyme NAD+ which can be regenerated by lactate dehydrogenase (LDH) catalyzing the reaction of pyruvate to lactate, which simultaneously converts NAD+ to NADH [22]. Notably, as lactate builds up and causes tissue acidosis, this inhibits ATP production through a negative feedback loop [23]. Ultimately, cytosolic ATP becomes depleted through maintenance of membrane potentials, and there is a build-up of intracellular sodium and calcium that draws water into the cells causing swelling [20, 21]. Increased intracellular calcium also activates calpain, a protease which converts xanthine dehydrogenase (XDH) to XO [24]. Phospholipases disrupt cellular membranes, leading to lipid peroxidation and increased circulating fatty acids [23].

Upon reperfusion, XO produces uric acid and superoxide (O_2^-) by degrading hypoxanthine [23]. O_2^- can then be converted to hydrogen peroxide (H_2O_2) and the hydroxyl radical (OH) which promotes further lipid peroxidation [23]. Lipid peroxidation releases arachidonic acid which is a primary substrate for production of prostaglandins [23]. In ischemia, prostaglandins typically cause vasodilation to increase blood flow, but in their absence, there is unopposed vasoconstriction leading to worsened ischemia [23]. Uric acid is a damage-associated molecular pattern (DAMP) which bind to inflammasomes and cause a cytokine storm in IRI, recruit neutrophils, and increased effector T-cells. This series of events following IRI demonstrates the role IRI may have in acute and chronic rejection. Lastly, reperfusion normalizes pH in the extracellular space and removes ions, leaving high intracellular osmolarity. Further water is drawn into cells, leading to further swelling and possible membrane rupture. Mitochondria, which incurred damage during the ischemic phase continue to produce ROS which cannot be eliminated due to antioxidant depletion (**Figures 1** and **2**).

In brief, at the onset of ischemia in the myocardium, reactive oxygen species (ROS) accumulate rapidly from various sources, including the mitochondrial electron transport chain (ETC) and oxidation of ferrous heme (Fe^{2+}) to ferric heme (Fe^{3+}) both of which result in the production of O_2^- [26]. Reperfusion causes additional ROS production by way of xanthine oxidase (XO) [20]. Following ischemia-reperfusion, neutrophils release toxic oxidants, leading to further damage of the myocardium [27]. Mitochondrial permeability transition pore (mPTP) opens in response to elevated ROS, increasing permeability of the membrane, and through various mechanisms leading to calcium overload, apoptosis, and necrosis of cells [28, 29]. It is believed that for this reason, although ischemic necrosis leads to significant cell death, reperfusion may lead to an additional 25–40% cell death in the myocardium [30].

The following sections will discuss differences in IRI in various tissues contained within free flaps and VCA, highlighting differences in mechanism, if applicable.

2.1 IRI in skin and subcutaneous tissue

2.1.1 Tolerance of ischemia in skin and subcutaneous tissue

IRI in the skin has been studied in the context of both VCA and flap surgery. It has been found that intracellular pH changes related to anoxia are reversible up to

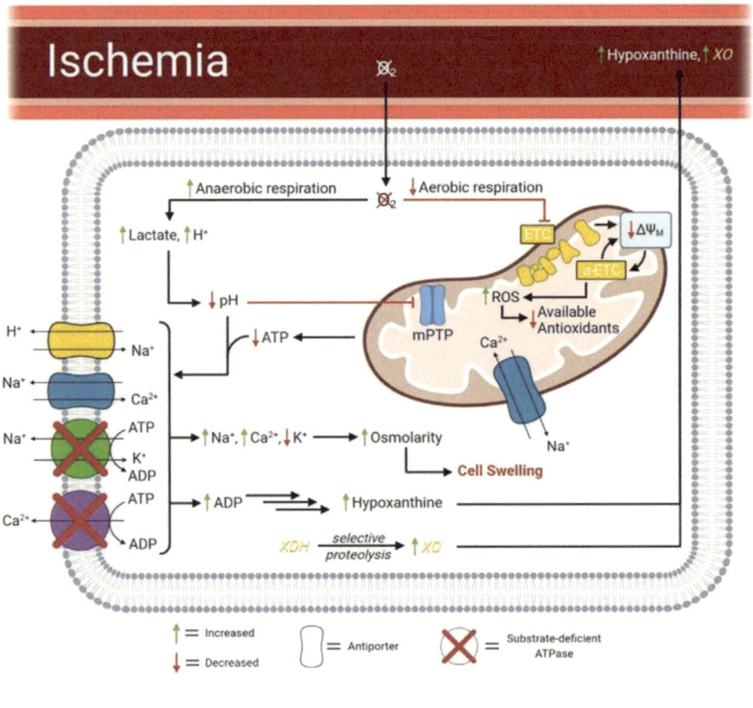

Figure 1.
Pathophysiology of ischemic injury [25].

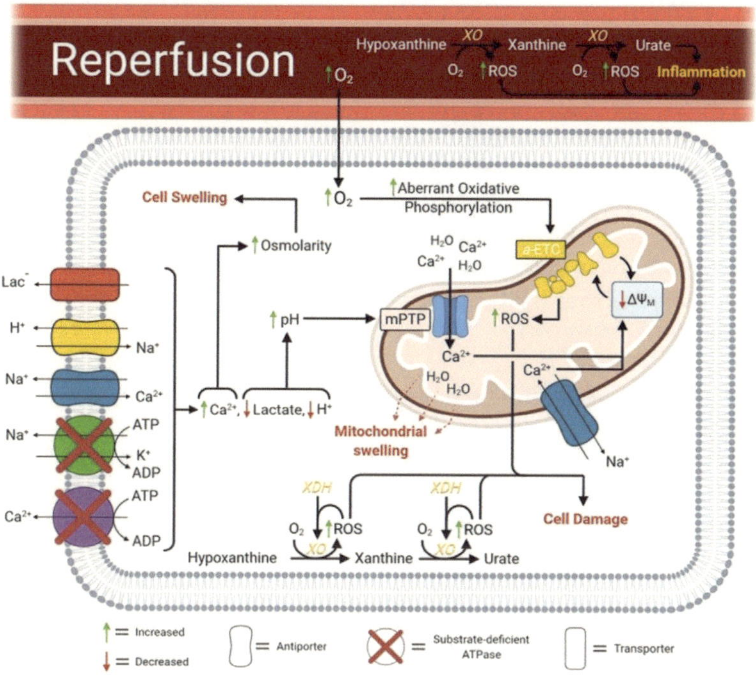

Figure 2.
Pathophysiology of reperfusion injury [25].

24 hours in both skin and subcutaneous tissue [31]. Notably, the effects of anoxia are worsened in warm and mitigated in cold environments [32]—several studies have cited that cooling flaps results in enhanced survival up to 48 hours [33]. In the setting of VCA, ischemic damage to the skin is negligible if warm or cold ischemia time is kept below 6 or 24 hours, respectively. Concern for IRI in skin and subcutaneous tissues is warranted beyond these time points.

2.1.2 IRI mechanistic considerations in skin and subcutaneous tissue

Ballestin, *et al.* showed that rat skin flaps which underwent ischemia-reperfusion (IR) had significantly higher inflammatory cell infiltration and increased necrosis [34]. They did not find significant changes in Th1/Th2 cytokine levels (i.e., IL-2, IL-4, IFN-y), but they did find overexpression of Arginase 1 which is released by M2 macrophages and shifts arginine metabolism to ornithine and urea [34]. This shift in metabolism is also known to happen in cardiac and renal IRI [18, 19]. Wang, *et al.* showed that like the myocardium, Drp1 mediates mitochondrial fission involved in IRI progression and that inhibiting Drp1 improves skin flap function [35, 36].

2.2 IRI in skeletal muscle

2.2.1 Tolerance of ischemia in skeletal muscle

It is widely appreciated that irreversible ischemic damage of skeletal muscle is 3 hours with no preservative intervention. When comparing rat muscle and skin flaps in cold (4°C) storage conditions, Wagh, *et al.* reported the critical ischemia time of muscle (16 hours) to be less than one third that of skin (3.5 days) [37]. This stark difference is sensible, as skeletal muscle is more metabolically active and will thus expend its energy stores more quickly [7]. Lactate production in skeletal muscle has been shown to occur continuously for up to 6 hours due to anaerobic respiration until it can no longer produce ATP to sustain the tissue [38]. Critical ischemia times in VCA models have yet to be sufficiently studied. Some articles suggest that muscle constituents have a warm critical ischemia time of less than 2 hours, which can be extended up to 8 hours when cooled [39]. The rapid susceptibility of muscle to ischemic insult implies that the ischemia time of VCA replants is largely dictated by skeletal muscle.

2.2.2 IRI considerations in different muscle fibres

IRI has also been shown to have differential effects in different muscle fibre types. In general, it has been found that Type II fibres exhibit more damage and necrosis than Type I fibres after IR—with Type II fast-twitch fibres sustaining the most damage to the mitochondria, sarcoplasmic reticulum, and myofibrils [40]. Type II fast-twitch fibres also demonstrated delayed recovery of function after IR compared to slow twitch fibres, indicating either more profound ischemic damage or a slower course of repair [41]. Hence, the predominant muscle fibre type in each free flap or composite tissue should be considered when estimating critical ischemia time.

2.2.3 Mechanistic considerations in skeletal muscle

The molecular mechanism of IRI in skeletal muscle is quite similar to the myocardium, though where XO is the primary source of ROS in cardiac muscle, NADPH oxidase (NOX) is located in sarcoplasmic reticulum is the most significant source of ROS in skeletal muscle (though both muscle types use both enzymes) [30]. Membrane disruption due to lipid peroxidation is quite pronounced in skeletal muscle as compared to the myocardium [40]. Neutrophils are recruited and release toxic oxidants, leading to changes to permeability of capillaries, increased interstitial fluid pressure and ultimately capillary compression [30]. An additional component of injury in the muscle is mediated by myeloperoxidase from neutrophils, an enzyme which converts hydrogen peroxide (H_2O_2) and chloride into hypochlorous acid (HOCl) which damage myocyte membranes and further peroxidation of lipids [42]. As a result, the muscle cannot get nutrients and is being directly attacked by enzymes. Another subtle difference includes that the subsarcolemmal mitochondria (SSM) are more sensitive to ischemia than interfibrillar mitochondria (IFM) of the myocardium because SSM release cytochrome c more readily in response to elevated calcium levels than IFM, leading to apoptosis of myocytes [43].

2.2.4 Clinical scenarios of IRI in skeletal muscle

Clinically, IRI in skeletal muscle can also be observed in acute compartment syndrome; intracompartmental pressure increases sufficiently to collapse capillaries and ultimately leads to cessation of tissue perfusion [40]. It can also be seen in acute limb ischemia where arterial blood flow is acutely interrupted to a limb. Both acute compartment syndrome and acute limb ischemia scenarios are surgical emergencies.

2.3 IRI in peripheral nerves

2.3.1 Tolerance of ischemia in peripheral nerves

Although not as well studied as some other tissue types, IRI in the peripheral nerve is an important consideration in tissue transplantation. Ischemia induced degeneration of nerve fibers has been reported in several studies—suggesting that reperfusion may result in microvascular or oxidative damage following anoxia [44, 45]. The critical ischemic time for nerve tissue at normal temperature is approximately 8 hours [40]. Iida, *et al.* also report that extended periods of reperfusion (42 days) permitted nerve fibre regeneration [44]. Studies have shown that early inhibition of inducible nitrous oxide synthase exhibited protection/reduction of IRI in the nerve [46].

2.3.2 Mechanistic considerations in peripheral nerves

In mild-moderate ischemia, restoration of blood flow can restore nerve action potentials rapidly [47]. It is hypothesized that the likely mechanism in ischemic fibre degeneration is due to oxidative stress and that in severe ischemia, there is a breakdown of the blood-nerve barrier, also mediated by xanthine oxidase production of hypoxanthine [47]. Nagamatsu, *et al.* showed a large increase in lipid hydroperoxides as well as blood-nerve barrier breakdown with ischemia, and therefore significant endoneurial edema [47]. In reperfusion, they showed worsening edema in the nerve [47]. Nagamatsu, *et al.* suggest that clinically, a bulk ischemia time during surgery (i.e., use of a tourniquet for an entire procedure) is more harmful than if there is periodic reperfusion at regular intervals throughout the procedure [47].

2.4 IRI in bone

2.4.1 Tolerance of ischemia in bone

In VCA, bone constituents may display relative resistance to ischemia. Still, increasing ischemia times result in appreciable changes to bone composition, ultrastructure, mechanical properties, and cellularity [48]. Messner, *et al.* note that on the 10th day following transplantation (cold ischemia = 10 hours), bones subject to ischemia were more brittle compared to controls in the rat model [48]. In addition, they note the formation of a lighter boney layer containing blood vessels and trabeculae superficial to the cortices of bones—the thickness of which was proportional to cold ischemia time [48]. Loss of osteocytes in the lacunar network and changes to the ultrastructure of the bone marrow were also observed 10 days following ischemia [48], though more precise analysis with electron microscopy revealed that osteocytes are irreversibly damaged within 4 hours, and lacunae were near-completely devoid of viable osteocytes within 24 hours [49]. Weiss, *et al.* conducted histomorphometric analysis of bone grafts after 4 and 8 hours of warm ischemia time revealed similar findings, with a drastic decrease in percentage of osteocyte-occupied lacunae [50]. Although osteocytes have been the subject of the aforementioned studies, all bone cell types, such as osteoblasts, osteoclasts, chondrocytes, and bone marrow cells are vulnerable to IRI [51].

Like other tissues, bone IRI is mitigated at decreased temperatures. It was found that after just 3–7 hours of ischemia at 37°C, growth and/or development of bone was effectively stunted [52]. Indeed, another study found that bones subject to just

6 hours of warm ischemia exhibited central areas of disorganization and complete destruction of the growth plate [53]. Decreasing temperatures to 0–5°C, however, can increase the critical ischemia time of bone to over 24 hours [52]. Albeit studies suggest that non-lethal changes can accrue in bone tissue at significantly shorter durations of ischemia [51].

2.4.2 Mechanistic considerations in bone

Information regarding mechanism of IRI in bone has not been extensively studied. It is notable that in contrast to other tissue types and organ ischemia studies, anoxia appears to readily induce bone cell apoptosis in the ischemic phase—rather than necrosis [51, 54]. No bone cell type appears to be particularly sensitive to ischemia compared to the others [51].

2.4.3 Clinical scenarios of IRI in bone

Bone IRI may occur in a variety of clinical circumstances, including bone compression, fractures, transplantation, thromboembolic events, and of course, vascular disruption [39]. Systemic diseases, such as Cushing's Disease and sickle cell anemia, may also result in IRI [55, 56].

2.5 IRI in vasculature

2.5.1 Tolerance of ischemia in vasculature

It is plausible to assume that any condition or event resulting in compromised blood flow will lead to ischemia of distal vessels and structures. The endothelium is particularly sensitive to IRI. Functions of the endothelium include controlling vascular tone and blood flow, participating in coagulation and inflammatory cascades, dictating the permeability of vessels to various macro- and micromolecules, forming new blood vessels, and facilitating immune response pathways [57]. As such, the endothelium is of utmost importance to preserve.

2.5.2 Mechanistic considerations in vasculature

Upon exposure to ischemia, the capacity for endothelium to facilitate vasodilation is particularly compromised [58]. This is a hallmark sign of arteriolar endothelial dysfunction following IRI and is at least in part due to decreased bioavailability of nitrous oxide, which decreases substantially during the reperfusion period [59]. Another potential mechanism for impaired vasodilation includes reduced shear forces or reduced endothelial nitrous oxide synthase activity caused by pH-dependent protein denaturation/proteolysis [59]. Impaired arteriole vasodilation as a result of IRI has been observed throughout the vasculature with varying severities [59]. While animal studies have shown that the renal vasculature is somewhat resilient to ischemia, cerebral vasculature shows signs of endothelial dysfunction even after minor insult [59].

When perfusion is re-established, free radicals are abundantly produced and complement proteins and WBCs are activated. In addition to producing ROS which exacerbate impairment of endothelium-dependent vasodilation, the inflammatory cascade results in activation of the endothelium itself [59, 60]. This leads to marked cell swelling, hypercoagulability, immune cell infiltration, and extravasation of fluid/proteases into the interstitium [59, 60]. While some posit that cell volume increases in response to disrupted membranes and/or ion channel dysregulation, others suggest that endothelial cell swelling is a direct result of increased cell packing from vasoconstriction [61]. Albeit less relevant in the context of IRI-related arteriolar dysfunction, leukocyte recruitment has also been shown to play a role at the arterial level. Neutrophils localize and become activated in response to enhanced adhesion molecule expression in arterioles, providing an additional source of ROS and resulting in injury upon reperfusion [59].

IRI can also be observed at the level of the capillary. Ischemic injury at this level is characterized by a decrease in the proportion of perfused capillaries and an increase in fluid filtration—a central mechanism of which has not been agreed upon in the literature. Decreased capillary perfusion can be attributed to a combination of 1) vessel congestion caused by platelet and leukocyte recruitment (leukocyte plugging), and 2) narrowing and compression of the vessels caused by barrier dysfunction-related interstitial edema [62]. It is hypothesized that ischemia-related barrier dysfunction is caused by decreased ATP stores and increased ROS production, wherein the endothelial cytoskeleton is interrupted, intercellular adhesion molecules are internalized, intercellular junctions are compromised [63], and finally, vessel permeability increases [64–66]. Barrier dysfunction may also be related to the recruitment and subsequent transendothelial migration of leukocytes, namely neutrophils [67]. The overall result of leukocyte plugging and vessel compression is significantly increased capillary bed resistance, even in the circumstance of restored systemic pressure.

Leukocyte activity in response to ischemic insult is the prominent mechanism of venule dysfunction in vascular IRI. Decreased oxygen in the setting of ischemia results in upregulated expression of adhesion molecules such as P-selectin or ICAM-1 in endothelial cells, promoting localization and activation of neutrophils, which can lead to increased vascular permeability as discussed above [68, 69]. Leukocyte-mediated damage can also be caused indirectly by way of interaction with other blood cells, such as platelets [70].

3. Strategies to combat IRI in flaps and VCA

Strategies to combat IRI in plastic surgery involve efforts that can be applied prior to ischemia (pre-ischemic period), during ischemia (ischemic period) and reperfusion (post-ischemic period). Some strategies are well developed and integrated into clinical practice, whilst others are still experimental and have not been translated into clinical practice (**Figure 3**).

3.1 Pre-ischemic period

3.1.1 Local and remote ischemic preconditioning

In 1986, Murry, *et al.* showed that inducing multiple brief periods of ischemia by clamping coronary arteries before a sustained ischemic insult reduces infarct size in a canine model [71]. This principle was first tested in skeletal muscle by Mounsey, *et al.* in latissimus dorsi flaps of pigs [72, 73]. In their initial study, a cycle of 30 minutes of pedicle clamping and 30 minutes of reperfusion prior to 4 hours of warm ischemia and 48 hour reperfusion resulted in 20% increased survival when compared to their warm ischemia-only control group [72, 73]. Pang, *et al.* also showed that three cycles

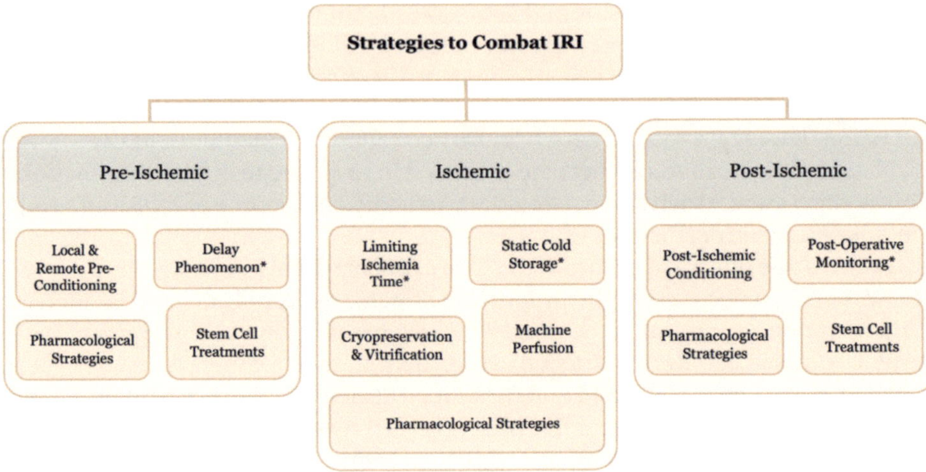

Figure 3.
*Overview of strategies to combat IRI in free flaps and VCA. *Indicates current use in clinical settings.*

of 10 minute ischemia/10 minute reperfusion significantly reduced IRI damage in both latissimus dorsi and gracilis muscles when conducted before the 4 hour sustained ischemia protocol [74]. This principle is called local ischemic preconditioning, and the potential mechanism was elucidated by Pang, *et al.* using adenosine receptor blockers and ATP-sensitive K channel blockers (see in Section 3.1.3, Pharmacological strategies) [74]. Despite the reduction of IRI, local ischemic preconditioning is impractical in clinical conditions because (1) it increases operative time, (2) each clamp cycle carries risk of damaging the pedicle, and (3) the workflow of a free flap procedure is generally already set-up in a way that the ischemia time is limited to time needed to perform anastomoses.

Oxman, *et al.* showed that inducing ischemia on a remote site can also reduce IRI at a distant organ [75]. This principle is called remote ischemic preconditioning. Oxman, *et al.* used a rat model to show that 10 minutes of limb ischemia through tourniquet application could precondition the myocardium against reperfusion injury [75]. Following success in this initial study, similar investigations were performed on skeletal muscle flaps. Addison, *et al.* applied three cycles of 10 minutes IR by applying a tourniquet to the hindlimbs of pigs and testing whether IRI was mitigated on the gracilis, rectus abdominis, and latissimus dorsi after 4 hours of ischemia and 48 hours of reperfusion [76]. Addison, *et al.* showed similar results to what was achieved with local ischemic preconditioning, however non-specific blockage of adenosine receptors did not reduce effects of preconditioning, though could be reversed by naloxone [76]. Furthermore, Moses, *et al.* demonstrated that inhibition of mitochondrial ATP-sensitive K channels resulted in abolition of effects of remote conditioning [77]. Moreover, opening these channels without remote preconditioning showed protective effects [77]. Interestingly, Kolbenschlag, *et al.* used remote ischemic preconditioning on both free and pedicled flap patients on post-operative day 1, 5, and 12 to assess oxygen saturation and flow to the flap after intervention [78]. Significant improvements were seen in free flaps, however effects were insignificant in pedicled flaps [78]. Although this method had shown effectiveness in experimental settings, a recent clinical trial of this technique by Krag, *et al.* in head and neck free flap reconstructions showed no significant effect on the complications and overall survival of the flap [79].

3.1.2 Delay phenomenon

Currently, the most noteworthy strategy in the pre-ischemic period is augmenting viability by surgical or vascular delay. The delay phenomenon is an experimentally and clinically proven form of preconditioning, also known as pre-injury conditioning, achieved by inflicting sublethal ischemia that causes permanent vascular changes in the flap [80]. This can be achieved by (1) surgically incising the flap boundaries without undermining, and/or by (2) dividing other source arteries or perforators that also nourish the intended flap area (vascular delay) 2 weeks before the definitive surgery [81]. Vascular delay results in two main events within the flap: a hypoxic state caused by reduced blood supply, and a hyperadrenergic state caused by severed sympathetic nerve endings [82]. This cascade of events results in hyperplasia, enlargement and re-orientation of the existing choke vessels that link individual skin perforator territories [83, 84]. It also drives angiogenesis within the flap via recruited progenitor cells with the effect of growth factors such as FGF and VEGF [82, 85, 86]. The HIF1a-VEGF (hypoxia) axis plays a central role in the delay phenomenon. An experimental study in rat skin flaps by Jiang, *et al.* showed that application of VEGFR antagonist significantly decreased the vascular enhancing effects of surgical delay [87]. Correspondingly, experimental studies employing VEGF as a pre-treatment showed "delay-like" vascular changes in the flap, albeit they were not as effective as actual surgical delay [88].

The merit of the surgical delay strategy has been known for several hundreds of years, traced back to the sixteenth century work of Tagliacozzi from his descriptions of staged nasal reconstruction using forearm flaps [89]. In current clinical practice, flap delay is used to enhance the flap area intended for transfer, mainly in pedicled flaps. It is used in various locations, including but not limited to the paramedian forehead flap for nasal reconstruction [90], the reverse sural flap for foot and ankle reconstruction [91], and the tensor fascia lata flap to cover extensive defects in the abdomen or lumbar region [92].

The transverse rectus abdominis myocutaneous (TRAM) flap classically demonstrates the concept of delay in the clinical setting [93]. TRAM incorporates the rectus abdominis as well as the overlying abdominal skin and fat. It is mainly used for autologous breast reconstructions. Employing the delay phenomenon by dividing the inferior pedicle and incising the flap boundaries opens the linking vessels between the two systems, thus increasing its vascularity with time, allowing a larger skin paddle to be transferred as if it were based on the inferior pedicle [83, 84]. Pedicled TRAM flaps are less frequently used now, having mostly been replaced by the deep inferior epigastric perforator (DIEP) flap sparing [94]. Even with advanced methods of pre-operative perforator selection [95], some flaps may show vascular compromise during dissection, or in some patients a larger flap may be needed. Delay procedures are helpful to increase vascularity and enhance flap volume (extended DIEP) [96].

3.1.3 Pharmacological strategies

Although pharmacological strategies have not yet seen clinical adoption, many studies have investigated their promise in reducing the effects of IRI. Commonly, the rationale of pharmacological treatment lies in preventing the generation of ROS and other inflammatory modulators, or by inducing signaling pathways that yield cell protection or neovascularization. For instance, free radical scavengers such as edavarone and sodium channel blockers such as riluzole have been investigated as protective agents for IRI in muscle [97, 98]. Treatment with vitamin C prior to ischemia has also been trialed for moderation of reperfusion injury, with positive findings in animal skeletal muscle [99, 100].

In the early 1990s, Pang, *et al.* demonstrated that, similar to preconditioning muscle with short-duration ischemia, pharmacological methods could be used to improve the tolerance of skeletal muscle to ischemic insult [74]. Preconditioning pig latissimus dorsi with 10 minutes of intravenous adenosine receptor agonist resulted in reduced muscle infarct after 4 hours of global ischemia [74]. This would allow for a more acute approach to achieving ischemic tolerance, and is thus termed acute (pharmacologic) ischemic preconditioning. Notably, the effects of pharmacologic preconditioning are sustained and do not require continuous treatment [74].

Vascular Endothelial Growth Factor (VEGF) is a potent mitogen implicated in the hypoxia signaling cascade [101]. Its expression is upregulated in the presence of HIF-1a, a factor which is constitutively expressed in the cell but otherwise ubiquitinated/degraded under normoxic conditions [101]. In the case of hypoxia, HIF-1a is stabilized and promotes the expression of VEGF, which stimulates vasculo- and angiogenesis [101]. Employing recombinant forms of VEGF for expedited angiogenesis in tissue healing (including myocardium- and ischemia-related applications) has thus been of increasing interest and widely studied in experimental research [102].

3.1.4 Stem cell treatment

Interestingly, treatment with bone marrow-derived and adipose-derived stem cells (BMSC and ADSC, respectively), prior to tissue ischemia may also hold promise in IRI reduction. These stem cells carry the potential to differentiate into endothelial cells [103], which can actively participate in neoangiogenesis and thus improve tissue survival in the ischemic environment [104, 105]. These stem cells also participate in cytoprotective cytokine and proangiogenic factor signaling [106], further potentiating their preventative effects in IRI [107]. Reichenberger, *et al.*, for example, suggest that ADSCs may downregulate intracellular TNF-alpha expression, thereby avoiding programmed cell death and promoting cell survival [108]. This claim is complicated by the observed upregulation of HIF-1alpha, VEGF-a, CCL4, and other factors that can also have pro-inflammatory, pro-angiogenic, and/or vasoactive effects [108, 109].

In 2009, Uysal *et al.* described the injection of ADSCs into random skin flaps prior to inducing 6 hours of global ischemia [105]. They found that flaps treated with stem cells showed statistically significant increases in vascular density, number of vessels, flap survival and number of endothelial cells compared to controls [105]. Similar methods and results have been reported by Ichioka, *et al.* [110]. Uysal, *et al.* posit that the observed improvements are a combination of not only enhanced angiogenesis and anti-inflammatory effects, but also upregulation of chemoattractants and other factors that induce in vivo migration, differentiation, and proliferation of ADSCs [105]. Improved blood supply at early time points in the postoperative period promote nutrition/oxygen delivery, sustaining the ischemic tissue until neovascularization is achieved.

Advantageously, adipose tissue containing ADSCs can be harvested in large quantities from the human body in a less invasive manner, with minimal donor site morbidity [105, 106]. It has also been suggested in the literature that ADSCs possess a similar level of potency and proliferative efficiency to that of BMSCs [105, 111]. In the future, this could present an avenue for personalized IRI prevention strategies. Data on this strategy in the context of skin flap protection, however, is limited [108].

3.2 Ischemic period

3.2.1 Limiting ischemia time

Clinically, the best predictor of flap and VCA survival is limiting ischemia time. Current research is targeted at strategies taken to prolong allowable ischemia time by various preservation methods when ischemia time must be extended. In free flap surgeries, the surgeon has control over the onset of ischemia time. The recipient bed, along with the recipient artery and veins are prepared, and molding of the flap is done (when necessary) before pedicle division. Taking this approach permits the surgeon to limit ischemia to the time needed to perform anastomoses. The resultant ischemia in this controlled setting is usually not significant enough to decrease the overall survival of the flap, but it may increase post-operative complications. Chang, *et al.* demonstrated that ischemia time greater than 5 hours was associated with greater complications and flap loss as compared to groups with ischemia time less than 3, 3–4, and 4–5 hours; they did so in osteocutaneous fibula flaps where they had 116 flaps for 114 patients undergoing head and neck reconstruction [112]. Interestingly, overall flap survival was not different across groups [112]. Marre, *et al.* divided their 182 patients who underwent DIEP flaps for breast reconstruction into 4 quartiles (P_{25}, P_{50}, P_{75}, P_{100}) according to intraoperative ischemia time (39–177 minutes) and found that increased ischemia time (above 100 minutes, P_{100}) was associated with increased complications such as venous/arterial thrombosis, skin slough and partial flap loss [113]. It was also found that ischemia time was an independent risk factor for microvascular complications on multivariate analysis [113]. Further, Lee, *et al.* showed that DIEP flap ischemia time over 100 minutes was significantly associated with ultrasound-diagnosed fat necrosis 3 months postoperatively [114].

Clinically, VCA ischemia time is seen in injuries leading to digital amputations. For digital replantations, 12 hours of warm ischemia or 24 hours of cold ischemia are generally considered to be safe [115, 116]. However, successful digital replantations have been reported even after 94 hours of ischemia [117]. As the amputation becomes more proximal, prompt intervention and more stringent ischemia times are necessary due to the proportion of muscle constituents. In major replantations (amputation level above the radiocarpal joint), for example, warm ischemia above 6 hours or expected cold ischemia above 12 hours may be considered a contraindication—especially for cases above the mid-forearm level—to replantation [115, 116]. In these situations, temporary vascular shunting by means of catheters can be performed in an attempt to reduce ischemia time until a stable bone fixation is achieved, radical debridement is completed, and the limb can be properly anastomosed [118]. A major clinical consideration in IRI with replantations is systemic reperfusion syndrome associated with hypotension, metabolic acidosis, hyperkalemia, myoglobinuria, and in some instances cardiovascular collapse and death [119].

3.2.2 Static cold storage

Currently, the gold standard method for preserving composite tissues is static cold storage (SCS). SCS decreases the temperature of the tissue, thereby decreasing metabolic demand and preserving energy stores during ischemia. For every 10°C decrease in temperature, a two-fold decrease in metabolic rate is observed [120]. Unlike in free flap surgery, where the workflow of the surgery is centered on minimizing ischemia time to time of microvascular anastomosis, VCA is often a transplant from donor to recipient and may need to be transported to different sites as is done with solid organ transplantation. As such, expanding ischemia time through various preservation methods is critical in advancement of clinical VCA accessibility. In SCS, the tissue is flushed with a preservation solution and stored at 4°C. The procured tissue is wrapped in moist gauze, then placed in a waterproof bag on ice until transfer to the recipient operating room [116]. The optimal preservation solution for VCA has yet to be defined. Thus, solutions for solid organ preservation are used [25]. To date, University of Wisconsin (UW) solution has been most commonly used for hand and face preservation [121–125]. Rostami, *et al.* compared 4 different preservation solutions, including Perfadex, HTK, UW, and heparinzied saline [126]. Heparinized saline showed the worst outcomes, HTK resulted in higher apoptotic cell count in nerve and skin, and Perfadex and UW were the preferred solutions [126]. Even with SCS, composite tissues used in plastic and reconstructive surgery are limited to the cold ischemia time of skeletal muscle of just 4–6 hours—this has bred the need to move away from SCS as the gold standard, and as such significant advancements have been made in more sophisticated preservation methods described in the following paragraphs.

3.2.3 Cryopreservation

Cryopreservation is a technique aimed at lowering the rate of metabolism, and ultimately function, in tissue using temperatures below −80°C. At this temperature, chemical activity and enzymatic activity are substantially reduced, but structure remains unchanged, allowing for indefinite preservation. Cryopreservation on its own is fatal to biological tissue without the use of cryoprotectant agents such as glycerol, dimethyl sulfoxide (DMSO), or ethylene glycerol [127]. Cryoprotectants reduce ice formation by increasing concentration of solutes in the tissue [127]. Although there are no human studies that have evaluated cryopreservation in VCA, studies have described single tissue and free flap responses to cryopreservation. Rinker, *et al.* show that 9/10 epigastric flaps in Lewis rats cryopreserved with DMSO and trehalose continued to be viable at 60 days and survival after transplant ranged 5–60 days [128]. Arav, *et al.* successfully cryopreserved then transplanted the above-knee rat hindlimb, which remained viable until their endpoint of 3 days [129]. Cryopreservation in free flaps and VCA continue to be limited by their composite nature as each tissue varies in its susceptibility to ischemia and IRI, as well as optimal cryoprotectants.

3.2.4 Vitrification

Vitrification is a process of cryopreservation which avoids the transition from liquid to crystalline structure, but rather shifts to a glass-like phase that behaves like a solid but avoids the ice crystals of cryopreservation [128]. Theoretically, vitrification allows for indefinite storage of tissues in this state. Vitrification contrasts from regular cryopreservation by transitioning from liquid to solid phase very quickly in order to suppress ice nucleation in the process, and in the vitrified state, viscosity prevents ice crystal formation [130]. Arav, *et al.* also vitrified 3 above-knee rat hindlimbs which similarly to their cryopreserved limbs remained viable for 3 days post-operatively, which was their endpoint [129]. Vitrification continues to be very limited due to the significant technical difficulty associated with rapid supercooling.

3.2.5 Machine perfusion

Machine perfusion has become a very popular research avenue in transplant research, particularly following success of ex vivo lung perfusion in the clinical setting. Ex vivo machine perfusion entails the connection of vasculature to an external pump capable of perfusing the tissue with a perfusion with a solution (+/− an oxygen carrier). Machine perfusion allows for constant delivery of oxygen, nutrients, removal of toxic metabolites such as lactate, and tissue viability testing. The first known perfusion of a composite tissue occurred in 1964, when Delorme, *et al.* perfused 6 lower extremities with autologous blood [131]. Since then, several landmark studies have furthered our understanding of the utility of machine perfusion in VCA preservation. In 2011, Constantinescu, *et al.* successfully perfused porcine forelimbs for 12 hours. The forelimbs exhibited retained functional capacity, evidenced by successful electrical stimulation of muscles as compared to loss of stimulation in the SCS control group [132]. Ozer, *et al.* furthered the porcine forelimb work by showing normal single-muscle fibre contractility after 12 hours of perfusion with autologous blood, and successful transplant of limbs to recipient pigs with normalized lactate levels post-reperfusion [133, 134]. Werner, *et al.* perfused 5 human upper limbs with a plasma-based perfusate for 24 hours, which resulted in normal electrical stimulation throughout and no histological myocyte damage [134]. Gok, *et al.* perfused rat hindlimbs for 6 hours with STEEN solution (perfusate optimized for lung perfusion) enriched with RBCs. They found that the muscles remained viable, with no evidence of ischemic necrosis on histology [135]. Krezdorn, *et al.* showed greater 7-day post-operative replantation survival and integrity of porcine forelimbs after 24 hours of perfusion with modified STEEN as compared to SCS control stored for 4 hours [136]. Burlage, *et al.* perfused rat hindlimbs with acellular perfusates (bovine serum albumin (BSA), with either polyethylene glycol or oxygen carrier HBOC-201 added) at subnormothermic temperatures for 6 hours and were successful in heterotopically transplanting the limbs, noting superiority of the group perfused with HBOC-201 in 30-day survival post-operatively [137].

Although the past decade has seen an explosion of research in use of machine perfusion, major limitations are still being explored. Most studies only follow-up post replantation for a maximum of 1 month. Due to heterotopic transplantation, there is a major automutilation confounder as well. A major clinical consideration is the extravasation of perfusate and subsequent edema and weight gain which may result in compartment syndrome necessitating fasciotomies to maintain tissue survival. There is thus a need to develop a perfusate which limits this adverse effect of machine perfusion by providing endothelial protection and adequate balance of hydrostatic and oncotic pressures. To-date, there is no perfusate that has been specifically designed and optimized for use in VCA; no study has been done to directly compare experimental outcomes of various perfusates currently in use for VCA perfusion. Datta, *et al.* reviewed preservation solutions currently used in literature and hypothesized that an ideal solution will reduce ROS production, thus attenuating IRI in VCA, but cautions that the significant diversity within VCA itself will likely give rise to the need to cater solutions to each type of VCA based on tissue subunit composition [25].

3.2.6 Pharmacological strategies

As discussed previously in pre-ischemic treatment methods, treatment with various agents during tissue ischemia may also improve survival upon reperfusion. In one study, bone grafts were exposed to varying durations of warm ischemia time prior to reperfusion. Just prior to anastomosis, the experimental group was treated with superoxide dismutase—which functioned to prevent the generation of reactive oxygen species when blood flow was re-established. Bone grafts treated with superoxide dismutase exhibited enhanced survival compared to controls [50]. A study by Tamura, *et al.* also achieved pronounced protection from IRI by administering a derivative of vitamin C prior to reperfusion in a rat hind limb model [53].

3.3 Post-ischemic period

3.3.1 Post-ischemic conditioning

The principle outlined in Section 3.1.1 (Local and remote ischemic preconditioning) also has a protective effect when applied just before sustained reperfusion—this is known as post-ischemic conditioning. This strategy was first described in myocardial tissue by Zhao, *et al.* where they showed three cycles of 30 second coronary artery clamping and 30 seconds of reperfusion applied just before the 3 hour reperfusion period following a 50 minute ischemic period resulted in significant reduction of infarct size compared to their control group [138]. Moreover, the protective effect was similar to the pre-conditioning group that they included in their study [138]. This strategy was again applied to muscle flaps. Park, *et al.* showed that six cycles of 15 second IR periods at the end of 3 hours of ischemia result in the attenuation of IRI in rat extensor digitorum longus [139]. The possible mechanistic explanation of this effect was studied by McAllister, *et al.* on pig latissimus dorsi muscle flaps [140]. They showed that intravenous injection of cyclosporine A, an inhibitor of the opening of mPTP after 4 hours of ischemia results in a similar effect to four cycles of 30 second IR [140]. They also found this effect could be reversed by actractyloside, an mPTP opener [140]. Moreover, McAllister, *et al.* showed that the application of cariporide, a Na^+/H^+ exchange inhibitor, effectively reduces the mitochondrial Ca^{2+} content and has protective effects like cyclosporine A [140]. Despite promising results, ischemic post-conditioning is currently not common clinical practice.

3.3.2 Monitoring for microvascular complications post-operatively

The reperfusion period starts upon the completion of proper anastomosis of vessels. It is critical to monitor the transplanted tissue hourly, particularly in the first 24 hours, as this is the period where most microvascular complications will arise due to arterial and/or venous insufficiency. Capillary refill time, temperature, color, and turgor are monitored [141, 142], blood flow is confirmed with a doppler, and oxygenation with a tissue oximeter [143, 144]. Short capillary refill time (<2 seconds), purple skin color, marked edema, and increased turgor are indications of venous insufficiency [142]. Long capillary refill (>3 seconds), pallor and cool temperature are indicators of arterial insufficiency [142]. Arterial insufficiency usually results from thrombosis within the anastomosis whilst global venous insufficiency may result from venous thrombosis, torsion in the pedicle, or hematoma around the pedicle [145, 146]. When these complications arise, the flap returns to an ischemic state and blood flow must be restored. Failure to recognize these changes, or late intervention are risks of losing the tissue entirely. As expected, time from the initial operation until salvage attempt negatively correlates with salvage success [147, 148].

3.3.3 Pharmacological strategies

Pharmacological treatment is usually initiated in the OR and continued post-operatively to decrease risk of thrombosis. Low molecular weight heparin, unfractionated heparin and aspirin are the most commonly used anticoagulant and anti-platelet agents [149]. However, there is no consensus on the optimal regime, and it is questionable whether they actually have any effect on overall survival [149, 150]. Treating muscle with copolymer surfactants—which have been shown to adsorb and seal damaged cell membranes—post-injury has also seen success in improving the survival of muscles in the rat [151]. Orfany, *et al.* describe a significant reduction of IRI using a mouse acute limb ischemia model with mitochondrial transplantation, leading to decreased apoptosis, infarct, and increasing viability and function post-IRI [152].

Treatments targeting IRI in the vasculature have also been explored. In a study by Ward, *et al.*, superoxide dismutase or Trolox (antioxidants) were used to prevent morphological endothelial cell changes characteristic of ischemic injury, such as cell swelling and bleb formation [153]. Another study found that incubating arterioles in sepiapterin, a BH4 precursor, or MH4, a BH4 analog, could restore endothelium-dependent vasodilation following a period of ischemia in the pig [154]. Although this work primarily sought to explain the mechanism by which endothelial function is blunted in IRI (depletion of cofactor BH4), this work paves the way for future reagent-based approaches to IRI prevention [154].

Although not a pharmacologic measure per se, Haapaniemi, *et al.* also suggest that by increasing the partial pressure of oxygen in the tissue, treatment with hyperbaric oxygen can effectively reduce IRI [155].

3.3.4 Stem cell treatment

Similarly discussed in the pre-ischemic section of this chapter, stem cells have also been investigated as a post-ischemic treatment strategy for IRI. Studies have shown that intravenous treatment of skin flaps with adipose derived stem cells exhibited enhanced flap survival, flap perfusion, and expression of pro-angiogenic and inflammatory genes in the rat [108]. Another study by Nakagami, *et al.* found enhanced blood flow and capillary density 4 weeks post-transplantation of adipose derived stem cells co-cultured with human aortic endothelial cells in the ischemic mouse hindlimb [156].

4. Conclusion

In conclusion, ischemia reperfusion injury is of critical concern in Plastic and Reconstructive Surgery as the highest complexity reconstructive options offered to patients are subject to ischemia. In contrast to ischemia of solid organs for transplant, Plastic Surgery must uniquely manage composite tissues with varying tolerances to ischemia and IRI. Various measures are employed to mitigate the adverse effects of IRI, some of which are present in clinical settings today whilst others have yet to be translated to human clinical trials. Firstly, in the pre-ischemic period, great effort is made to work with well-vascularized tissues through pre-operative planning whenever possible and strategies such as delay can be employed. Significant benefits have been described through local and remote pre-conditioning methods, and with pharmacological and stem cell treatments in the pre-clinical setting. Secondly, the ischemic period occurs after division of the pedicle which is currently the target of most research efforts. Currently, SCS is the gold standard of storage, but it has limits and research has shown promising outcomes with freezing methods and machine perfusion. Thirdly, in the post-ischemic, or reperfusion period, rigorous post-operative monitoring of both the patient and the transplanted tissue to promptly address any complications that may arise. Some post-conditioning and pharmacological treatments have been described in the pre-clinical setting with promise to enhance the reperfusion period. Altogether, there have been significant advances in IRI implications in Plastic and Reconstructive Surgery, and in order to continue increasing accessibility to these advanced reconstructive options for patients with significant tissue loss, research must be continued with ultimate translation to clinical studies in the near future.

Conflict of interest

The authors declare no conflict of interest.

Author details

Nina Hadzimustafic[1,2], Andrew D'Elia[1,2], Cagdas Duru[1] and Siba Haykal[1,2,3*]

1 Latner Thoracic Surgery Laboratories, University Health Network, Toronto General Hospital, Toronto, ON, Canada

2 Temerty Faculty of Medicine, University of Toronto, Toronto, ON, Canada

3 Division of Plastic and Reconstructive Surgery, Department of Surgery, University of Toronto, Toronto, ON, Canada

*Address all correspondence to: siba.haykal@uhn.ca

References

[1] Ali A, Wang A, Ribeiro RVP, et al. Static lung storage at 10°C maintains mitochondrial health and preserves donor organ function. Science Translational Medicine. 2021;**13**:7601

[2] Hess NR, Ziegler LA, Kaczorowski DJ. Heart donation and preservation: Historical perspectives, current technologies, and future directions. Journal of Clinical Medicine. 2022;**11**:5762

[3] Nieto-Ríos JF, Ochoa-García CL, Serna-Campuzano A, et al. Time of cold ischemia and delayed graft function in a cohort of renal transplant patients in a reference center. Indian Journal of Nephrology. 2019;**29**:8

[4] Sibulesky L, Li M, Hansen RN, et al. Impact of cold ischemia time on outcomes of liver transplantation: A single center experience. Annals of Transplantation. 2016;**21**:145-151

[5] Khouri RK. Free flap surgery. The second decade. Clinics in Plastic Surgery. 1992;**19**:757-761

[6] Hallock GG. The complete classification of flaps. Microsurgery. 2004;**24**:157-161

[7] Kerrigan CL, Stotland MA. Ischemia reperfusion injury: A review. Microsurgery. 1993;**14**:165-175

[8] Khouri RK. Avoiding free flap failure. Clinics in Plastic Surgery. 1992;**19**:773-781

[9] Honrado CP, Murakami CS. Wound healing and physiology of skin flaps. Facial Plastic Surgery Clinics of North America. 2005;**13**:203-214

[10] Deramo P, Rose J. Flaps: Muscle and Musculocutaneous. StatPearls. 2023. Available from: https://www.ncbi.nlm.nih.gov/books/NBK546581/ [Accessed: August 1, 2023]

[11] Lee MG, Kim JS, Lee DC, et al. Fascial free flap for reconstruction of the dorsolateral hand and digits: The advantage of a thin contour. Archives of Plastic Surgery. 2016;**43**:551

[12] Boretto JG, Cicco FL De. Fasciocutaneous Flaps. StatPearls. 2022. Available from: https://www.ncbi.nlm.nih.gov/books/NBK562280/ [Accessed: August 1, 2023]

[13] Kearns M, Ermogenous P, Myers S, et al. Osteocutaneous flaps for head and neck reconstruction: A focused evaluation of donor site morbidity and patient reported outcome measures in different reconstruction options. Archives of Plastic Surgery. 2018;**45**:495

[14] Wells MW, Rampazzo A, Papay F, et al. Two decades of hand transplantation: A systematic review of outcomes. Annals of Plastic Surgery. 2022;**88**:335-344

[15] Diep GK, Berman ZP, Alfonso AR, et al. The 2020 facial transplantation update: A 15-year compendium. Plastic and Reconstructive Surgery. Global Open. 2021;**9**:e3586. Epub ahead of print 2 April 2021. DOI: 10.1097/GOX.0000000000003586

[16] Lopez CD, Girard AO, Lake IV, et al. Lessons learned from the first 15 years of penile transplantation and updates to the Baltimore criteria. Nature Reviews Urology. 2023;**20**:294-307

[17] Jones BP, Williams NJ, Saso S, et al. Uterine transplantation in transgender women. BJOG. 2019;**126**:152

[18] Schlüter K-D, Schulz R, Schreckenberg R. Arginase induction and activation during ischemia and reperfusion and functional consequences for the heart. Frontiers in Physiology. 2015;**6**. Epub ahead of print 11 March 2015. DOI: 10.3389/FPHYS.2015.00065

[19] Ansermet C, Centeno G, Lagarrigue S, et al. Renal tubular arginase-2 participates in the formation of the corticomedullary urea gradient and attenuates kidney damage in ischemia-reperfusion injury in mice. Acta Physiologica. 2020;**229**:e13457

[20] Paradis S, Charles AL, Meyer A, et al. Chronology of mitochondrial and cellular events during skeletal muscle ischemia-reperfusion. American Journal of Physiology. Cell Physiology. 2016;**310**:C968

[21] Kalogeris T, Baines CP, Krenz M, et al. Cell biology of ischemia/reperfusion injury. International Review of Cell and Molecular Biology. 2012;**298**:229-317

[22] Yang Y, Sauve AA. NAD+ metabolism: Bioenergetics, signaling and manipulation for therapy. Biochimica et Biophysica Acta. 2016;**1864**:1787

[23] Cowled P, Fitridge R. Pathophysiology of reperfusion injury. In: Mechanisms of Vascular Disease: A Reference Book for Vascular Specialists. Adelaide, AU: University of Adelaide Press; 2011. pp. 331-350

[24] Granger DN, Kvietys PR. Reperfusion injury and reactive oxygen species: The evolution of a concept. Redox Biology. 2015;**6**:524-551

[25] Datta S, Fitzpatrick AM, Haykal S. Preservation solutions for attenuation of ischemia–reperfusion injury in vascularized composite allotransplantation. SAGE Open Medicine. 2021;**9**:205031212110349. DOI: 101177/20503121211034924

[26] Zhou T, Chuang CC, Zuo L. Molecular characterization of reactive oxygen species in myocardial ischemia-reperfusion injury. BioMed Research International. 2015;**2015**:864946. Epub ahead of print 2015. DOI: 10.1155/2015/864946

[27] Vinten-Johansen J. Involvement of neutrophils in the pathogenesis of lethal myocardial reperfusion injury. Cardiovascular Research. 2004;**61**:481-497

[28] Crompton M. Mitochondrial intermembrane junctional complexes and their role in cell death. Journal of Physiology. 2000;**529**:11-21

[29] Kim JS, Jin Y, Lemasters JJ. Reactive oxygen species, but not Ca2+ overloading, trigger pH- and mitochondrial permeability transition-dependent death of adult rat myocytes after ischemia-reperfusion. American Journal of Physiology. Heart and Circulatory Physiology. 2006. Epub ahead of print May 2006;**290**:H2024-H2034. DOI: 10.1152/AJPHEART.00683.2005

[30] Zhou T, Prather ER, Garrison DE, et al. Interplay between ROS and Antioxidants during ischemia-reperfusion injuries in cardiac and skeletal muscle. International Journal of Molecular Sciences. 2018;**19**:417

[31] Serafin D, Georgiade NG, Mullen RY, et al. Transcutaneous PO2 monitoring for assessing viability and predicting survival of skin flaps: Experimental and clinical correlations. Journal of Microsurgery. 1981;**2**:165-178

[32] Donski PK, Franklin JD, Hurley JV, et al. The effects of cooling on experimental free flap survival. British Journal of Plastic Surgery. 1980;**33**:353-360

[33] Cooley BC, Hansen FC, Dellon AL. The effect of temperature on tolerance to ischemia in experimental free flaps. Microsurgery. 1981;**3**:11-14

[34] Ballestín A, Casado JG, Abellán E, et al. Ischemia-reperfusion injury in a rat microvascular skin free flap model: A histological, genetic, and blood flow study. PLoS One. 2018;**13**:e0209624

[35] Wang Y, Wu Y, Zhou M, et al. GRK2 deletion improves the function of skin flap following ischemia-reperfusion injury by regulating Drp1. American Journal of Translational Research. 2021;**13**:223

[36] Zepeda R, Kuzmicic J, Parra V, et al. Drp1 loss-of-function reduces cardiomyocyte oxygen dependence protecting the heart from ischemia-reperfusion injury. Journal of Cardiovascular Pharmacology. 2014;**63**:477-487

[37] Wagh M, Pantazi G, Romeo R, et al. Cold storage of rat skeletal muscle free flaps and pre-ischemic perfusion with modified UW solution. Microsurgery. 2000;**20**(7):343-349

[38] Harris K, Walker PM, Mickle DAG, et al. Metabolic response of skeletal muscle to ischemia. The American Journal of Physiology. 1986;**250**:H213-H220. Epub ahead of print 1986. DOI: 10.1152/AJPHEART.1986.250.2.H213

[39] He J, Khan UZ, Qing L, et al. Improving the ischemia-reperfusion injury in vascularized composite allotransplantation: Clinical experience and experimental implications. Frontiers in Immunology. 2022;**13**:998952

[40] Gillani S, Cao J, Suzuki T, et al. The effect of ischemia reperfusion injury on skeletal muscle. Injury. 2012;**43**:670-675

[41] Woitaske MD, McCarter RJM. Effects of fiber type on ischemia-reperfusion injury in mouse skeletal muscle. Plastic and Reconstructive Surgery. 1998;**102**:2052-2063

[42] Klebanoff SJ, Kettle AJ, Rosen H, et al. Myeloperoxidase: A front-line defender against phagocytosed microorganisms. Journal of Leukocyte Biology. 2013;**93**:185

[43] Lesnefsky EJ, Chen Q, Tandler B, et al. Mitochondrial dysfunction and myocardial ischemia-reperfusion: Implications for novel therapies. Annual Review of Pharmacology and Toxicology. 2017;**57**:535-565

[44] Iida H, Schmelzer JD, Schmeichel AM, et al. Peripheral nerve ischemia: Reperfusion injury and fiber regeneration. Experimental Neurology. 2003;**184**:997-1002

[45] Saray A, Can B, Akbiyik F, et al. Ischaemia-reperfusion injury of the peripheral nerve: An experimental study—Saray—1999—Microsurgery—Wiley Online Library. Microsurgery. 1999;**19**(8):374-380. Available from: https://onlinelibrary.wiley.com/doi/abs/10.1002/%28SICI%291098-2752%281999%2919%3A8%3C374%3A%3AAID-MICR5%3E3.0.CO%3B2-A [Accessed: July 28, 2023]

[46] Shin SJ, Qi WN, Cai Y, et al. Inhibition of inducible nitric oxide synthase promotes recovery of motor function in rats after sciatic nerve ischemia and reperfusion. The Journal of Hand Surgery. 2005;**30**:826-835

[47] Nagamatsu M, Schmelzer JD, Zollman PJ, et al. Ischemic reperfusion causes lipid peroxidation and fiber degeneration. Muscle & Nerve. 1996;**19**:37-47

[48] Messner F, Hautz T, Blumer MJF, et al. Critical ischemia times and the

effect of novel preservation solutions HTK-N and TiProtec on tissues of a vascularized tissue Isograft. Transplantation. 2017;**101**:e301-e310

[49] James J, Steijn-Myagkaya GL. Death of osteocytes: Electron microscopy after in vitro ischaemia. Journal of Bone and Joint Surgery—Series B. 1986;**68**:620-624

[50] Weiss APC, Moore JR, Randolph MA, et al. Preventing oxygen free-radical injury in ischemic revascularized bone grafts. Plastic and Reconstructive Surgery. 1988;**82**:486-495

[51] De Groot H. Ischemia-reperfusion injury. A phenomenon, that also occurs in the bone. Materwiss Werksttech. 2007;**38**:965-968

[52] Berggren A, Weiland AJ, Dorfman H. The effect of prolonged ischemia time on osteocyte and osteoblast survival in composite bone grafts revascularized by microvascular anastomoses. Plastic and Reconstructive Surgery. 1982;**69**:290-298

[53] Tamura Y, Inoue G, Miura T, et al. Reperfusion injury in bone: Effects of CV-3611, a free radical scavenger, on ischemic revascularized bone grafts in rats. Journal of Reconstructive Microsurgery. 1992;**8**:471-479

[54] Sato M, Sugano N, Ohzono K, et al. Apoptosis and expression of stress protein (ORP150, HO1) during development of ischaemic osteonecrosis in the rat. Journal of Bone and Joint Surgery. British Volume (London). 2001;**83-B**:751-759

[55] Hasenmajer V, Sbardella E, Sciarra F, et al. The immune system in Cushing's syndrome. Trends in Endocrinology and Metabolism. 2020;**31**:655-669

[56] Hebbel RP, Belcher JD, Vercellotti GM. The multifaceted role of ischemia/reperfusion in sickle cell anemia. The Journal of Clinical Investigation. 2020;**130**:1062-1072

[57] Nordling S, Brännström J, Carlsson F, et al. Enhanced protection of the renal vascular endothelium improves early outcome in kidney transplantation: Preclinical investigations in pig and mouse. Scientific Reports. 2018;**8**:5220. Epub ahead of print 1 December 2018. DOI: 10.1038/S41598-018-21463-1

[58] Aboo Bakkar Z, Fulford J, Gates PE, et al. Prolonged forearm ischemia attenuates endothelium-dependent vasodilatation and plasma nitric oxide metabolites in overweight middle-aged men. European Journal of Applied Physiology. 2018;**118**:1565-1572

[59] Seal JB, Gewertz BL. Vascular dysfunction in ischemia-reperfusion injury. Annals of Vascular Surgery. 2005;**19**:572-584

[60] Stewart DJ, Pohl U, Bassenge E. Free radicals inhibit endothelium-dependent dilation in the coronary resistance bed. American Journal of Physiology. 1988;**255**:H765-H769. Epub ahead of print 1988. DOI: 10.1152/AJPHEART.1988.255.4.H765

[61] Ward BJ, McCarthy A. Endothelial cell 'swelling' in ischaemia and reperfusion. Journal of Molecular and Cellular Cardiology. 1995;**27**:1293-1300

[62] Harris AG, Steinbauer M, Leiderer R, et al. Role of leukocyte plugging and edema in skeletal muscle ischemia-reperfusion injury. The American Journal of Physiology. 1997;**273**:H989-H996. Epub ahead of print 1997. DOI: 10.1152/AJPHEART.1997.273.2.H989

[63] Alexander JS, Alexander BC, Eppihimer LA, et al. Inflammatory mediators induce sequestration of VE-cadherin in cultured human endothelial cells. Inflammation. 2000;**24**:99-113

[64] Hinshaw DB, Sklar LA, Bohl B, et al. Cytoskeletal and morphologic impact of cellular oxidant injury. The American Journal of Pathology. 1986;**123**:454

[65] Hinshaw DB, Burger JM, Miller MT, et al. ATP depletion induces an increase in the assembly of a labile pool of polymerized actin in endothelial cells. American Journal of Clinical Pathology. 1993;**264**:454-464. Epub ahead of print 1993. DOI: 101152/ajpcell19932645C1171, 10.1152/AJPCELL.1993.264.5.C1171

[66] Kevil CG, Ohno N, Gute DC, et al. Role of cadherin internalization in hydrogen peroxide-mediated endothelial permeability. Free Radical Biology & Medicine. 1998;**24**:1015-1022

[67] Marcus BC, Hynes KL, Gewertz BL. Loss of endothelial barrier function requires neutrophil adhesion. Surgery. 1997;**122**:420-427

[68] Kurose I, Anderson DC, Miyasaka M, et al. Molecular determinants of reperfusion-induced leukocyte adhesion and vascular protein leakage. Circulation Research. 1994;**74**:336-343

[69] Sawaya DE, Zibari GB, Minardi A, et al. P-selectin contributes to the initial recruitment of rolling and adherent leukocytes in hepatic venules after ischemia/reperfusion. Shock. 1999;**12**:227-232

[70] Oliver MG, Specian RD, Perry MA, et al. Morphologic assessment of leukocyte-endothelial cell interactions in mesenteric venules subjected to ischemia and reperfusion. Inflammation. 1991;**15**:331-346

[71] Murry CE, Jennings RB, Reimer KA. Preconditioning with ischemia: A delay of lethal cell injury in ischemic myocardium. Circulation. 1986;**74**:1124-1136

[72] Mounsey RA, Pang CY, Boyd JB, et al. Augmentation of skeletal muscle survival in the latissimus dorsi porcine model using acute ischemic preconditioning. The Journal of Otolaryngology. 1992;**21**(5):315-320

[73] Mounsey RA, Pang CY, Forrest C. Preconditioning: A new technique for improved muscle flap survival. Otolaryngology–Head and Neck Surgery. 1992;**107**:549-552

[74] Pang CY, Yang RZ, Zhong A, et al. Acute ischaemic preconditioning protects against skeletal muscle infarction in the pig. Cardiovascular Research. 1995;**29**(6):782-788

[75] Oxman T, Arad M, Klein R, et al. Limb ischemia preconditions the heart against reperfusion tachyarrhythmia. The American Journal of Physiology. 1997;**273**:H1707-H1712. Epub ahead of print 1997. DOI: 10.1152/AJPHEART.1997.273.4.H1707

[76] Addison PD, Neligan PC, Ashrafpour H, et al. Noninvasive remote ischemic preconditioning for global protection of skeletal muscle against infarction. American Journal of Physiology. Heart and Circulatory Physiology. 2003;**285**:H1435-H1443. Epub ahead of print 1 October 2003. DOI: 10.1152/AJPHEART.00106.2003

[77] Moses MA, Addison PD, Neligan PC, et al. Mitochondrial KATP channels in hindlimb remote ischemic preconditioning of skeletal muscle against infarction. American Journal of Physiology. Heart and Circulatory Physiology. 2005;**288**:H559-H567. Epub ahead of print February 2005. DOI: 10.1152/AJPHEART.00845.2004

[78] Kolbenschlag J, Sogorski A, Kapalschinski N, et al. Remote ischemic conditioning improves blood flow and

oxygen saturation in Pedicled and free surgical flaps. Plastic and Reconstructive Surgery. 2016;**138**:1089-1097

[79] Krag AE, Hvas AM, Hvas CL, et al. Remote ischemic preconditioning in microsurgical head and neck reconstruction: A randomized controlled trial. Plastic and Reconstructive Surgery. Global Open. 2020;**8**:e2591. Epub ahead of print 21 January 2020. DOI: 10.1097/GOX.0000000000002591

[80] Hamilton K, Wolfswinkel EM, Weathers WM, et al. The delay phenomenon: A compilation of knowledge across specialties. Craniomaxillofacial Trauma & Reconstruction. 2014;**7**:112-118

[81] Dhar SC, Taylor GI. The delay phenomenon: The story unfolds. Plastic and Reconstructive Surgery. 1999;**104**:2079-2091

[82] Ghali S, Butler PEM, Tepper OM, et al. Vascular delay revisited. Plastic and Reconstructive Surgery. 2007;**119**:1735-1744

[83] Taylor GI, Palmer JH. The vascular territories (angiosomes) of the body: Experimental study and clinical applications. British Journal of Plastic Surgery. 1987;**40**:113-141

[84] Taylor GI, Corlett RJ, Dhar SC, et al. The anatomical (angiosome) and clinical territories of cutaneous perforating arteries: Development of the concept and designing safe flaps. Plastic and Reconstructive Surgery. 2011;**127**:1447-1459

[85] Wong MS, Erdmann D, Sweis R, et al. Basic fibroblast growth factor expression following surgical delay of rat transverse rectus abdominis myocutaneous flaps. Plastic and Reconstructive Surgery. 2004;**113**:2030-2036

[86] Tepper OM, Capla JM, Galiano RD, et al. Adult vasculogenesis occurs through in situ recruitment, proliferation, and tubulization of circulating bone marrow-derived cells. Blood. 2005;**105**:1068-1077

[87] Jiang Z, Gong X. Reply: Effect of endogenous vascular endothelial growth factor on flap surgical delay in a rat flap model. Plastic and Reconstructive Surgery. 2019;**144**:1117e. Epub ahead of print 1 December 2019. DOI: 10.1097/PRS.0000000000006220

[88] Khan A, Ashrafpour H, Huang N, et al. Acute local subcutaneous VEGF165 injection for augmentation of skin flap viability: Efficacy and mechanism. American Journal of Physiology. Regulatory, Integrative and Comparative Physiology. 2004;**287**:R1219-R1229. Epub ahead of print November 2004. DOI: 10.1152/AJPREGU.00143.2004

[89] Zimbler MS. Gaspare Tagliacozzi (1545-1599): renaissance surgeon. Archives of Facial Plastic Surgery: Official Publication for the American Academy of Facial Plastic and Reconstructive Surgery, Inc and the International Federation of Facial Plastic Surgery Societies. 2001;**3**:283-284

[90] Itani Y, Yotsuyanagi T, Yamauchi M, et al. The laterally extended Paramedian forehead flap for nasal reconstruction: The delay technique revisited. Plastic and Reconstructive Surgery. Global Open. 2020;**8**:E2871

[91] Kareh AM, Felder JM. Successful use of delayed reverse sural artery flap in single vessel legs with severe atherosclerotic disease and venous insufficiency. Plastic and Reconstructive Surgery. Global Open. 2023;**11**:E4740

[92] De Luna GD, Cárdenas Salomon CM, Barrera García G, et al. Bilateral fascia Lata flap: An alternative for massive Abdominal Wall defect repair. Plastic and Reconstructive Surgery. Global Open.

2020;**8**:e4740. Epub ahead of print 2020. DOI: 10.1097/GOX.0000000000002577

[93] Hartrampf CR, Scheflan M, Black PW. Breast reconstruction with a transverse abdominal island flap. Plastic and Reconstructive Surgery. 1982;**69**:216-224

[94] Blondeel PN, Boeckx WD. Refinements in free flap breast reconstruction: The free bilateral deep inferior epigastric perforator flap anastomosed to the internal mammary artery. British Journal of Plastic Surgery. 1994;**47**:495-501

[95] Rozen WM, Bhullar HK, Hunter-Smith D. How to assess a CTA of the abdomen to plan an autologous breast reconstruction. Gland Surgery. 2019;**8**:S291-S296

[96] Beugels J, Levine JL, Vasile JV, et al. The delay procedure in deep inferior epigastric artery perforator flap breast reconstruction. Plastic and Reconstructive Surgery. 2023. Available from: https://pubmed.ncbi.nlm.nih.gov/37335555/# [Accessed: July 28, 2023]

[97] Li RW, Deng Y, Pham HN, et al. Riluzole protects against skeletal muscle ischaemia-reperfusion injury in a porcine model. Injury-International Journal of The Care of The Injured. 2020;**51**:178-184

[98] Yokoyama H, Tsujii M, Iino T, et al. Inhibitory effect of edaravone on systemic inflammation and local damage in skeletal muscles following long-term ischemia to murine hind limb. Journal of Orthopaedic Surgery (Hong Kong). 2019;**27**. Epub ahead of print 1 September 2019. DOI: 10.1177/2309499019874470

[99] Kyriakides C, Wang Y, Austen WG, et al. Moderation of skeletal muscle reperfusion injury by a sLe(x)-glycosylated complement inhibitory protein. American Journal of Physiology. Cell Physiology. 2001;**281**:C224-C230. Epub ahead of print 2001. DOI: 10.1152/AJPCELL.2001.281.1.C224

[100] Kearns SR, Daly AF, Sheehan K, et al. Oral vitamin C reduces the injury to skeletal muscle caused by compartment syndrome. Journal of Bone and Joint Surgery. British Volume (London). 2004;**86**:906-911

[101] Zachary I. Vascular endothelial growth factor. The International Journal of Biochemistry & Cell Biology. 1998;**30**:1169-1174

[102] Neumeister MW, Song YH, Mowlavi A, et al. Effects of liposome-mediated gene transfer of VEGF in ischemic rat gracilis muscle. Microsurgery. 2001;**21**:58-62

[103] Planat-Benard V, Silvestre JS, Cousin B, et al. Plasticity of human adipose lineage cells toward endothelial cells. Circulation. 2004;**109**:656-663

[104] Rafii S, Lyden D. Therapeutic stem and progenitor cell transplantation for organ vascularization and regeneration. Nature Medicine. 2003;**9**:702-712

[105] Uysal AC, Mizuno H, Tobita M, et al. The effect of adipose-derived stem cells on ischemia-reperfusion injury: Immunohistochemical and ultrastructural evaluation. Plastic and Reconstructive Surgery. 2009;**124**:804-815

[106] Meliga E, Strem BM, Duckers HJ, et al. Adipose-derived cells. Cell Transplantation. 2007;**16**:963-970. DOI: 103727/096368907783338190

[107] AndersonCD,Heydarkhan-HagvallS, Schenke-Layland K, et al. The role of cytoprotective cytokines in cardiac ischemia/reperfusion injury. The Journal of Surgical Research. 2008;**148**:164-171

[108] Reichenberger MA, Heimer S, Schaefer A, et al. Adipose derived stem cells protect skin flaps against ischemia-reperfusion injury. Stem Cell Reviews and Reports. 2012;**8**:854-862

[109] Ashrafpour H, Huang N, Neligan PC, et al. Vasodilator effect and mechanism of action of vascular endothelial growth factor in skin vasculature. American Journal of Physiology. Heart and Circulatory Physiology. 2004;**286**:946-954

[110] Ichioka S, Kudo S, Shibata M, et al. Bone marrow cell implantation improves flap viability after ischemia-reperfusion injury. Annals of Plastic Surgery. 2004;**52**:414-418

[111] Tobita M, Uysal AC, Ogawa R, et al. Periodontal tissue regeneration with adipose-derived stem cells. Tissue Engineering Part A. 2008;**14**:945-953. Available from: https://home.liebertpub.com/tea

[112] Chang SY, Huang JJ, Tsao CK, et al. Does ischemia time affect the outcome of free fibula flaps for head and neck reconstruction? A review of 116 cases. Plastic and Reconstructive Surgery. 2010;**126**:1988-1995

[113] Marre D, Hontanilla B. Increments in ischaemia time induces microvascular complications in the DIEP flap for breast reconstruction. Journal of Plastic, Reconstructive & Aesthetic Surgery. 2013;**66**:80-86

[114] Lee KT, Lee JE, Nam SJ, et al. Ischaemic time and fat necrosis in breast reconstruction with a free deep inferior epigastric perforator flap. Journal of Plastic, Reconstructive & Aesthetic Surgery. 2013;**66**:174-181

[115] Woo SH. Practical tips to improve efficiency and success in upper limb replantation. Plastic and Reconstructive Surgery. 2019;**144**:878E-911E

[116] Maricevich M, Carlsen B, Mardini S, et al. Upper extremity and digital replantation. Hand (N Y). 2011;**6**:356-363

[117] Wei FC, Chang YL, Chen HC, et al. Three successful digital replantations in a patient after 84, 86, and 94 hours of cold ischemia time. Plastic and Reconstructive Surgery. 1988;**82**:346-350

[118] Ince B, Dadaci M, Altuntas Z. Use of a temporary shunt as a salvage technique for distal extremity amputations requiring repair by vessel grafting during critical ischemia. Archives of Plastic Surgery. 2016;**43**:544

[119] Tantry TP, Shetty P, Shetty R, et al. The anesthetic considerations while performing supraclavicular brachial plexus block in emergency surgical patients using a nerve stimulator. Anesthesia, Essays and Researches. 2015;**9**:276

[120] Jing L, Yao L, Zhao M, et al. Organ preservation: From the past to the future. Acta Pharmacologica Sinica. 2018;**39**(5):845-857

[121] Jones JW, Gruber SA, Barker JH, et al. Successful hand transplantation. One-year follow-up. Louisville hand transplant team. The New England Journal of Medicine. 2000;**343**:468-473

[122] Pei G, Xiang D, Gu L, et al. A report of 15 hand allotransplantations in 12 patients and their outcomes in China. Transplantation. 2012;**94**:1052-1059

[123] Barret JP, Serracanta J, Collado JM, et al. Full face transplantation organization, development, and results—The Barcelona experience: A case report. Transplantation Proceedings. 2011;**43**:3533-3534

[124] Guo S, Han Y, Zhang X, et al. Human facial allotransplantation: A 2-year follow-up study. Lancet. 2008;**372**:631-638

[125] Devauchelle B, Badet L, Lengelé B, et al. First human face allograft: Early report. Lancet. 2006;**368**:203-209

[126] Rostami S, Xu M, Datta S, et al. Evaluation of early markers of ischemia-reperfusion injury and preservation solutions in a modified Hindlimb model of vascularized composite Allotransplantation. Transplantation direct. 2021;**8**:e1251. Epub ahead of print 13 December 2021. DOI: 10.1097/TXD.0000000000001251

[127] Pegg DE. Principles of cryopreservation. Methods in Molecular Biology. 2015;**1257**:3-19

[128] Rinker B, Cui XD, Cibull ML, et al. Cryopreservation of composite tissue transplants. Hand (N Y). 2008;**3**:17-23

[129] Arav A, Friedman O, Natan Y, et al. Rat Hindlimb cryopreservation and transplantation: A step toward "organ banking". American Journal of Transplantation. 2017;**17**:2820-2828

[130] Finger EB, Bischof JC. Cryopreservation by vitrification: A promising approach for transplant organ banking. Current Opinion in Organ Transplantation. 2018;**23**:353-360

[131] Delorme TL, Shaw RS, Austen WG. Musculo-skeletal functions in the amputated perfused human being limb. Surgical Forum. 1964;**15**:450-452

[132] Constantinescu MA, Knall E, Xu X, et al. Preservation of amputated extremities by extracorporeal blood perfusion; a feasibility study in a porcine model. The Journal of Surgical Research. 2011;**171**:291-299

[133] Ozer K, Rojas-Pena A, Mendias CL, et al. Ex situ limb perfusion system to extend vascularized composite tissue allograft survival in swine. Transplantation. 2015;**99**:2095-2101

[134] Werner NL, Alghanem F, Rakestraw SL, et al. Ex situ perfusion of human limb allografts for 24 hours. Transplantation. 2017;**101**:e68-e74

[135] Gok E, Alghanem F, Moon R, et al. Development of an ex-situ limb perfusion system for a rodent model. ASAIO Journal. 2019;**65**:167-172

[136] Krezdorn N, Macleod F, Tasigiorgos S, et al. Twenty-four-hour ex vivo perfusion with acellular solution enables successful replantation of porcine forelimbs. Plastic and Reconstructive Surgery. 2019;**144**:608e-618e

[137] Burlage LC, Lellouch AG, Taveau CB, et al. Optimization of ex vivo machine perfusion and transplantation of vascularized composite allografts. Journal of Surgical Research. 2022;**270**:151-161

[138] Zhao ZQ, Corvera JS, Halkos ME, et al. Inhibition of myocardial injury by ischemic postconditioning during reperfusion: Comparison with ischemic preconditioning. American Journal of Physiology. Heart and Circulatory Physiology. 2003;**285**:H579-H588. Epub ahead of print 1 August 2003. DOI: 10.1152/AJPHEART.01064.2002

[139] Park JW, Kang JW, Jeon WJ, et al. Postconditioning protects skeletal muscle from ischemia-reperfusion injury. Microsurgery. 2010;**30**:223-229

[140] McAllister SE, Ashrafpour H, Cahoon N, et al. Postconditioning for salvage of ischemic skeletal muscle from reperfusion injury: Efficacy and mechanism. American Journal of Physiology. Regulatory, Integrative and Comparative Physiology. 2008. Epub ahead

of print August 2008;**295**:R681-R689. DOI: 10.1152/AJPREGU.90303.2008

[141] Lovetinska V, Sukop A, Klein L, et al. Free-flap monitoring: Review and clinical approach. Acta Chirurgiae Plasticae. 2020;**61**(1-4):16-23

[142] Roehl KR, Mahabir RC. A practical guide to free tissue transfer. Plastic and Reconstructive Surgery. 2013;**132**:147e-158e. Epub ahead of print July 2013. DOI: 10.1097/PRS.0B013E3182910FBA

[143] Sultan DL, Atamian E, Tarr J, et al. A prospective cohort study Re-examining tissue oximetry monitoring in microsurgical breast reconstruction. Annals of Plastic Surgery. 2023;**90**:580-584

[144] Malik MS, Akoh JA, Houlberg K. The use of the implantable Doppler probe as a blood flow monitoring device in clinical settings: A narrative review of the evidence. Experimental and Clinical Transplantation. 2023;**21**:83-92

[145] Chiu YH, Chang DH, Perng CK. Vascular complications and free flap salvage in head and neck reconstructive surgery: Analysis of 150 cases of Reexploration. Annals of Plastic Surgery. 2017;**78**:S83-S88

[146] Boissiere F, Gandolfi S, Riot S, et al. Flap venous congestion and salvage techniques: A systematic literature review. Plastic and Reconstructive Surgery. Global Open. 2021;**9**:e3327

[147] Shen AY, Lonie S, Lim K, et al. Free flap monitoring, salvage, and failure timing: A systematic review. Journal of Reconstructive Microsurgery. 2021;**37**:300-308

[148] Odorico SK, Reuter Muñoz K, J. Nicksic P, et al. Surgical and demographic predictors of free flap salvage after takeback: A systematic review. Microsurgery. 2023;**43**:78-88

[149] Lee KT, Mun GH. The efficacy of postoperative antithrombotics in free flap surgery: A systematic review and meta-analysis. Plastic and Reconstructive Surgery. 2015;**135**:1124-1139

[150] Dawoud BES, Kent S, Tabbenor O, et al. Does anticoagulation improve outcomes of microvascular free flap reconstruction following head and neck surgery: A systematic review and meta-analysis. The British Journal of Oral & Maxillofacial Surgery. 2022;**60**:1292-1302

[151] Murphy AD, McCormack MC, Bichara DA, et al. Poloxamer 188 protects against ischemia-reperfusion injury in a murine hind-limb model. Plastic and Reconstructive Surgery. 2010;**125**:1651-1660

[152] Orfany A, Arriola CG, Doulamis IP, et al. Mitochondrial transplantation ameliorates acute limb ischemia. Journal of Vascular Surgery. 2020;**71**:1014-1026

[153] Ward BJ, Scoote M. Antioxidants attenuate Postischemic endothelial cell swelling and luminal membrane Blebbing in cardiac capillaries. Microvascular Research. 1997;**53**:179-186

[154] Tiefenbacher CP, Chilian WM, Mitchell M, et al. Restoration of endothelium-dependent vasodilation after reperfusion injury by tetrahydrobiopterin. Circulation. 1996;**94**:1423-1429

[155] Haapaniemi T, Nylander G, Sirsjö A, et al. Hyperbaric oxygen reduces ischemia-induced skeletal muscle injury. Plastic and Reconstructive Surgery. 1996;**97**:602-607

[156] Nakagami H, Maeda K, Morishita R, et al. Novel autologous cell therapy in ischemic limb disease through growth factor secretion by cultured adipose tissue–derived stromal cells. Arteriosclerosis, Thrombosis, and Vascular Biology. 2005;**25**:2542-2547

Chapter 8

Advancement in Reperfusion Injury Awareness and Mitigation

Vashisth Bhavsar, Ashish Patel, Shantilal Padhiyar, Tejas B. Patel and Vipul Prajapati

Abstract

Understanding reperfusion damage, raising knowledge of its underlying processes, and creating measures to lessen its negative consequences have all seen significant progress over time. The developing knowledge of the pathophysiological processes, such as oxidative stress, inflammation, calcium excess, and mitochondrial dysfunction, that lead to reperfusion damage. Clinicians may now identify biomarkers and use modern imaging techniques to identify reperfusion damage in its early phases, allowing for prompt treatment and better patient outcomes. Real-time evaluation of tissue viability during reperfusion is now possible thanks to the development of non-invasive monitoring techniques, which supports clinical judgment. The use of pharmaceutical substances that target certain pathways, such as antioxidants, anti-inflammatory substances, and calcium homeostasis regulators. Additionally, cutting-edge approaches like therapeutic hypothermia and remote ischemia conditioning have demonstrated promise in lowering reperfusion damage and enhancing patient prognosis. Our knowledge of the underlying processes has considerably increased thanks to improvements in reperfusion injury recognition and mitigation, which have also created new opportunities for therapeutic intervention. These developments are anticipated to result in more efficient methods for reducing reperfusion damage and eventually enhance patient outcomes in a variety of therapeutic situations via continuing study and cooperation.

Keywords: awareness, mitigation, reperfusion, injury, oxidative, inflammatory

1. Introduction

When blood flow is restored to tissues or organs after a time of insufficient blood supply, damage to the afflicted region results. This process is known as ischemia-reperfusion injury (IRI). This phenomena may have important effects on a number of medical disorders, such as trauma, organ transplantation, stroke, and heart attack. In order to reduce tissue damage and enhance patient outcomes, it is essential to understand the processes driving IRI.

Ischemia means reduced blood flow to a tissue or organ, causing a lack of essential nutrients and oxygen needed for normal operation. Several factors like blocked blood vessels, narrowed arteries, or decreased heart output can lead to this reduced blood flow. Ischemia can have severe effects as tissues need a constant supply of oxygen and nutrients for their proper functioning [1].

Reperfusion is the process of restoring blood flow to ischemic tissue when a deficiency in blood supply has occurred. Reperfusion, however important to stop irreversible tissue damage, paradoxically can also cause more harm. A series of biochemical and cellular changes that take place after the blood flow is restored and the successive damage which will occur is, known as ischemia-reperfusion damage [2].

Adenosine triphosphate (ATP) is produced through the process of glycolysis when there is an oxygen shortage, which occurs during ischemia. This method is less effective. It leads to the elevation of metabolic waste products including lactate and reactive oxygen species (ROS). The quick rush of oxygen that occurs during reperfusion when blood flow is restored sets off a chain of events that exacerbates cellular damage [3].

The production of ROS, which includes superoxide anions, hydrogen peroxide, and hydroxyl radicals, is one of the main processes underpinning IRI. ROS are very reactive chemicals that harms lipids, proteins, and DNA as well as other biological components. Overwhelming antioxidant defense systems caused by excessive ROS generation result in oxidative stress and the start of inflammatory pathways [4].

After the rise of ROS it accompanies the increased inflammatory response is which is very critical. Tumor necrosis factor-alpha (TNF-alpha) and other pro-inflammatory cytokines are released after reperfusion, activating immune cells and drawing leukocytes to the site of damage. This inflammatory reaction is amplified by the immune cell invasion, leading to tissue dysfunction and damage [5].

Beyond this there is excessive release of excitatory amino acids like glutamate brought on by reperfusion damage. When too much glutamate binds to its receptors on neurons, such as NMDA receptors, AMPA receptors, and kainate receptors excitotoxicity happens. This results in an influx of calcium ions and eventual neuronal cell death. This mechanism is very important when it comes to stroke and brain damage [5].

Depending on the tissue or organ involved, ischemia-reperfusion damage may have different effects. IRI, for instance, can cause myocardial infarction, arrhythmias, and even myocardial stunning in the heart. IRI can lead to acute kidney injury and renal dysfunction in the kidneys. Similar to this, IRI can reduce liver graft function and raise the possibility of organ rejection.

The development of prospective treatment strategies has been made possible by our growing understanding of IRI's underlying processes. In experimental investigations, methods for lowering oxidative stress, controlling the inflammatory response, and avoiding excitotoxicity have showed promise. Aside from that, protective benefits have been shown for strategies such ischemic preconditioning, which applies small bouts of ischemia prior to the protracted ischemic insult [6].

IRI takes place when blood flow is restored to ischemic tissues or organs, a complicated pathological. It involves a series of actions that lead to tissue damage, such as oxidative stress, inflammation, and excitotoxicity. To improve patient outcomes for different medical conditions, we might find the answer in understanding the hidden processes and developing specific treatments that can reduce the negative effects of IRI.

2. Advanced pathological causes of ischemia reperfusion injury

When blood flow is restored to previously ischemic (lack of blood supply) tissue, harm known as ischemia-reperfusion occurs. It may have an impact on the heart, brain, liver, and kidneys, among other bodily organs. Ischemia-reperfusion damage has complicated underlying mechanisms that include several pathogenic processes. Advanced pathogenic causes of ischemia-reperfusion damage include the following:

1. Oxidative stress: The abrupt return of oxygen during reperfusion of ischemic tissue results in the production of reactive oxygen species (ROS). Cell injury and death can result from ROS-induced oxidative damage to cellular components such lipids, proteins, and DNA [7].

2. Inflammation: Ischemia-reperfusion causes an inflammatory reaction that is characterized by the discharge of pro-inflammatory chemicals, the attraction of immune cells, and the activation of several signaling pathways. Excessive inflammation can increase the damage brought on by ischemia-reperfusion and lead to tissue injury [8].

3. Ischemia disturbs the normal calcium equilibrium in cells, resulting in calcium excess. When blood flow is resumed, there is a sudden inflow of calcium, which causes an excess of intracellular calcium. The degradation of cellular membranes and proteins by enzymes such phospholipases and proteases, which are activated by high calcium levels, can lead to cell death [9].

4. Mitochondrial impairment: Mitochondrial function may be impaired by ischemia-reperfusion damage. The absence of oxygen causes diminished ATP synthesis and a buildup of metabolic waste products during ischemia. The abrupt return of oxygen once blood flow has been restored might cause mitochondrial enlargement, reduced ATP synthesis, and increased ROS production, aggravating cellular damage [10].

5. Endoplasmic reticulum stress: Ischemia-reperfusion may impair ER function, resulting in the buildup of unfolded or improperly folded proteins within the ER

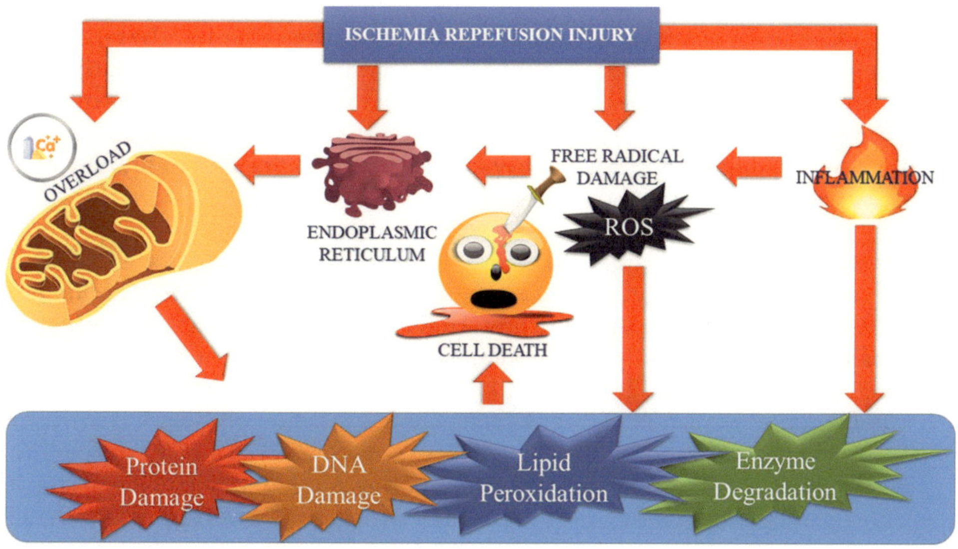

Figure 1.
Reperfusion.

lumen. This results in ER stress and the unfolded protein response (UPR), which can cause tissue damage and cell death [11].

6. Autophagy dysregulation: Autophagy is a cellular mechanism that breaks down and recycles damaged proteins and organelles. The normal control of autophagy can be upset by ischemia-reperfusion, which can result in either excessive autophagy (autophagic cell death) or deficient autophagy (accumulation of damaged cellular components), both of which can cause tissue damage [12].

These are a few of the more complex pathological causes of harm from ischemia and reperfusion. It's crucial to keep in mind that these processes are linked and may interact, enhancing the total harm done to the afflicted tissue. In order to reduce the effects of ischemia-reperfusion damage, treatment techniques can be developed with the aid of an understanding of these processes (**Figure 1**).

3. Therapeutic advancement and mitigation in treatment of ischemia reperfusion injury

Medical research is currently investigating improvements in therapy techniques and mitigation strategies for IRI. The following are some areas of concentration and prospective treatments that have made progress:

3.1 Mitochondrial-targeted therapies

Mitochondria play a critical role in IRI. Recent studies have focused on developing therapies that specifically target and protect mitochondria during reperfusion. To alleviate mitochondrial malfunction and lessen tissue damage, these strategies include antioxidants, peptides, and medications that specifically target the mitochondria [13]. The so-called "powerhouses of cells," mitochondria, are essential for sustaining cellular energy metabolism and controlling cell death pathways. The lack of oxygen and nutrients during ischemia causes mitochondrial malfunction and the buildup of reactive oxygen species (ROS), both of which eventually result in cell death [14]. Reperfusion causes an increase in ROS due to the abrupt restoration of oxygen, aggravating the damage. Mitochondrial-targeted medicines seek to reduce IRI by targeting oxidative stress and mitochondrial malfunction directly. In this field, a number of strategies have been investigated:

1. Mitochondrial antioxidants: To remove ROS and lessen oxidative stress, these substances directly target the mitochondria. Examples include SS-31, MitoQ, and MitoTEMPO. These antioxidants are able to reduce cell death pathways and enhance tissue repair by lowering mitochondrial oxidative damage.

2. Mitochondrial pore modulators: A crucial process that results in cell death is the opening of the mitochondrial permeability transition pore (mPTP) during IRI. Medications like sanglifehrin A and cyclosporine A target the mPTP and stop it from opening, maintaining mitochondrial function and lowering cell death [15].

3. Mitochondrial biogenesis inducers: Improving mitochondrial biogenesis, the process of creating new mitochondria, has demonstrated potential as a defense

against IRI. A number of substances, including resveratrol, PGC-1 activators, and exercise mimics, stimulate mitochondrial biogenesis and enhance cellular energetics, improving tissue lifespan [16].

4. Stabilizers of the mitochondrial membrane: The mitochondrial membrane's integrity is essential for preserving mitochondrial activity. The mitochondrial membrane is stabilized by substances like TRO40303 and elamipretide, preventing IRI from rupturing it and sustaining mitochondrial activity.In preclinical and early clinical investigations, these mitochondrial-targeted treatments have showed promise, highlighting their potential to lower IRI and improve patient outcomes [17]. To improve treatment plans, identify the most efficient therapeutic agents and doses, and evaluate long-term safety, further study is still required. Therapies that target the mitochondria provide a precise and cutting-edge way to reduce ischemia-reperfusion harm. These treatments have the potential to considerably enhance patient outcomes in a variety of medical illnesses where IRI plays a key role by particularly treating mitochondrial malfunction and oxidative stress. To fully grasp these interventions' therapeutic potential and turn them into successful patient treatments, more clinical trials and research are required [18].

3.2 Ischemic conditioning

Before the major ischemic event, tissues are subjected to small bouts of ischemia and reperfusion. This process is known as ischemic conditioning. Techniques for pre- and post-conditioning have showed promise in lowering IRI. The damaged organ is subjected to cycles of brief durations of ischemia and reperfusion using these techniques, which activates adaptive mechanisms and provides protection from further IRI.

1. Preconditioning is the process of introducing a protective state into a tissue or organ before an ischemia event takes place. This tactic entails exposing the tissue to numerous pharmacological stimuli or substances for brief intervals of sublethal ischemia [19]. Preconditioning aims to activate endogenous protective pathways and defensive systems that offer protection from ensuing protracted ischemia. Preconditioning is caused by a number of intricate processes, including signaling pathways involving adenosine, nitric oxide, protein kinases, and reactive oxygen species. These pathways set off a series of actions that eventually promote tissue healing after reperfusion, boost cellular survival, and reduce inflammation. Preconditioning has been investigated in different organs, including the heart, brain, liver, and kidneys, and has shown promising results in reducing IRI and improving functional outcomes [20].

2. On the other hand, postconditioning entails putting preventative measures in place right away once blood flow has been restored. This method seeks to interfere in the crucial early reperfusion phase, when damage processes are either begun or enhanced. A series of short cycles of ischemia and reperfusion or the injection of certain pharmacological substances are frequently used in postconditioning [21]. Interrupting harmful processes including oxidative stress, calcium excess, inflammation, and cell death pathways that are brought on by reperfusion is the aim. Postconditioning methods enable the reduction of tissue damage, maintenance of organ function, and improvement of damaged tissue healing [17].

3. Techniques for preconditioning and postconditioning both have the potential to lessen ischemia reperfusion damage and enhance patient outcomes. These methods have been thoroughly investigated in preclinical models and have proved effective in testing. The intricacy of the underlying systems, the need for more clinical studies, and other variables have made it difficult to translate these ideas into clinical practice. Nevertheless, current research continues to develop and examine these methods in an effort to create efficient therapies that can prevent ischemia reperfusion harm to organs and tissues and enhance patient outcomes in a variety of clinical contexts [22].

4. Certain receptors, including those for A3 adenosine, δ opioids, α_1 norepinephrine, β_2 bradykinin, UCN, and APN-BPN, up-regulate the mitochondrial permeability transition pore (mPTP) during the preconditioning phase. This causes an excess production of porins, which damages DNA and reduces the production of crucial proteins. In the preconditioning phase, prosurvival kinases like Akt and Erk1/2 are activated, which reduces the damage sustained after IRI damage [23] (**Figure 2**).

Techniques for pre- and post-conditioning are crucial tactics in the study of ischemia reperfusion damage. These methods have a great deal of promise for minimizing tissue injury, promoting tissue repair, and boosting patient outcomes in a variety of therapeutic settings. These methods will be improved by additional research and developments in our knowledge of the underlying systems, which will also open the door for their application in clinical settings [4, 11].

3.3 Pharmacological interventions

The ability of several pharmacological treatments to lower IRI has been researched. Adenosine receptor agonists, bradykinin receptor agonists, nitric oxide

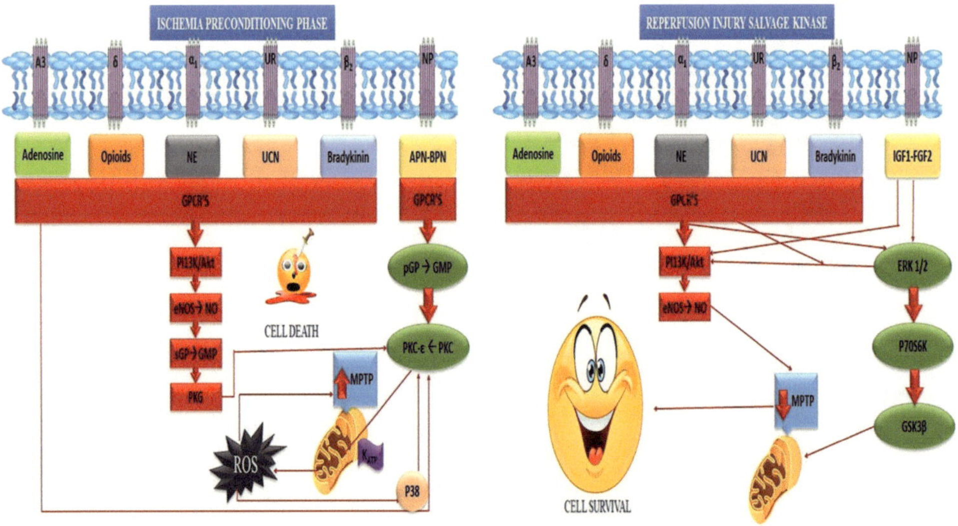

Figure 2.
Advantages preconditioning and postconditioning.

donors, and anti-inflammatory medications are a few examples. These medications work by minimizing oxidative stress, decreasing inflammation, and enhancing blood flow, among other IRI-related processes.

1. Opponents of the adenosine receptor An endogenous nucleoside known as adenosine interacts with the body's A1, A2A, A2B, and A3 receptors. In several organs, including the heart, liver, and kidneys, adenosine receptor agonists have shown protective benefits against IRI [24]. These agonists work by decreasing inflammation, encouraging vasodilation, and preventing the production of mediators that cause inflammation. These substances can lessen tissue damage brought on by IRI by triggering adenosine receptors [25].

2. Bradykinin, a peptide that regulates pain and inflammation, has antagonists for its receptor [26]. Vasodilation, enhanced vascular permeability, and the release of anti-inflammatory chemicals have all been linked to bradykinin receptor activation. In the context of cardiovascular disorders, bradykinin receptor agonists have been studied for their ability to mitigate IRI-induced damage. These agonists can aid in the defense against IRI by encouraging vasodilation and decreasing inflammation [16].

3. Donors of Nitric Oxide: Nitric oxide (NO) is a signaling molecule that plays a role in a number of physiological processes, such as vasodilation, anti-inflammation, and the inhibition of platelet aggregation [27]. NO has been demonstrated to have protective benefits in the setting of IRI by increasing blood flow, lowering oxidative stress, and preventing leukocyte activation. Compounds that release nitric oxide (NO) gradually are known as nitric oxide donors. It has been investigated if certain donors, such as organic nitrates and nitrovasodilators, can reduce IRI by increasing NO bioavailability and exerting vasoprotective and anti-inflammatory effects [28].

4. Anti-inflammatory medications: IRI is characterized by inflammation, and treating this inflammatory response has been the main goal of treatment approaches [29]. Anti-inflammatory medications have been researched for their ability to lessen IRI, including corticosteroids, nonsteroidal anti-inflammatory drugs (NSAIDs), and immunomodulatory therapies. These medications can reduce immune cell activation, limit the synthesis of inflammatory mediators, and lessen the tissue damage brought on by IRI. Anti-inflammatory medications have the potential to improve IRI in multiple organs by modifying the inflammatory response [30].

Anti-inflammatory medications, nitric oxide donors, adenosine receptor agonists, and bradykinin receptor agonists have shown promise in preventing ischemia-reperfusion damage. These pharmacological medicines can aid in preventing tissues and organs from suffering injury as a result of ischemia and subsequent reperfusion by specifically targeting IRI-related pathways such inflammation, vasoconstriction, and oxidative stress. To investigate their efficacy, ideal dosage, and potential adverse effects in various therapeutic circumstances, more investigation and clinical trials are required.

3.4 Stem cell therapy

Therapies based on stem cells have demonstrated promise in reducing IRI. In particular, the capacity of mesenchymal stem cells (MSCs) to control inflammation, encourage tissue repair, and improve angiogenesis has received substantial research. In preclinical research and early clinical trials for IRI in multiple organs, MSCs have shown encouraging outcomes.

1. Modulation of Inflammation: MSCs' immunomodulatory abilities allow them to control the immune system and lessen inflammation. They can influence the activity and performance of immune cells such T cells, B cells, natural killer (NK) cells, and macrophages [31, 32].

2. MSCs can develop into a variety of cell types, including osteoblasts, chondrocytes, adipocytes, and myocytes, therefore promoting tissue repair. They also release a variety of bioactive chemicals, including growth factors, cytokines, chemokines, and extracellular vesicles, that aid in tissue healing [33, 34].

3. Angiogenesis is boosted: MSCs have pro-angiogenic qualities and can encourage the growth of new blood vessels. They release angiogenic substances such fibroblast growth factor (FGF), hepatocyte growth factor (HGF), and vascular endothelial growth factor (VEGF), which promote endothelial cell migration, proliferation, and the development of capillary-like structures [35, 36].

4. MSCs have extraordinary capacities to control inflammation, encourage tissue healing, and boost angiogenesis. Due to these qualities, they are promising therapeutic agents in regenerative medicine and have a huge potential for the treatment of a wide range of ailments, wounds, and tissue damage.

3.5 Remote ischemic conditioning (RIC)

In RIC, a remote organ or tissue is subjected to brief episodes of ischemia and reperfusion, which causes the target organ to activate defense systems. IRI has been successfully decreased by RIC in a variety of organs, including the heart, kidney, and liver. It is a non-invasive method that can be economical and have several uses in clinical practice [37]. In RIC, a blood pressure cuff is repeatedly inflated and deflated on a limb, causing momentary episodes of ischemia and reperfusion. The temporary ischemia episodes trigger a protective response in distant organs, improving tolerance for ischemic assaults in the future. The possibility of RIC to lessen tissue damage during cardiac surgery, heart attacks, strokes, organ transplantation, and other ischemia-related disorders has been studied. Pharmacological RIC: In order to duplicate the preventive benefits of RIC without requiring physical treatments, researchers are investigating the use of pharmacological medicines [38]. For instance, the capacity of medications like adenosine, erythropoietin, and distant ischemic preconditioning (RIPerC) mimetic compounds to pharmacologically produce RIC-like effects has been studied.

1. Remote ischemia Preconditioning (RIPC) is a technique for preventing further ischemia damage by administering RIC before the ischemic stimulus. To improve RIPC protocols, novel strategies have been devised, such as figuring out the appropriate conditioning time, cycles, and length.Researchers are examining the

synergistic benefits of integrating remote ischemic conditioning (RIC) with different treatment modalities. Examples include combining RIC with stem cell therapy, therapeutic hypothermia, and medication therapies in an effort to increase the overall protective benefits [39].

2. The value of RIC Cardiovascular Health: RIC has demonstrated potential in lowering the extent of myocardial infarctions, enhancing heart function, and minimizing negative outcomes in patients having cardiac surgeries. Patients with heart failure, coronary artery disease, and other cardiovascular disorders could possibly benefit from it. Neuroprotection: In stroke patients, RIC has shown potential neuroprotective benefits that may lessen ischemic brain damage and enhance neurological outcomes [40]. The best RIC protocols for various stroke subtypes are still being investigated, as is the use of RIC in neurodegenerative illnesses. Renal Protection: RIC has been investigated for its capacity to safeguard the kidneys from ischemia harm after heart surgery and kidney transplantation. The ability to lessen acute kidney damage and enhance renal function has been demonstrated. Other Potential Applications: RIC is being investigated in a number of other domains, including limb ischemia, sepsis, spinal cord damage, and liver transplantation, among others [36, 41, 42].

4. Limitations and challenges in the treatment of ischemia reperfusion injury

Although ischemia–reperfusion damage therapies have come a long way, there are still certain restrictions and difficulties. A few of these are:

1. Duration sensitivity: Treatments for ischemia-reperfusion damage must be effective quickly. The damage after reperfusion will be more severe the longer the ischemia phase lasts. Rapid response is essential, however in some circumstances, it might not be possible because of delays in identifying the issue or getting medical help [21].

2. There is a limited therapeutic window for effectively treating ischemia-reperfusion damage [43]. In order to avoid excessive damage without running the danger of negative side effects, therapies must be given at the proper time. This might be difficult, especially in urgent situations or uncertain clinical settings.

3. The absence of particular remedies despite the fact that there are broad steps to reduce ischemia-reperfusion harm is still a problem. It is still difficult to create treatments or medications that prevent reperfusion damage without sacrificing the positive outcomes of reperfusion [44].

4. Patients may be more vulnerable to ischemia-reperfusion damage if they have pre-existing medical problems like diabetes or cardiovascular disease [45]. The intricacy of the healing process is increased by managing these underlying issues at the same time as treating the injury.

5. Additional considerations include patient variability, which makes it difficult to develop therapies that work for everyone and forces the use of individualized

strategies for better results. IRI severity can vary greatly across persons and various organs [46]. IRI is a multi-factorial, intricate process that uses a number of different paths and processes. Trying to address each of these issues at once is challenging. Therapies that focus on particular components of the injury might not be enough to produce the best results [47].

5. Conclusions and future prospective

The management and treatment of many medical diseases have significantly improved as a result of the development in reperfusion injury knowledge and mitigation. Reperfusion damage can have negative consequences and impair patient outcomes because it happens when blood flow is restored to tissues after an interval of ischemia. Healthcare professionals have made outstanding strides in reducing reperfusion damage and enhancing patient outcomes, nevertheless, because to considerable research, cutting-edge technologies, and improved treatment approaches.

The greater comprehension of its underlying processes is one of the most important developments in the knowledge of reperfusion damage. Deeper understanding of the intricate molecular and cellular mechanisms that take place during reperfusion damage has been attained by scientists and researchers [48]. This information has made it possible to create tailored interventions and treatments.

Numerous methods have been investigated in terms of mitigating measures. Antioxidants, anti-inflammatory drugs, and adenosine receptor agonists are a few examples of pharmacological therapies that have demonstrated promising outcomes in lowering reperfusion injury and limiting tissue damage [49]. Reperfusion harm has also been lessened as a result of improvements in medical technology, such as better imaging methods, fresh surgical techniques, and inventive medication delivery systems.

Additionally, better detection and prompt response have resulted from healthcare professionals' greater understanding of reperfusion damage. When individuals at risk for reperfusion injury are identified early, preventative interventions can be done, which lessens the degree and amount of tissue damage [50]. The sharing of information and expertise has been enhanced by multidisciplinary cooperation between doctors, surgeons, pharmacologists, and researchers, resulting in more efficient treatment plans.

However, difficulties continue to persist despite these tremendous gains. Reperfusion damage is still a complicated phenomenon, and further investigation is required to completely understand it [51]. Additionally, meticulous assessment and validation are needed for the conversion of laboratory results into clinical practice. To evaluate the safety and effectiveness of novel medicines and interventions, clinical trials and long-term research are essential.

The improvement of patient outcomes has showed significant promise with awareness and mitigation. Healthcare personnel are now better able to prevent, identify, and treat reperfusion damage because to a mix of scientific advancements, technology advancements, and cooperative efforts [52]. Our capacity to lessen the destructive effects of reperfusion damage and raise the standard of patient care will be further enhanced by ongoing research and the incorporation of new information into clinical practice.

In order to better patient outcomes in the face of this disorder, researchers and physicians continue to focus on creating targeted medicines and understanding the underlying processes [21].

It is unclear why numerous cytoprotective treatments, although showing promise in animal models of acute myocardial IRI, have failed to improve clinical outcomes in IRI patients. As a result, novel mitochondrial targets both inside and outside the particular tissue under IRI need to be the focus of creative techniques in order to enhance the translation of cytoprotective medicines into the clinical context for the benefit of patients. Targeting cytoprotective therapy to the ischemic tissues using nanoparticles and mitochondria with chemical alteration (such as MitoQ and MitoSNO) may increase the effectiveness of tissue protection. Additionally, the identification of the MPTP as well as other mitochondrial channels such as mitochondrial calcium unipors and Na^{+}/Ca^{2+} exchanger may lead to the development of brand-new cytoprotective treatments. Finally, research is required to determine how aging and co-morbid conditions affect the effectiveness of cytoprotective treatments.

Acknowledgements

We extend our heartfelt appreciation to all the individuals who have made invaluable contributions to the completion of this book chapter. Their unwavering support, expertise, and dedication have greatly enhanced the quality and depth of our work. We would like to express our gratitude to:

First and foremost, we are immensely grateful to our esteemed co-authors, Dr. Vashisth P. Bhavsar and Mr. Shantilal P. Padhiyar. Their intellectual prowess, insightful perspectives, and tireless efforts have been instrumental in shaping this chapter into its final form. Their expertise and commitment to excellence have significantly enriched the content and overall coherence of our work.

We owe a profound debt of gratitude to our mentor and advisor, Dr. Tejas B. Patel and Dr. Ashish D. Patel for their exceptional guidance and wisdom throughout the writing process. Their invaluable feedback, critical insights, and unwavering support have been pivotal in steering our research in the right direction.

We would also like to extend our appreciation to Dr. Vipul Prajapati for their assistance in data collection, analysis, and research coordination. Their diligence, meticulousness, and dedication have contributed significantly to the depth and accuracy of our findings.

Our sincere thanks go to Faculty of Pharmacy. Dharmsinh Desai University for providing us with the necessary resources, facilities, and research support. Their continued investment in academic pursuits has enabled us to pursue this endeavor with passion and commitment.

We would like to acknowledge the contributions of our colleagues and friends who have offered their valuable insights and feedback during the various stages of this writing process. Their constructive criticism, stimulating discussions, and encouragement have been invaluable in refining our ideas and arguments.

Furthermore, we express our gratitude to the anonymous reviewers whose meticulous examination and thoughtful suggestions have greatly improved the overall quality of this chapter. Their expertise and attention to detail have undoubtedly elevated the significance and credibility of our work.

Last but not least, we extend our heartfelt appreciation to our families and loved ones for their unwavering support, patience, and understanding throughout this endeavor. Their love, encouragement, and sacrifices have provided us with the motivation and strength to pursue our academic goals.

We humbly acknowledge the contributions of all individuals involved, whether mentioned explicitly or not, as this collective effort has brought this chapter to fruition. Without their assistance, this work would not have been possible.

Conflict of interest

The authors declare no conflict of interest.

Notes/thanks/other declarations

I am truly grateful for the time and effort you invested in reviewing and providing feedback on the initial draft. Your constructive criticism and thoughtful comments have helped me refining my ideas and present them more effectively. I sincerely appreciate your willingness to share your expertise and collaboration with me on this project. Your contribution have been invaluable, and I am immensely grateful for the opportunity to work with you all.

Appendices and nomenclature

ATP	Adenosine Triphosphate
ROS	Reactive oxygen species
TNF-α	Tumor Necrosis Factor-alpha
ER	Endoplasmic Reticulum
MitoTEMPO	(2- (2,2,6,6-Tetramethylpiperidin-1-oxyl-4-ylamino)-2-oxoethyl) triphenylphosphonium chloride
mPTP	Mitochondrial Permeability Transition pore
PGC-1α	Peroxisome proliferator-activated receptor-γ coactivator 1α
NO	Nitric oxide
NSAIDs	Nonsteroidal Anti-Inflammatory Drugs
HGF	Hepatocyte Growth Factor
FGF	Fibroblast Growth Factor
VEGF	Vascular Endothelial Growth Factor
RIC	Remote Ischemic Conditioning
RIPerC	Remote Ischemic Preconditioning
MCU	Mitochondrial Calcium Unipors
NCX	Na^{+}/Ca^{2+} exchanger

DOI: http://dx.doi.org/10.5772/intechopen.112732

Author details

Vashisth Bhavsar[1*], Ashish Patel[2], Shantilal Padhiyar[3], Tejas B. Patel[4] and Vipul Prajapati[3]

1 Department of Pharmacology, Dharamsinh Desai University, Gujarat, India;

2 Department of Chemistry, Charusat University, Changa, Nadiad, Gujarat, India

3 Department of Pharmaceutical Chemistry, Dharamsinh Desai University, Gujarat, India

4 Department of Pharmaceutics, Dharamsinh Desai University, Gujarat, India

*Address all correspondence to: vashisthbhavsar@gmail.com

References

[1] Tsang A, Hausenloy DJ, Yellon DM. Myocardial Postconditioning: Reperfusion injury revisited. American Journal of Physiology-Heart and Circulatory Physiology. 2005;**289**(1):H2-H7. DOI: 10.1152/ajpheart.00091.2005

[2] Bolli R, Becker LB, Gross GJ, Mentzer RM, Balshaw DM, Lathrop DA. Myocardial protection at a crossroads. Circulation Research. 2004;**95**(2): 125-134. DOI: 10.1161/01.res.0000137171.97172.d7

[3] Eltzschig HK, Eckle T. Ischemia and reperfusion—From mechanism to translation. Nature Medicine. 2011;**17**(11):1391-1401. DOI: 10.1038/nm.2507

[4] Kalogeris T, Baines CP, Krenz M, Korthuis RJ. Cell biology of ischemia/reperfusion injury. International Review of Cell and Molecular Biology. 2012;**298**(298):229-317. DOI: 10.1016/b978-0-12-394309-5.00006-7

[5] Bhavsar V, Vaghasiya J, Suhagia BN, Thaker P. Protective effect of Eichhornia Crassipes against cerebral ischemia reperfusion injury in Normal and diabetic rats. Journal of Stroke and Cerebrovascular Diseases. 2020;**29**(12):105385. DOI: 10.1016/j.jstrokecerebrovasdis.2020.105385

[6] Tasoulis M, Douzinas EE. Hypoxemic reperfusion of ischemic states: An alternative approach for the attenuation of oxidative stress mediated reperfusion injury. Journal of Biomedical Science. 2016;**23**:7. DOI: 10.1186/s12929-016-0220-0

[7] Wei H, Frenkel K. Relationship of oxidative events and DNA oxidation in SENCAR mice to in vivo promoting activity of Phorbol Ester-type tumor promoters. Carcinogenesis. 1993;**14**(6):1195-1201. DOI: 10.1093/carcin/14.6.1195

[8] Chen L, Deng H, Cui H, Fang J, Zuo Z, Deng J, et al. Inflammatory responses and inflammation-associated diseases in organs. Oncotarget. 2017;**9**(6):7204-7218. DOI: 10.18632/oncotarget.23208

[9] Rajadurai M, Prince SM, P. Preventive effect of Naringin on isoproterenol-induced cardiotoxicity in Wistar rats: An in vivo and in vitro study. Toxicology. 2007;**232**(3):216-225. DOI: 10.1016/j.tox.2007.01.006

[10] Silva-Platas C, Villegas CA, Oropeza-Almazán Y, Carrancá M, Torres-Quintanilla A, Lozano O, et al. Ex vivo cardiotoxicity of antineoplastic casiopeinas is mediated through energetic dysfunction and triggered mitochondrial-dependent apoptosis. 2018;**2018**:1-13. DOI: 10.1155/2018/8949450

[11] Ruan Y, Zeng J, Jin Q, Chu M, Ji K, Wang Z, et al. Endoplasmic reticulum stress serves an important role in cardiac ischemia/reperfusion injury (review). Experimental and Therapeutic Medicine. 2020;**20**(6):1-1. DOI: 10.3892/etm.2020.9398

[12] Ryter SW, Cloonan SM, Choi AMK. Autophagy: A critical regulator of cellular metabolism and homeostasis. Molecules and Cells. 2013;**36**(1):7-16. DOI: 10.1007/s10059-013-0140-8

[13] Marin W, Marin D, Ao X, Liu Y. Mitochondria as a therapeutic target for cardiac ischemia-reperfusion injury (review). International Journal of Molecular Medicine. 2020;**47**(2):485-499. DOI: 10.3892/ijmm.2020.4823

[14] Checa J, Aran JM. Reactive oxygen species: Drivers of physiological and pathological processes. Journal of Inflammation Research. 2020;**13**: 1057-1073. DOI: 10.2147/JIR.S275595

[15] Bernardi P, Carraro M, Lippe G. The mitochondrial permeability transition: Recent progress and open questions. The FEBS Journal. Nov 2022;**289**(22):7051-7074. DOI: 10.1111/febs.16254

[16] Yang N, Guan Q-W, Chen F-H, Xia Q-X, Yin X-X, Zhou H-H, et al. Antioxidants targeting mitochondrial oxidative stress: Promising Neuroprotectants for epilepsy. Oxidative Medicine and Cellular Longevity. 2020;**2020**:1-14. DOI: 10.1155/2020/6687185

[17] Clemente-Suárez VJ, Martín-Rodríguez A, Yáñez-Sepúlveda R, Tornero-Aguilera JF. Mitochondrial transfer as a novel therapeutic approach in disease diagnosis and treatment. International Journal of Molecular Sciences. 2023;**24**(10):8848. DOI: 10.3390/ijms24108848

[18] Eirin A, Lerman A, Lerman LO. Enhancing mitochondrial health to treat hypertension. Current Hypertension Reports. 2018;**20**(10):89. DOI: 10.1007/s11906-018-0889-4

[19] Jang M-H, Kim D-H, Han J-H, Kim J, Kim J-H. A single bout of remote ischemic preconditioning suppresses ischemia-reperfusion injury in asian obese young men. International Journal of Environmental Research and Public Health. 2023;**20**(5):3915. DOI: 10.3390/ijerph20053915

[20] Stetler RA, Leak RK, Gan Y, Li P, Hu X, Jing Z, et al. Preconditioning provides neuroprotection in models of CNS disease: Paradigms and clinical significance. Progress in Neurobiology. 2014;**0**:58-83. DOI: 10.1016/j.pneurobio.2013.11.005

[21] Soares ROS, Losada DM, Jordani MC, Évora P, Castro-e-Silva O. Ischemia/reperfusion injury revisited: An overview of the latest pharmacological strategies. International Journal of Molecular Sciences. 2019;**20**(20):5034. DOI: 10.3390/ijms20205034

[22] Smith BR, Edelman ER. Nanomedicines for cardiovascular disease. Nature Cardiovascular Research. 2023;**2023**:1-17. DOI: 10.1038/s44161-023-00232-y

[23] Hausenloy DJ, Tsang A, Yellon DM. The reperfusion injury salvage kinase pathway: A common target for both ischemic preconditioning and postconditioning. Trends in Cardiovascular Medicine. 2005;**15**(2):69-75. DOI: 10.1016/j.tcm.2005.03.001

[24] Effendi WI, Nagano T, Kobayashi K, Nishimura Y. Focusing on adenosine receptors as a potential targeted therapy in human diseases. Cells. 24 Mar 2020;**9**(3):785. DOI: 10.3390/cells9030785

[25] Marceau F, Bachelard H, Bouthillier J, Fortin J-P, Morissette G, Bawolak M-T, et al. Bradykinin receptors: Agonists, antagonists, expression, Signaling, and adaptation to sustained stimulation. International Immunopharmacology. 2020;**82**:106305. DOI: 10.1016/j.intimp.2020.106305

[26] Rex DAB, Vaid N, Deepak K, Dagamajalu S, Prasad TSK. A comprehensive review on current understanding of bradykinin in COVID-19 and inflammatory diseases. Molecular Biology Reports. Oct 2022;**49**(10):9915-9927. DOI: 10.1007/s11033-022-07539-2

[27] Lundberg JO, Weitzberg E. Nitric oxide Signaling in health and disease. Cell. 2022;**185**(16):2853-2878. DOI: 10.1016/j.cell.2022.06.010

[28] Vaghasiya J, Sheth N, Bhalodia Y, Manek R. Sitagliptin protects renal ischemia reperfusion induced renal damage in diabetes. Regulatory Peptides. 2011;**166**(1-3):48-54. DOI: 10.1016/j.regpep.2010.08.007.

[29] Delbaere Q, Chapet N, Huet F, Delmas C, Mewton N, Prunier F, et al. Anti-Inflammatory drug candidates for prevention and treatment of cardiovascular diseases. Pharmaceuticals (Basel). 4 Jan 2023;**16**(1):78. DOI: 10.3390/ph16010078

[30] English K. Mechanisms of mesenchymal stromal cell immunomodulation. Immunology & Cell Biology. 2012;**91**(1):19-26. DOI: 10.1038/icb.2012.56

[31] Alcayaga-Miranda F, Cuenca J, Martin A, Contreras L, Figueroa FE, Khoury M. Combination therapy of menstrual derived mesenchymal stem cells and antibiotics ameliorates survival in Sepsis. Stem Cell Research & Therapy. 2015;**6**(1). DOI: 10.1186/s13287-015-0192-0

[32] Caplan AI. Mesenchymal stem cells: Time to change the name! Stem Cells Translational Medicine. 2017;**6**(6):1445-1451. DOI: 10.1002/sctm.17-0051

[33] Gnecchi M, Zhang Z, Ni A, Dzau VJ. Paracrine mechanisms in adult stem cell signaling and therapy. Circulation Research. 2008;**103**(11):1204-1219. DOI: 10.1161/circresaha.108.176826

[34] Kinnaird T, Stabile E, Burnett MS, Lee CW, Barr S, Fuchs S, et al. Marrow-derived stromal cells express genes encoding a broad spectrum of arteriogenic cytokines and promote in vitro and in vivo arteriogenesis through paracrine mechanisms. Circulation Research. 2004;**94**(5):678-685. DOI: 10.1161/01.res.0000118601.37875.ac

[35] Rafii S, Lyden D. Therapeutic stem and progenitor cell transplantation for organ vascularization and regeneration. Nature Medicine. 2003;**9**(6):702-712. DOI: 10.1038/nm0603-702

[36] Hausenloy DJ, Yellon DM. Remote ischaemic preconditioning: Underlying mechanisms and clinical application. Cardiovascular Research. 2008;**79**(3):377-386. DOI: 10.1093/cvr/cvn114

[37] Li D, Liu W, Wang G, Shi X. Impact of combined ischemic preconditioning and remote ischemic Perconditioning on ischemia-reperfusion injury after liver transplantation. Scientific Reports. 2018;**8**(1). DOI: 10.1038/s41598-018-36365-5

[38] Perrin C, Athersuch K, Elder G, Martin M, Alsalhani A. Recently developed drugs for the treatment of drug-resistant tuberculosis: A Research and Development case study. BMJ Global Health. 2022;7(4):e007490. DOI: 10.1136/bmjgh-2021-007490

[39] Rahman M, Islam M, Islam M, Harun-Or-Rashid M, Islam M, Abdullah S, et al. Stem cell transplantation therapy and neurological disorders: Current status and future perspectives. Biology. 2022;**11**(1):147. DOI: 10.3390/biology11010147

[40] Paul S, Candelario-Jalil E. Emerging neuroprotective strategies for the treatment of ischemic stroke: An overview of clinical and preclinical studies. Experimental Neurology. 2021;**335**:113518. DOI: 10.1016/j.expneurol.2020.113518

[41] Przyklenk K, Whittaker P. Remote ischemic preconditioning: Current knowledge, unresolved questions, and future priorities. Journal of Cardiovascular Pharmacology and Therapeutics. 2011;**16**(3-4):255-259. DOI: 10.1177/1074248411409040

[42] Heusch G, Rassaf T. Time to give up on cardioprotection? Circulation Research. 2016;**119**(5):676-695. DOI: 10.1161/circresaha.116.308736

[43] Trujillo-Rangel WÁ, García-Valdés L, Méndez-Del Villar M, Castañeda-Arellano R, Totsuka-Sutto SE, García-Benavides L. Therapeutic targets for regulating oxidative damage induced by ischemia-reperfusion injury: A study from a pharmacological perspective. Oxidative Medicine and Cellular Longevity. 11 Apr 2022;**2022**:8624318. DOI: 10.1155/2022/8624318

[44] Naito H, Nojima T, Fujisaki N, Tsukahara K, Yamamoto H, Yamada T, et al. Therapeutic strategies for ischemia reperfusion injury in emergency medicine. Acute Medicine & Surgery. 13 Apr 2020;**7**(1):e501. DOI: 10.1002/ams2.501

[45] Leon BM, Maddox TM. Diabetes and cardiovascular disease: Epidemiology, biological mechanisms, treatment recommendations and future research. World Journal of Diabetes. 2015;**6**(13):1246. DOI: 10.4239/wjd.v6.i13.1246

[46] Masior Ł, Grąt M. Methods of attenuating ischemia-reperfusion injury in liver transplantation for hepatocellular carcinoma. International Journal of Molecular Sciences. 30 Jul 2021;**22**(15): 8229. DOI: 10.3390/ijms22158229

[47] Li Y, Gao Y, Li G. Preclinical multi-target strategies for myocardial ischemia-reperfusion injury. Frontiers in Cardiovascular Medicine. 2022;**2022**:9. DOI: 10.3389/fcvm.2022.967115

[48] Schirone L, Forte M, D'Ambrosio L, Valenti V, Vecchio D, Schiavon S, et al. An overview of the molecular mechanisms associated with myocardial ischemic injury: State of the art and translational perspectives. Cell. 2022;**11**(7):1165. DOI: 10.3390/cells11071165

[49] Montecucco F, Nathoe H. How to manage the abundant COVID-19 submissions to a peer-reviewed Scientific Journal. European Journal of Clinical Investigation. Jun 2021;**51**(6):e13569. DOI: 10.1111/eci.13569

[50] Ibáñez B, Heusch G, Ovize M, Van de Werf F. Evolving therapies for myocardial ischemia/reperfusion injury. Journal of the American College of Cardiology. 2015;**65**(14):1454-1471. DOI: 10.1016/j.jacc.2015.02.032

[51] Granger DN, Kvietys PR. Reperfusion injury and reactive oxygen species: The evolution of a concept. Redox Biology. 2015;**6**:524-551. DOI: 10.1016/j.redox.2015.08.020

[52] Widimsky P, Snyder K, Sulzenko J, Hopkins LN, Stetkarova I. Acute ischaemic stroke: Recent advances in reperfusion treatment. European Heart Journal. 7 Apr 2023;**44**(14):1205-1215. DOI: 10.1093/eurheartj/ehac684

Section 4

Biomarkers and Molecular Mechanisms

Chapter 9

Perspective Chapter: Role of Caspase-3 as Neonatal Hypoxic Ischemic Encephalopathy Biomarker

Johnny Lambert Rompis and Natharina Yolanda

Abstract

Neonatal hypoxic-ischemic encephalopathy (HIE) is a severe form of neonatal brain damage caused by decreased cerebral blood flow and hypoxia and can cause various serious irreversible neurological sequelae. An early diagnosis of HIE is essential for subsequent treatment and prognosis. Caspase, a protease enzyme that has an essential role in the apoptosis of programmed cell death, is one of the promising biomarkers for diagnosing HIE. Caspase-3 is recognized for its activated proteolytic apoptosis role in cells responding to specific extrinsic or intrinsic inducers of this mode of cell death. Caspase-3 is activated within 1 to 3 hours after neonatal hypoxic-ischemia and is a principal executioner of apoptosis. The role of caspase-3 in apoptosis, pyroptosis, necroptosis, and autophagy might be more profound than its role in cell death. Such functions of caspase-3 require further exploration, however, as there are still many possibilities for its roles in clinical diagnosis and treatment.

Keywords: apoptosis, biomarker, caspase-3, hypoxic-ischemic encephalopathy, cell death

1. Introduction

Neonatal hypoxic-ischemic encephalopathy (HIE) is a severe form of neonatal brain damage caused by decreased cerebral blood flow and hypoxia, leading to asphyxia as a clinical sign. HIE is a diffuse disruption of brain function and structure; the development of hypoxic-ischemia can cause a variety of serious irreversible neurological sequelae, including epilepsy, delayed growth and development, cognitive impairment, intelligence disturbance, cerebral palsy, and even neonatal death. Hypoxic-ischemic insults may lead to necrosis or apoptosis of brain cells, depending on the severity of the insults and the cell's maturity [1].

Perinatal asphyxia occurs two times per 1000 live births in wealthy nations, although it can happen up to 10 times more frequently in underdeveloped nations. Up to 25% of afflicted newborns survive with lifelong neurologic abnormalities, and 15–20% of affected infants die during the neonatal period [2, 3]. An early diagnosis

IntechOpen

of HIE is essential for subsequent treatment and prognosis. There are several known biomarkers studied in relation to HIE, but their usefulness is limited (S100 protein, interleukin-6, and glial fibrillary acidic protein [GFAP]) [4] or does not correspond to prognosis (blood pH, serum lactate, aspartate aminotransferase [AST], alanine transaminase [ALT], prothrombin time [PT], activated thromboplastin time [APTT], creatinine, urea, troponin T, and fibrinogen) [5]. Caspase is one of the promising newer biomarkers for diagnosing HIE. A family of protease enzymes known as caspase plays a crucial part in apoptosis, or "programmed cell death." Caspase is short for cysteine-dependent aspartate-directed protease. There are 12 caspases in humans, and these are categorized into three subtypes based on their function: Initiator caspases (caspase 2, 8, 9, and 10) signal apoptosis; executioner caspase (caspase 3, 6, and 7) leads to apoptosis; and inflammatory caspases (caspase 1, 4, 5, 11, and 12) organize inflammatory cytokine signaling and pyroptosis [6].

Caspase-3 is one of the most important components in programmed cell death as it catalyzes the specific cleavage of many essential cellular proteins. By understanding the role and mechanism of caspase-3 in neonates with HIE, it might be possible to use caspase-3 as a biomarker to diagnose HIE and/or even prevent and treat HIE promptly.

2. Pathophysiology of hypoxic-ischemic encephalopathy

Intermediate anoxia or acute hypoxia in neonatal encephalopathy leads to decreased cerebral perfusion. A biphasic process of primary and secondary energy failure at the cellular level distinguishes systemic hypoxemia and cerebral hypoperfusion. The initial phase consists of triggering the hypoxic-ischemic interval that leads to primary energy failure (a reduction in high-energy phosphorylated metabolites and intracellular pH). This phase may be severe, resulting in permanent brain injury or subacute brain injury if the case is responsive to resuscitation [7].

The phases in hypoxic-ischemic encephalopathy consist of primary energy failure, latent phase, secondary energy failure, and tertiary phase. First, an immediate primary neuronal injury occurs due to the brain's interruption of oxygen and glucose. The associated decrease in adenosine triphosphate (ATP) production results in the failure of the ATP-dependent Na-K pump. Sodium enters cells followed by water causing cell edema, widespread depolarization, and cell death. Cell death and lysis cause the release of glutamate, an excitatory amino acid, which causes an increase in intracellular calcium influx and further cell death [7, 8].

The acute phase, also known as primary energy failure, is characterized by anaerobic metabolism, oxidative stress, neuronal cell death, and excitotoxicity. In the process of excitotoxicity, an excessive amount of the excitatory amino acid, glutamate, leads to overstimulation of the 2-(aminomethyl)phenylacetic acid (AMPA), kainite (KA), and N-methyl-D-aspartate (NMDA) receptors. Overstimulation of AMPA and KA causes an influx of sodium (Na+) and chloride (Cl−), which leads to an increased cellular osmolality. Overstimulation of NMDA triggers the influx of calcium (Ca2+), which leads to apoptosis and necrosis. The mitogen-activated protein kinase (MAPK) signaling pathway is overactivated after the hypoxic-ischemic event, leading to further neuronal apoptosis. Prostanoids also play a role in the hypoxic-ischemic event: Stimulating prostanoid receptors may be neuroprotective and prevent cerebellar neuronal injury. A partial recovery with reperfusion happens 30 to 60 minutes after the hypoxic-ischemic event in a penumbra of the brain, depending on the length of reduced perfusion and the presence or absence of medical intervention [8, 9].

The severity of the original energy failure influences how badly the secondary energy failure phase will be. Necrosis may result in neuronal cell death if the hypoxic-ischemic insult is severe. There is a brief time of recuperation when blood flow has been restored. Normal brain metabolism is present throughout this brief time of recuperation, known as the latent phase. The hypoxic-ischemic insult's intensity and magnitude are hypothesized to have an impact on the latent period. The latent period shortens with increasing injury severity. It is currently uncertain exactly when the latent period, the secondary energy failure phase, and the primary energy failure phase start and terminate. The ideal time for therapeutic treatments is thought to be during the latent phase [9]. The latent phase may last 1 to 6 hours. This latent phase is characterized by neuroinflammation and the continuation of an activated apoptotic cascade. In neonates with moderate to severe HIE, the latent phase is followed by the secondary phase, also known as secondary energy failure [8].

Neuronal cell death may be immediate or delayed and results from neuronal apoptosis or necrosis. Activation of proteases and endonucleases, neuronal apoptosis, microglial activation, reduction of growth factors and protein synthesis, and accumulation of excitatory neurotransmitters happened within approximately 6 to 15 hours. This secondary phase also caused cytotoxic edema, excitotoxicity, and cerebral hyperperfusion. The tertiary phase occurs in the weeks or months following primary energy failure. It involves remodeling the injured brain, astrogliosis, and late cell death [8–11].

The most important molecular trigger of apoptosis is an influx of Ca2+ and the generation of reactive oxygen species (ROS). These membrane perturbations involve the release of ceramide from sphingomyelin, translocation of the mitochondrion of proapoptotic member Bc1-2 family formation of the mitochondrial permeability pore, and release from the mitochondrion of cytochrome c and apoptosis-inducing factor and of caspases, especially caspase-3 by cytochrome c [8–10].

3. Role of Caspase-3 in programmed cell death

Caspase-3 is a lysosomal enzyme involved in the apoptotic pathway. It is a caspase protein that is encoded by the CASP3 gene. Caspase-3 is recognized for its activated proteolytic apoptosis role in cells responding to specific extrinsic or intrinsic inducers of this mode of cell death [12].

All caspases are initially created as dormant zymogens (known as procaspases), which are later transformed to activation by a variety of distinct internal and/or external cues. Procaspase-3 is made up of two subunits, one big and one small, known as p20 and p10, respectively, as well as an N-terminal prodomain. These two components work together to form the mature protease's catalytically active pocket [13].

Caspase-3 is synthesized as an inactive 32 kDa proenzyme and is processed during apoptosis generating two subunits of 17 and 12 kDa. Caspase-9 cleaves and activates caspase-3, which is present in the cell as an inactive proenzyme. Caspase-3 is activated within 1 to 3 hours after neonatal hypoxia-ischemia and is a principal executioner of apoptosis [10].

The particular cleavage of several cellular proteins is catalyzed by caspase-3, a death protease that is regularly activated. Whether reliant or independent of mitochondrial cytochrome c release and caspase-9 action, pathways to caspase-3 activation have been discovered. Caspase-3 is essential for apoptotic chromatin condensation and DNA fragmentation in all cell types, as well as for other classic apoptotic markers, throughout normal brain development [14].

4. Caspase-dependent mechanisms of apoptotic cell death

Cell death may be achieved by various mechanisms. During development and throughout life in cell renewal tissues, cells are continuously eliminated by mechanisms that induce apoptosis. Caspases play a crucial role in programmed cell death (apoptosis). Two main pathways have evolved for activating the caspase cascade: The mitochondrial pathway (intrinsic pathway) and the death receptor pathway (extrinsic pathway) [13].

A hypoxic event initiates the intrinsic pathway. The permeabilization of the mitochondrial outer membrane (MOMP) is one of the important stages in this process. The Bcl-2 family members provide the main function in MOMP. These proteins are classified as proapoptotic (Bax, Bak, etc.) and antiapoptotic (Bcl-2, Bcl-XL, etc.) proteins based on whether they include one or more Bcl-2 homolog (BH) domains. Subgroups of proapoptotic members have also been established: The BH3-only proteins and the BH1, BH2, and BH3-containing proteins. Bax and Bak are prone to conformational changes and oligomerization as a result of apoptotic stimuli, and they produce MOMP by disrupting the lipid bilayer, either creating pores or interacting with channels. Bax and Bak are counteracted by Bcl-2 antiapoptotic members, which are present in the outer membrane. In this regulation, BH3-only proteins have an essential role. A consequence of such proapoptotic cellular stressors is the permeabilization of the mitochondrial outer membrane and the release of apoptogenic factors such as cytochrome c into the cytoplasm. Cytochrome c molecules bind to an adaptor protein, apoptotic protease activating factor 1 (APAF-1), which recruits initiator caspase-9. This leads to the formation of the APAF1-containing macromolecular complex called the apoptosome [15–17].

Mature caspase-9 remains bound to the apoptosome, recruiting and activating executioner caspase-3 and caspase-7. This complex, in turn, binds and activates procaspase 9. Inhibitors of apoptosis (IAPs), of which x-linked IAP (XIAP) is the sole direct caspase-3 inhibitor, block the activation of caspase-3 and -7, while Smac/Diablo and Omi/HtrA2, which are released from the intermembrane space when mitochondria are injured, can also block this process [15, 17].

The extrinsic pathway includes cell surface receptor signaling. Death receptor-like Fas or Fas ligand (FasL) binding leads to receptor trimerization and recruitment of specific adaptor proteins. The Fas receptor contains a death domain (DD) in its cytoplasmic region that interacts with the adaptor protein. Extracellularly-mediated ligand binding to death receptors causes caspase-8 to bind to the Fas-associated death domain (FADD) adaptor protein, thereby forming a death-inducing signaling complex (DISC). FADD contains a death effector domain (DED), which recruits the DED-containing procaspase-8 into the DISC [16, 17].

Procaspase-8 is proteolytically activated to the enzymatically active caspase-8, activating downstream effector caspases. The oligomerization and activation of DISC are facilitated by the recruitment of caspase-8, which self-cleaves. The ultimate steps of apoptotic cell death are then brought about by the activation of downstream effector caspases, which is caused by cleaved caspase-8 [15].

The death receptor and mitochondrial-associated death pathways may interact in some cell types. In this instance, the proapoptotic Bcl-2 family member Bid is cleaved by caspase-8, activating the mitochondrial pathway. Truncated Bid (t-Bid) translocate to the mitochondria after being cleaved, where they cause the release of cytochrome c, an important step in the mitochondrial process. [16, 17].

Together with other effector caspases (including caspase-7 and -6), the extrinsic and intrinsic pathways come together at caspase-3 to plan the destruction of certain cell structures through the cleavage of a particular substrate. These caspase-mediated cleavages produce phenotypic changes in the apoptotic cell [15].

5. Caspase-independent mechanisms of apoptotic cell death

Caspase-independent cell death (CICD) ensues when a signal generally induces apoptosis and fails to activate caspases. Activation of caspases can occur after the ligation of death receptors or after the release of proapoptotic factors from mitochondria. Bcl-2 family proteins control the latter pathway. The APAF-1 binds to the caspase recruitment domain (CARD) in this pathway, triggering the activation of caspase-9 as the initiator. The proapoptotic factor cytochrome c causes caspase-9 and Apaf-1 to associate, leading to the development of apoptosomes. This component is found in the intermembrane gap of mitochondria, which also contributes to electron transport during respiration [13, 18].

Cytochrome c is released from the intermembrane gap during apoptosis as a result of increased permeability of the mitochondrial outer membrane. This process is triggered and controlled by pro- and antiapoptotic Bcl-2 family proteins [13, 18].

In cells lacking apoptosome-mediated caspase activation due to a lack of caspase-3, caspase-9, or Apaf-1, excessive Bax and Bak stimulation can cause mitochondrial dysfunction-triggered death. Bax and Bak must both be activated for this mitochondrial step because neither can start the intrinsic apoptotic pathway by itself [17].

Mitochondria, however, can release multiple factors that may trigger caspase-independent cell death. Moreover, cell death may be caused by altered mitochondrial energetics directly due to the loss of cytochrome c.

Numerous mitochondrial intermembrane space proteins are produced during MOMP in the absence of caspase activation, precipitating loss of mitochondrial function and potentially causing cell death. The simultaneous activation of mitochondrial fusion and inactivation of mitochondrial fission causes a disruption in mitochondrial morphology. CICD is influenced by these occurrences. The mechanism by which MOMP can follow CICD is through either a general decline in mitochondrial function or the release of mitochondrial proteins that can induce CICD [13, 18].

6. Necrotic cell death mediated by caspases

The following is the necrosis mechanism mediated by inflammatory caspase. The proinflammatory subfamily of caspases, counting caspase-1, caspase-4, caspase-5, and caspase-11, is known to intercede in a type of necrotic cell passing named pyroptosis (Greek roots pyro, connecting with fire or fever), which is portrayed by cell enlarging, lysis, and arrival of proinflammatory cytokines and intracellular substance [19].

When stimulated by pathogens such as bacteria, viruses, or their byproducts such as lipopolysaccharide (LPS) and viral DNA, phagocytes such as macrophages, monocytes, and dendritic cells (DCs), as well as other cell types (such as T cells), undergo pyroptosis. Like apoptosis, the critical execution mechanism of pyroptosis involves cleavage events mediated by caspases. The ability of inflammatory caspases to promote cell lysis involves gasdermin D (GSDMD) cleavage to promote membrane formation. Inflammasomes may activate inflammatory caspases mediating pyroptosis. The inflammasome pathways include the canonical inflammasomes that mediate the activation of caspase-1 and the noncanonical inflammasome that promotes the activation of caspase-4, 5, and [13, 19, 20].

Human caspase-1, caspase-4, and caspase-5 are identified as gene clusters on chromosome 11. Caspase-1, the enzyme directly involved in the processing of pro-IL-1β, is subject to regulation by caspase-4, -5, and -11 [18]. The activation of pyroptosis is proinflammatory as opposed to apoptosis, which largely has anti-inflammatory effects. This is due to the processing and release of mature IL-1 and IL-18, which have strong proinflammatory activity in promoting vasodilation and extravasation of immune cells, the generation of IL-17-producing helper T cells-mediated (Th17) response, and the production of interferon- (IFN-) by NK and Th1 cells [19, 21]. Additionally, this is due to the rapid loss of cell membrane integrity and release of cytosolic contents.

Caspases also play a role in the program of cell death through necrosis. For this necrotic cell death, however, caspase-3 plays a direct role. Several studies have shown a relationship between caspase-3 and the process of necrosis. It is known that LPS is a highly induced proinflammatory caspase for mediating sepsis but also capable of mediating the cleavage of downstream caspases such as caspase-3/-7. It was likewise found that caspase-3 severs the GSDMD-related protein DFNA5 after Asp270 to produce a necrotic DFNA5-N section that causes the plasma layer to instigate optional rot/pyroptosis [22, 23].

The role of caspase-3 might be more profound than explained above; we need to explore more of its role in apoptosis, pyroptosis, necroptosis, and autophagy. There is emerging evidence that caspase-3 also has a pivotal role in regulating the growth and homeostatic maintenance of both normal and malignant cells and tissues in multicellular organisms. There are still many vast possibilities for the role of caspase-3 and its use in the clinical identification and treatment.

7. Conclusions

Caspase-3 is one of the most essential components in programmed cell death due to its catalyzing the specific cleavage of many essential cellular proteins. Caspase-3 is activated within 1 to 3 hours after neonatal hypoxic-ischemia and is a principal executioner of apoptosis. Pathways to caspase-3 activation have been identified whether dependent or independent of mitochondrial cytochrome c release and caspase-9 function.

Conflict of interest

The authors declare no conflict of interest.

List of abbreviations

AMPA	2-(aminomethyl)phenylacetic acid
APAF-1	apoptotic protease activating factor 1
ALT	alanine transaminase
APTT	activated partial thromboplastin time
AST	aspartate aminotransferase
ATP	adenosine triphosphate
BH	Bcl-2 homolog
DD	death domain
CARD	caspase recruitment domain
CICD	caspase-independent cell death
DC	dendritic cells
DED	death effector domain
DISC	death-inducing signaling complex
FADD	Fas-associated death domain
GFAP	glial fibrillary acidic protein
GSDMD	gasdermin D
HIE	hypoxic-ischemic encephalopathy
IAP	inhibitors of apoptosis
IFN	interferon
KA	kainite
LPS	lipopolysaccharide
MAPK	mitogen-activated protein kinase
MOMP	mitochondrial outer membrane
NMDA	N-methyl-D-aspartate
PT	prothrombin time
t-Bid	truncated Bid
ROS	reactive oxygen species
XIAP	x-linked inhibitors of apoptosis

Author details

Johnny Lambert Rompis* and Natharina Yolanda
Faculty of Medicine, Department of Child Health, University of Sam Ratulangi, Manado, Indonesia

*Address all correspondence to: albmalon@yahoo.com

References

[1] Gluckman PD, Wyatt JS, Azzopardi D, Ballard R, Edwards AD, Ferriero DM, et al. Selective head cooling with mild systemic hypothermia after neonatal encephalopathy: Multicentre randomised trial. Lancet. 2005;**365**:663-670

[2] Odd D, Heep A, Luyt K, Draycott T. Hypoxic-ischemic brain injury. Planned delivery before intrapartum events. Journal of Neonatal-perinatal Medicine. 2017;**10**(4):347-353

[3] Hagberg H, Mallard C, Ferriero DM, Vannucci SJ, Levison SW, Vexler ZS, et al. The role of inflammation in perinatal brain injury. Nature Reviews. Neurology. 2015;**11**:192-208

[4] Douglas-Escobar M, Weiss MD. Biomarkers of hypoxic-ischemic encephalopathy in newborns. Frontiers in Neurology. 2012;**3**:144

[5] Michiniewicz B, Szpecht D, Sowinska A, Sibiak R, Syzmankiewicz M, Gadzinowski J. Biomarkers in newborns with hypoxic-ischemic encephalopathy treated with therapeutic hypothermia. Child's Nervous System. 2020;**36**(12):2981-2988

[6] Yuan J, Nafajov A, Py B. Role of caspases in neurotic cell death. Cell. 2016;**167**(7):1193-1704

[7] Kleuskens DG, Costa FG, Annink KV, van den Hoogen A, Alderliesten T, Groenendaal F, et al. Pathophysiology of cerebral hyperperfusion in term neonates with hypoxic-ischemic encephalopathy: A systemic review for future research. Frontiers in Paediatrics. 2021;**9**:631258

[8] Allen KA, Brandon DH. Hypoxic-ischemic encephalopathy: Pathophysiology and experimental treatments. Newborn and Infant Nursing Reviews. 2011;**11**(3):125-133

[9] Inder TE, Volpe JJ. Pathophysiology: General principles. In: Volpe's Neurology of the Newborn. 6th ed. Amsterdam: Elsevier; 2017

[10] Bennet L, Roelfsema V, Pathipati P, Quaedackers JS, Gunn AJ. Relationship between evolving epileptiform activity and delayed loss of mitochondrial activity after asphyxia measured by near-infrared spectroscopy in preterm fetal sheep. The Journal of Physiology. 2006;**572**:141-154. DOI: 10.1113/jphysiol.2006.105197

[11] Qin X, Cheng J, Zhing Y, Mahgoub OK, Akter F, Fan Y, et al. Mechanism and treatment related to oxidative stress in neonatal hypoxic-ischemic encephalopathy. Frontiers in Molecular Neuroscience. 2019;**12**:88. DOI: 10.3389/fnmol.2019.00088

[12] Ponder KG, Boise LH. The prodomain of caspase-3 regulates its own removal and caspase activation. Cell Death Discovery. 2019;**5**:56. DOI: 10.1038/s41420-019-0142-1

[13] Porter AG, Janicke RU. Emerging roles of caspase-3 in apoptosis. Cell Death and Differentiation. 1999;**6**:99-104

[14] Alenzi FQ, Lotfy M, Wyse R. Swords of cell death: Caspase activation and regulation. Asian Pacific Journal of Cancer Prevention: APJCP. 2010;**11**:271-280

[15] Thornton C, Hagberg H. Role of mitochondria in apoptotic and necroptotic cell death in developing brain. Clinica Chimica Acta. 2015;**451**: 35-38. DOI: 10.1016/j.cca.2015.01.026

[16] Vekrellis K, McCarthy MJ, Watson A, Whitfield J, Rubin LL, Ham J. Bax promotes neuronal cell death and is downregulated during the development of the nervous system. Development. 1997;**124**:1239-1249

[17] Wang X, Han W, Du X, Zhu C, Carlsson Y, Mallard C, et al. Neuroprotective effect of Bax-inhibiting peptide on neonatal brain injury. Stroke. 2010;**41**:2050-2055

[18] Rodriguez J, Li T, Xu Y, Sun Y, Zhu C. Role of apoptosis-inducing factor in perinatal hypoxic-ischemic brain injury. Neural Regeneration Research. 2021;**16**(2):205-213

[19] Yuan J, Najafov A, Py B. Roles of caspases in necrotic cell death. Cell. 2016;**167**(7):1693-1604

[20] Shi J, Zhao Y, Wang K, Shi X, Wang Y, Huang H, et al. Cleavage of GSDMD by inflammatory caspases determines pyroptotic cell death. Nature. 2015;**526**:660-665

[21] Russo HM, Rathkey J, Boyd-Tressler A, Katsnelson MA, Abbott DW, Dubyak GR. Active Caspase-1 induces plasma membrane pores that precede Pyroptotic lysis and are blocked by lanthanides. Journal of Immunology. 2016;**197**:1353-1367

[22] Rogers C, Fernandes-Alnemri T, Mayes L, Alnemri D, Cingolani G, Alnemri ES. Cleavage of DNFNA5 by caspase-3 during apoptosis mediates progression to secondary necrotic/pyroptotic cell death. Nature Communications. 2016;**8**:14128. DOI: 10.1038/ncomms14128

[23] Shi J, Zhao Y, Wang Y, Gao W, Ding J, Li P, et al. Inflammatory caspases are innate immune receptors for intracellular LPS. Nature. 2014;**514**:187-192

Chapter 10

Exosomes in Reperfusion Injuries: Role in Pathophysiology and Perspectives as Treatment

Maritza G. Verdugo-Molinares, Marco Ku-Centurion and Zesergio Melo

Abstract

This chapter focuses on the emerging field of exosomes in the context of reperfusion injuries. Exosomes, nano extracellular vesicles with diverse cargo, play a crucial role in cell-to-cell communication. Exosome quantity and content changes have been implicated in various pathologies, including kidney, brain, heart, and liver ischemia-reperfusion injury. Particularly, exosomes derived from mesenchymal stem cells (MSCs) have shown promising potential as a treatment approach. This chapter aims to provide a comprehensive understanding of exosome biogenesis, the role of organ-specific exosomes in reperfusion injury pathophysiology, and the advantages and prospects of exosome-based treatments. By exploring the multifaceted aspects of exosomes in reperfusion injuries, this chapter will contribute to the advancement of knowledge in this field.

Keywords: exosomes, reperfusion, kidney, heart, brain cells, liver

1. Introduction

Exosomes are small extracellular vesicles released by various cell types in different cell conditions, including those involved in tissue repair and regeneration. These particles have been linked to a variety of biological phenomena, including immune responses, viral pathogenicity, pregnancy, diseases related to pregnancy, cardiovascular diseases, diseases related to the central nervous system, and the progression of cancer [1]. They play a crucial role in cell-to-cell communication by transferring bioactive macromolecules, such as proteins, nucleic acids, and lipids, between cells [2]. Exosomes have gained significant attention in physiology due to their unique formation process within cells [3], which is thought to play a crucial role in determining composition and potential functions after they are released into the extracellular space. In the context of reperfusion injuries, the potential protective effects of exosomes have garnered considerable attention.

Reperfusion injury refers to tissue damage that occurs when blood supply returns to previously ischemic tissue. While restoring blood flow, it is necessary to prevent further damage; re-establishing oxygen and nutrients can also lead to the generation of reactive oxygen species (ROS) and inflammatory responses, which can exacerbate tissue injury. Acute damage caused by reperfusion is characterized by cellular injury, upregulation of cytokines, infiltration of leukocytes, and the formation of neutrophil extracellular traps (NETs) among other cellular and tissue changes.

The study of exosomes has gained high importance given their potential use in different areas of biology and health, which will be described in this book chapter. Some of the topics most currently addressed are:

Exosomes as rich source of biomarkers: Exosomes can carry specific proteins, nucleic acids, and miRNAs that are indicative of cellular stress, injury, or regenerative processes. Studying the composition and content of exosomes released during reperfusion injuries can help identify potential biomarkers for early detection, prognosis, and monitoring of the extent of tissue damage.

Exosomes in cellular communication and cytoprotection: Exosomes released by certain cell types, such as endothelial cells, cardiomyocytes, and stem cells, have been shown to promote cell survival, reduce inflammation, and protect against reperfusion injury. Understanding the molecular cargo and mechanisms of exosomal transfer can provide insights into intercellular signaling and potential therapeutic targets.

Regenerative potential of exosomes content: Exosomes derived from stem cells, including mesenchymal stem cells (MSCs), have been reported to exhibit regenerative properties and promote tissue repair. These exosomes can transfer regenerative factors and modulate inflammatory responses, thereby enhancing the regenerative potential of damaged tissues after reperfusion injury.

Therapeutic Applications: Harnessing the therapeutic potential of exosomes is an active area of research. Researchers are exploring strategies to engineer exosomes with specific cargo or modify their composition to enhance their protective effects. Exosomes could be utilized as targeted delivery vehicles for therapeutic agents, such as anti-inflammatory drugs or regenerative factors, to mitigate reperfusion injury.

In this book chapter, we will review from the biological basis of exosome formation and structure to the physiology and involvement of exosomes in reperfusion damage. We will also analyze the most important studies that to date have given insights into the best techniques for isolating these particles. Finally, we will explore a series of future perspectives that involve the use of exosomes as possible tools for treatments in complicated pathologies.

2. Biogenesis of exosomes

2.1 Definition and characteristics of exosomes

Exosomes are a group of biomolecules between 50 to 100 nanometers in diameter. They have a density of 1.13–1.19 g/mL and exhibit characteristic morphology when viewed under a transmission electron microscope. Among their main protein markers, we find tetraspanins, TSG101, and Hsp70 primarily [4].

Exosomes are the smallest characterized molecules after exomeres [5]. With a size ranging from 30 to 200 nm, they are formed by a membrane system that contains the same biological structures as a cell, including nucleic acids, proteins, lipids, amino acids, and metabolites, see **Figure 1**. These components can reflect their cellular origin. This particular architecture exhibits an important array of membrane-associated, oligomeric proteins, resulting in protein heterogeneity [6].

An important role of exosomes is to communicate information between distant and different cells while also participating in the microenvironmental remodeling

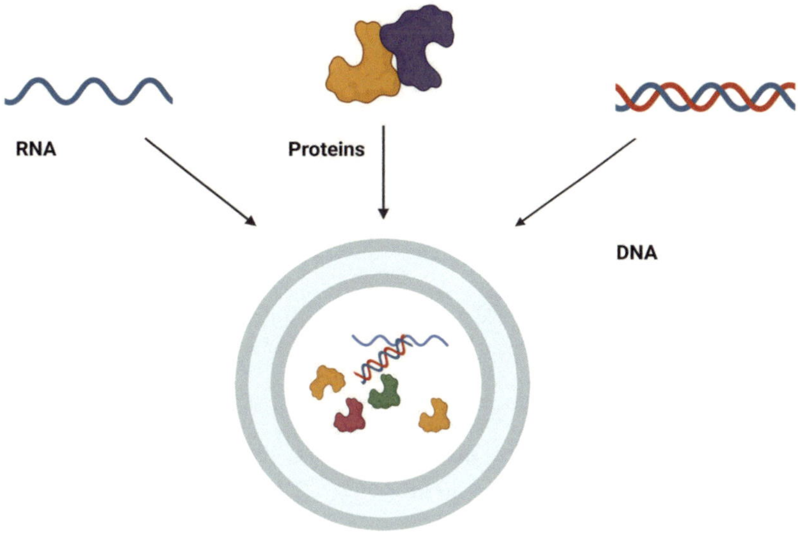

Figure 1.
Biogenesis of the exosomes.

of the extracellular matrix. The size of exosomes has been determined using various laboratory techniques; however, each of these techniques provides different size variations. The techniques used to determine the size of exosomes include single-particle interferometric reflectance (SPIR) imaging, fluorescence microscopy, nanotracking particle analysis, and resistive pulse sensing [6, 7]. Transmission electron microscopy is a technique that only determines the diameter of the exosome membrane. For this reason, when determining the diameter of these particles, we consider the method used for measurement. This measurement can be affected by different variables, including shrinking, swelling, or flattening. These processes are susceptible to affecting our samples.

Exosomes can originate from various sources, such as urine, blood, saliva, or even tears. The main role of great interest for which exosomes have been studied in recent years is their mediation of cell communication in both health and disease processes, directly affecting cell physiology [8].

2.2 Mechanisms of exosome formation and cargo loading

The process for the formation of exosomes is called biogenesis. This process describes how exosomes are formed inside cells and involves a crucial role of the plasma membrane in creating multivesicular bodies (MVBs). Exosomes are released from these MVBs out of the cell [4]. The process begins within an early endosome, containing endocytosed components. This early endosome can undergo three fates: it can either proceed toward the Golgi network, continue maturing as a late endosome, or recycle through endosome-lysosome fusion (**Figure 2**) [9].

MVBs are characterized by being formed as biological structures through the creation of cell membranes. Vesicles captured by these structures are deposited inside as intraluminal vesicles (ILVs). These vesicles, present within this newly formed component, are released outside the cell through the fusion of the intraluminal vesicles with the plasma membrane. This is how exosomes are released outside the

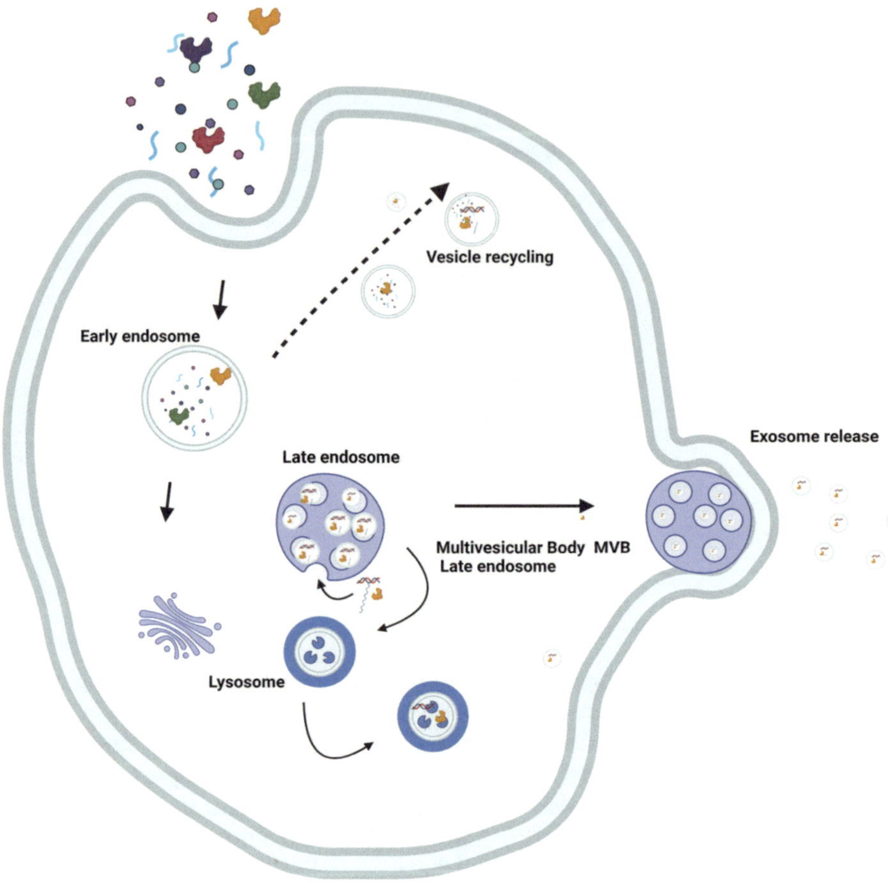

Figure 2.
Exosomes cargo.

cell [8]. The formed body has three potential destinations: one leads to the lysosomal pathway, where proteins are recycled through lysosomes [10], while the other involves the exocytic pathway, allowing newly formed exosomes to be released outside the cell (see **Figure 3**) [8].

Exosome formation involves a crucial role played by various proteins, including Rab GTPases and ESCRT proteins. Additionally, specific molecules can serve as markers for exosomes, including CD9, CD81, CD63, flotillin, TSG101, ceramide, and Alix [8]. Regarding the components present on the surfaces of these vesicles, tetraspanins, integrins, immunomodulatory proteins, and others can be mentioned [11]. In the process of exosome formation, various molecules are associated with the endosomal sorting complex required for transport (ESCRT). Generally, the proteins involved in this process can be divided into two categories: ESCRT-dependent and ESCRT-independent. ESCRT is a group of proteins responsible for coordinating and deforming membranes through its multi-protein machinery. This machinery facilitates the generation of new exosomes within intraluminal vesicles. ESCRT has the capability to form four distinct complexes: ESCRT 0, I, II, and III [12].

An important role of ESCRT 0 to II is direct participation in sorting cargo. This process occurs through the formation of microdomains on the vesicle's surface. These

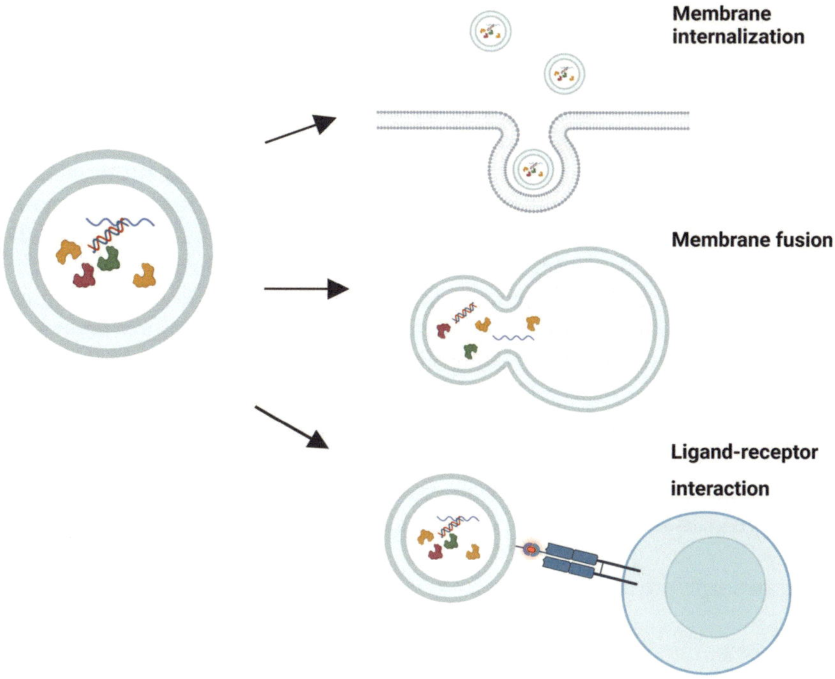

Figure 3.
Exosomes internalization.

domains act as organizing centers, facilitating signal transduction within the vesicle's interior. Following this, ESCRT manages the budding and cleavage of these domains to generate intraluminal vesicles (ILVs). Vps4 (Vacuolar protein sorting-associated protein 4) assists in dissociating ESCRT III after the membrane scission process is completed. The SNF7/CHMP4 protein complex plays a role in contributing to membrane formation by inducing inward budding and generating ILVs. This is achieved through the polymerization of the mentioned complex, resulting in the formation of spirals that accumulate potential energy. This accumulated energy enables the creation of negative curvature, leading to the generation of exosomes [13].

The second group of molecules involved in the process of exosome formation consists of those that are independent of ESCRT. These molecules can be either lipids or proteins. Among the most crucial for this process are tetraspanins, which play various roles in the pathway of exosome generation. Tetraspanins play a direct role in loading compounds into multivesicular bodies. They enhance the secretion of specific compounds into exosomes and enable the compartmentalization of the exosomal membrane into functional domains enriched with these proteins [14]. There are other lipid compounds strongly associated with promoting exosome formation, including ceramides, membrane sphingolipids, cholesterol, and lipid raft microdomains. These compounds induce spontaneous negative curvature of the membrane, facilitating the generation of intraluminal vesicles independently of ESCRT [15].

The process by which the contents of exosomes are introduced is referred to as cargo sorting. This process ensures that the relevant content is loaded inside the vesicles. The cargo can encompass various components, including amino acids, proteins, metabolites, lipids, as well as different types of RNA such as messenger RNA (mRNA), microRNA (miRNA), long noncoding RNA (lncRNA), circular RNA (circRNA), PIWI-interacting RNA (piRNA), and DNA [16]. The mechanisms to load these components have a different nature as shown in **Figure 2**. The process initiates with a signal that enables proteins to enter the endosomal pathway. This signal involves monoubiquitination, which allows the cargo to be recognized and bound by the ubiquitin-interacting motif (UIM) domain of the ESCRT 0 Vps27/Hrs protein [17].

Ubiquitination is recognized for facilitating the direct entry of proteins into exosomes. However, the precise mechanism for nonprotein compounds remains unclear. For instance, in the case of microRNA, the exact mechanism is not fully understood. It is known that microRNA can enter exosomes through selective binding to heterogeneous nuclear ribonucleoprotein A2B1 (hnRNA2B1), which is expressed on the exosome membrane [18]. The cellular state in which exosomes are generated plays a crucial role in determining the content of the generated exosomes. Furthermore, the protein content can be influenced by both ESCRT-dependent and ESCRT-independent factors, including but not limited to ESCRT-III, Alix, Syntenin-1, and ceramides. These factors contribute to shaping the composition of exosomes [19]. Finally, prior to sealing the vesicle that gives rise to the exosome, a deubiquitination process takes place to remove ubiquitin from the proteins associated with the cargo [20].

2.3 Release and uptake of exosomes by recipient cells

Released exosomes can engage with the plasma membranes of neighboring or remote cells, facilitating the internalization and subsequent release of their contents. This intricate process involves SNARE proteins, which play a pivotal role in mediating membrane fusion to enable exosome release [21].

The transportation of multivesicular bodies (MVBs) to the plasma membrane, facilitating the release of exosomes, is orchestrated by the cytoskeleton. Specifically, actin filaments and microtubules play a pivotal role in transporting MVBs, ultimately enabling the release of exosomes [19]. An essential aspect to consider regarding exosome distribution is that while exosomes can be present within the organism, their biodistribution is influenced by various factors. These factors include considerations such as their retention in lymph nodes and bone tissue, as well as potential competition with exosomes secreted by other cells. After exosomes have reached their recipient cell, they can engage in three distinct modes of interaction with the target cell. These interaction modes encompass internalization, membrane fusion, and binding to receptor ligands such as MHC and TNF ligands. These binding interactions can subsequently trigger the initiation of signaling cascades [22].

3. Isolation, characterization, and cargo analysis of exosomes

To comprehend the content of exosomes, various laboratory tests are essential to ascertain the internal composition of these vesicles. The initial step involves isolation, which determines their origin. As previously mentioned, the source can vary, encompassing cell cultures, plasma, sweat, tears, urine, and other bodily fluids. Characterization of exosomes involves assessing their physical attributes such as size, protein-lipid ratio, density, and other physicochemical parameters. Additionally, this characterization extends to quantitatively determining the contents of proteins, lipids, carbohydrates, and nucleic acids within the exosomes. Given the diverse range of tests that can be conducted on exosomes, it is crucial to discern which characteristics are the most pivotal parameters for addressing the specific questions we seek to answer.

3.1 Methods for isolating exosomes from different biological sources

The methods and techniques used to isolate exosomes can be categorized into conventional and novel approaches. Within conventional techniques, we encounter ultracentrifugation-based separation, size-based separation, and precipitation.

Ultracentrifugation stands as the primary technique employed for exosome isolation. This method exploits centrifugal force to create gradients within the sample. Notably, ultracentrifugation boasts simplicity, cost-effectiveness, high purity, and the potential for protocol standardization [23]. The second technique used is the separation based on size; this technique combines ultracentrifugation with size-exclusion chromatography; the advantages that this technique offers allow obtaining large amounts of exosomes with high purity; with this technique, urinary exosomes and those from platelets can be obtained [24]. The third technique involves precipitation using agents such as polyethylene glycol. While this method offers relative simplicity and speed in isolation, it comes with higher costs and inadequate specificity. This technique is applicable for extracting exosomes from serum, plasma, or cell supernatants [25].

On the other hand, novel isolation techniques offer technical advantages for exosome extraction; however, ensuring specificity and purity demands careful attention. Several of these techniques include:

Immunoaffinity Separation: This method relies on antigen-antibody interactions within a conjugated platform featuring specific antibodies on the exosome surface. It is a straightforward and specific technique, although it tends to be expensive [26]. Magnetic separation method involves employing magnetic beads conjugated with antibodies. Like immunoaffinity separation, magnetic separation offers the benefits of specificity and ease of execution. Nonetheless, it comes with a higher cost [27].

The subsequent category of techniques for exosome isolation involves separation based on their physical properties, particularly their size. These methods often utilize specialized membranes that serve as filters, akin to molecular exclusion chromatography. This type of technique offers a wide range of applications for exosome extraction [28].

Lipid-mediated separation: The most used technique involves the lipid nanoprobe coupled with high-affinity silica-based TiO_2. This approach offers the advantage of causing minimal damage to extracellular structures, thereby facilitating effective and efficient isolation. However, potential interference due to contamination remains a consideration with this method [29].

Thermophoretic enrichment: This method is both simple and quick to apply, utilizing thermophoresis to achieve efficient isolation of extracellular vesicles [30].

Microfluidic-based acoustics: It employs acoustic radiation as an active means to separate extracellular vesicles, effectively facilitating the efficient separation of exosomes [31].

3.2 Techniques for exosome characterization and cargo analysis

More contemporary techniques for exosome characterization encompass diverse approaches for their detection. The first approach employs colorimetric detection utilizing a reaction between hydrogen peroxide and TMB (3,3′,5,5′-Tetramethylbenzidine). Sample volumes required typically span from 100 to 500 μL. This method has been employed to evaluate exosomes sourced primarily from breast cancer cells, prostate cells, and urine [16]. The second characterization technique involves fluorescence-based detection. It is applicable to a variety of samples, including plasma, cell supernatants, and blood samples. Fluorophores are utilized, detectable by electronic equipment, with a detection limit ranging from 21 exosomes to 4 million particles per microliter of sample [16]. Electrochemical detection constitutes another technique, often using sample volumes ranging from 10 to 30 μL. Detection is achieved through specific biosensors and antibody microarray sensors [16].

Surface plasmon resonance detection methods (SPR-detection) involve utilizing specific antibodies to target antigens within exosomes. This method can be applied to exosomes from sources such as breast cancer cells (HER2 positive), lung cell lines, plasma, and urine samples from lung cancer patients. Sample volumes may range from 250 to 1500 μL [16].

Surface-Enhanced Raman Scattering (SERS) is a characterization technique utilizing sample volumes ranging from less than 1 to 400 μL. This technique enhances the Raman signal of small molecules attached to a rough metal surface through electromagnetic and chemical mechanisms. Exosomes for this method can originate from various sources including plasma, cell cultures, serum samples, and lung cells [16].

3.3 Relevance of cargo analysis in understanding exosome-mediated effects

It is very important to know the content of the exosomes to determine biomolecule profiles that it contains inside; it is important because it has been verified through these analyses that their content is different between the cells in the organism, even according to the physiological state of each of them specially in cancer [28]. Furthermore, research has shown that dysregulation of exosome-related proteins can contribute to the development and progression of disease states, highlighting their potential as diagnostic and therapeutic targets [32].

Various research teams have recognized exosomes as valuable sources of potential markers or biomarkers. These include applications for early diagnosis of various pathologies across different organs, including the kidneys. Consequently, thorough characterization and analysis of the content within these vesicles provide a means to comprehensively understand the intricate molecular and cellular mechanisms underpinning the pathophysiology of diverse diseases. This knowledge has the potential to revolutionize our understanding of disease development and progression and potentially aid in the development of novel diagnostic and therapeutic approaches.

4. Exosomes in reperfusion injury pathophysiology

The role of exosomes has been extensively investigated in various diseases such as cancer, neurodegenerative diseases, and heart failure. Additionally, pathogens exploit exosomes to infect host cells [33]. Numerous studies have highlighted augmented exosome release and alterations in their contents in hypoxic conditions [34]. Keeping up with the advancements in the study of reperfusion injury pathophysiology includes a comprehensive understanding of exosomes and their potential involvement in this phenomenon.

4.1 Kidney-derived exosomes and their role in reperfusion injury

The proximal tubule is considered the most sensitive cellular entity to ischemia, hypoxia, or nephrotoxic damage. This sensitivity is largely related to the high metabolic rate and strong reliance on oxidative phosphorylation of these cells [35]. Exosomes released by proximal tubular epithelial cells are believed to play a significant role in the context of ischemia-reperfusion injury. Many studies have demonstrated that these cells increased the production of exosomes under hypoxic conditions [36].

In a model of ischemia-reperfusion injury, exosomes demonstrated a significant role in mediating epithelial–mesenchymal communication (EMC) during fibrinogenesis. Another interesting observation was that the renal proximal tubular epithelium shows the major release of exosomes. The upregulation in exosome production was not limited to the model of ischemia-reperfusion injury; it was also observed in cases of unilateral obstruction and partial nephrectomy, showing its importance in different models of kidney damage [37].

A study of tubular epithelial cells (TECs) under hypoxic conditions revealed the capacity of exosomes to facilitate the activation of fibroblasts. Exosomes play a role in cell-to-cell communication with protein transport and mRNA transfer. The delivery of TGF-β1 mRNA *via* TECs exosomes to fibroblasts implicates rapid TGF-β1 production and autocrine signaling [38]. This mechanism could be applied to any mRNA transported by exosomes, not only for exacerbating damage but also for preparing cells for ischemic insult. The use of exosomes as an option for ischemia preconditioning (IPC) was analyzed by Dominguez et al. where they found that ischemic exosomes from adult renal cells improve renal function in rats with ischemic renal injury. Their findings suggest that the abundant ribosomal transcripts in ischemic exosomes help cells enhance their restoration after renal ischemia [39].

The capacity of exosomes to transport miRNA is also important. A comparison between renal tissue samples with and without ischemia-reperfusion identified upregulation of miR-150p that promotes fibroblast activation [40]. MiR-374b-5p found in exosomes of TECs is related to promoted macrophage activation in IR and increased kidney damage [40]. Both miRNAs are related to the inhibition of the suppressor of cytokine signaling (SOCS-1), which is a negative regulator of NF-κB signaling pathways [41].

Several well-known proteins that play a significant role in ischemia-reperfusion can be encapsulated within exosomes [42]. One way to study proteins around pathophysiology or as biomarkers of kidney disease is the study of urinary exosomes. This gives us a view of what is happening in the kidney, and it became an important part of kidney study. Increased fetuin-A and decrease of $Na+/H+$ exchanger isoform 3 (NHE3) and aquaporin 1 are examples of changes observed in urinary exosomes after ischemia-reperfusion [43].

4.2 Brain-derived exosomes: implications for ischemic stroke and reperfusion injury

Brain cells such as neurons, astrocytes, oligodendrocytes, endothelial cells, and microglia are capable of releasing exosomes [44]. Under pathologic conditions, neuron exosomes mediate nutritional metabolic support, nerve regeneration, inflammation, and propagation of toxic components, while exosomes released by astrocytes and microglia exert neuroprotective effects [45].

In a model of oxygen and glucose deprivation, astrocyte-derived exosomes inhibited neuron apoptosis and autophagy. The same results were found *in vivo* [46]. Also, *in vitro* and *in vivo* models of ischemia-reperfusion showed M2 microglia-derived exosomes attenuated damage, promoting neuronal survival *via* exosomal miR-124 [47].

Moreover, neuronal exosomes transfer miR-124 to astrocytes; this transmission is critical for neuronal activity; in fact, serum miR-124 is downregulated in ischemic stroke patients [48].

Microglia exosomal miRNA-317 has a protective effect after ischemic injury with Notch-1 as a target [49]. Additionally, microglia exosomes release miRNA-137 and -34a, both of which are capable of inhibiting Notch-1 [50].

The study of exosomal miRNA in the plasma of patients after ischemic stroke has associated miRNAs-9, −124, −134, −152-3p, and −223 with stroke severity and miRNAs-134 and -223 with poor prognosis [51].

Use of exosomes derived from plasma of a murine model of ischemic preconditioning decreases the damage in a cellular model of oxygen–glucose deprivation and restoration of N2a. The study identified miR-451a as a protective factor through Rac1 inactivation [52]. Rac1 suppression reduced infarction volume and promoted neural stem cell activity in brain ischemia-reperfusion [53].

Exosomes have different roles in angiogenesis, neurogenesis, autophagy, and blood–brain barrier during ischemic stroke, which made them a good source of biomarkers for diagnosis and prognostic of this neurological disease [54].

4.3 Cardiac exosomes: involvement in myocardial ischemia and reperfusion injury

The heart is another organ affected by ischemia-reperfusion. Myocardium ischemia-reperfusion injury involves mechanisms such as oxidative stress, intracellular calcium overload, energy metabolism disorder, apoptosis, endoplasmic reticulum stress autophagy, pyroptosis, ferroptosis, and necroptosis [55]. Cardiomyocytes can uptake exosomes from various cell types. Cardiac fibroblast exosomes can be internalized by cardiomyocytes. During ischemia-reperfusion injury, exosomes derived from cardiac fibroblasts elevate the levels of miR-133a, which has the capability to mitigate cardiomyocyte pyroptosis [56]. Additionally, cardiomyocytes are capable of uptaking exosomes released by polymorphonuclear neutrophils (PMNs). Exosomes originating from PMNs that have been stimulated with the calcium-sensing receptor (CaSR) demonstrate the capacity to mitigate ischemia-reperfusion damage in cardiomyocytes [57]. Cardiomyocytes can also take exosomes released by endothelial cells [58].

Angiogenesis is one of the most vital pathways involved in ischemia-reperfusion, playing a crucial role in the recovery following the insult. Therapeutic angiogenesis has emerged as a significant alternative for treating ischemic heart disease [59]. Pro-angiogenic miRNAs have been detected in exosomes such as miR-126-3, −125, −30c, −126, −17, and 19a/b [60].

Use of exosomes as a therapy of ischemic preconditioning is also considered in the heart. We have found cardioprotective proteins in cardiomyocyte exosomes such as IL-6 and heat shock proteins [61]. Serum exosomes of ischemic preconditioning rats have a protective effect in ischemia-reperfusion injury activating PI3K/AKT signaling pathway [62]. The cardioprotective effects of ischemic preconditioning (IPC) exosomes have also been attributed to the presence of miR-126a-3p, which influences Akt and Erk1/2 signaling pathways [63].

4.4 Liver-derived exosomes and their contribution to hepatic reperfusion injury

Hepatic ischemia-reperfusion injury (HIRI) arises during liver surgery and transplantation. Oxidative stress and inflammation are among the cellular and biochemical factors contributing to liver damage during IR. However, the complete process is still under study [64]. Liver cells are capable of releasing and taking exosomes. This included hepatocytes, Kupffer cells, and hepatic stellate cells, as well as biliary epithelial cells and endothelial cells [65]. One of the mechanisms involving hepatocyte exosomes promoting cell proliferation has been identified *via* sphingosine 1-phosphate (S1P) [66].

The liver can sustain damage during intestinal ischemic reperfusion due to the ability of intestinal cell exosomes to migrate and impact the liver. Zhao et al. conducted a study to investigate the potential influence of these exosomes on the liver. The study's findings indicated that exosomes generated after intestinal ischemia-reperfusion (IR) contributed to liver damage by polarizing M1 macrophages. Suppressing the release of exosomes resulted in a reduction of hepatic injury [67]. Indeed, this is an interesting perspective of how exosomes' effects extend beyond the cells of their originating organ.

5. Mesenchymal stem cell-derived exosomes as a potential treatment

The use of mesenchymal stem cells (MSCs) in immunomodulation and regenerative medicine is not new. Like all the cells that we have mentioned, MSCs are capable of producing exosomes. These exosomes have intrinsic characteristics of protein and miRNA that could have an effect in targets cells and also could be interesting vehicles of genes, drugs, enzymes, or RNA [68]. Another important characteristic is that MSCs are easy to be cultured and manipulated [69].

Exosomes have emerged as an important therapeutic option for several reasons. Their biological origin ensures that their components are easily metabolized by cells, and they possess low immunogenicity due to this inherent compatibility [70]. They also possess great stability and low toxicity [71]. In the context of brain, exosomes represent an excellent option of therapy and drug delivery for their capacity to cross BBB [72]. The use of MSC-derived exosomes shows promise as a treatment for ischemia-reperfusion injuries. Angiogenic factors like VEGF, FGF, Ang-1, and Ang-2, among others can be found in MSC exosomes. Also, important angiogenic miRNA as −107, −31, −126, 26a, and -20b-5p [73]. Their anti-inflammatory and immunomodulatory properties made them capable to regulate macrophage polarization [74, 75].

The origin of MSCs determines their cargo and effects on target cells. Even the exosomes from bone marrow MSCs (BMSCs) contain mRNA that is relevant to cell transcription and the regulation of proliferation; exosomes from human liver stem cells contain specific mRNA related to liver metabolism and its proliferation [76].

The *in vivo* following of MSC exosomes demonstrated their capacity to migrate to ischemic lesion after intravenously injected in a stroke animal model. These exosomes effectively promoted angiogenesis and neurogenesis [77].

MSC-derived exosomes have been tested in ischemia reperfusion with interesting results. MSCs for bone, adipose tissue, placental, kidney, and umbilical cord have been tried in clinical models of kidney ischemia reperfusion. In preclinical studies, these exosomes have demonstrated being anti-inflammatory and anti-fibrotic, as well as decreased tubular damage, creatinine, BUN, and proteinuria [78]. MSC exosomes in ischemic stroke have shown promoted angiogenesis, neurogenesis, oligodendrogenesis, and astrogenesis in experimental therapy [79].

6. Challenges and future perspectives

One of the primary challenges in exosome research is the isolation and purification of exosomes from complex biological samples. Existing isolation methods, such as ultracentrifugation, immunomagnetic bead isolation kits, and density gradient separation, have limitations in terms of yield, purity, and scalability [80]. Standardization of isolation protocols and characterization methods is essential to ensure consistency and comparability among studies; however, at present, there is still no consensus on the most efficient and effective method of extraction [81].

The therapeutic potential of exosomes heavily depends on their ability to carry and deliver specific cargo molecules, such as miRNAs, siRNAs, metabolites, and proteins, to target organs [82]. Nevertheless, efficiently loading therapeutic cargo into exosomes remains a challenge. Moreover, targeted delivery to affected tissues and cells needs improvement, as the passive targeting of exosomes may not always suffice for optimal therapeutic outcomes. These exosome-based therapies demand large-scale production to meet clinical demand. Cost-effective and scalable manufacturing processes that maintain the integrity and biological activity of exosomes are still under development [83]. In the same order of ideas, establishing Good Manufacturing Practice guidelines for exosome production is crucial for ensuring product quality and safety.

Understanding the *in vivo* behavior of exosomes, including biogenesis, distribution, clearance, and pharmacokinetics, is crucial for optimizing dosing regimens and predicting therapeutic outcomes. Robust and noninvasive imaging techniques are needed to track exosome distribution and uptake in real time. Considering all these biological features, exosomes may possess distinct immunogenicity profiles, potentially triggering immune responses upon administration [84]. Long-term safety assessments, including the potential for off-target effects and tumorigenicity, must be rigorously evaluated before advancing exosome-based therapies to the clinic [85].

Currently, bioengineering approaches offer exciting possibilities for exosome modification and optimization. Engineering exosomes with specific surface ligands or coatings can enhance their targeting ability and cargo-loading efficiency, enabling precise therapeutic interventions [86]. It is very interesting to think about combined therapies that include exosomes with other treatment modalities. Combining exosomes with drugs, gene therapy, or nanoparticles holds promise for synergistic effects and improved treatment outcomes. The synergistic potential of these combination therapies must be thoroughly investigated in preclinical and clinical studies.

Due to the variability in individuals, the goal of medicine in the present and into the future is to implement personalized treatments. The ability to derive patient-specific exosomes and make therapeutic approaches accordingly is an area of significant interest too. Personalized exosome-based therapies may enhance treatment efficacy and reduce the risk of adverse reactions. Preconditioning of donor cells, through either genetic modifications or exposure to specific stimuli, can influence the cargo content and therapeutic efficacy of exosomes [87]. These strategies could enhance the therapeutic potential of exosomes for reperfusion injuries.

To establish a future where exosomes are properly used in health, it is important to establish regulatory considerations for their correct commercialization. The regulatory landscape for exosome-based therapies is complex and dynamically evolving [88, 89]. Close collaboration between researchers, clinicians, and regulatory agencies is essential to establish appropriate guidelines for preclinical testing, clinical trials, and eventual approvals. In the same way, it is critical to protect intellectual property rights to incentivize investment in exosome research and development. Clear guidelines and policies related to patenting and licensing of exosome-based therapies are necessary to advance innovation.

7. Conclusions

Exosomes represent a promising avenue for addressing the challenges posed by reperfusion injuries, providing novel and targeted therapeutic options. However, several hurdles, including isolation standardization, cargo loading, scalability, safety, and regulatory approvals, must be overcome to realize their full potential. Emerging trends in engineering, combination therapies, personalized medicine, and *in vivo* tracking offer exciting possibilities for future developments in exosome-based therapies. Collaboration between researchers, clinicians, regulatory authorities, and industry stakeholders is essential to drive the field forward, ultimately benefiting patients worldwide. By addressing the current limitations and leveraging emerging trends, exosome-based therapies may revolutionize the treatment landscape for reperfusion injuries, offering hope for improved patient outcomes and enhanced quality of life.

Acknowledgements

We would like to express our gratitude to all those who have contributed to the creation of this book chapter. We extend our appreciation to all scientists of CIBO and CIATEJ for their valuable collaboration. And our families to be always with us, thanks.

Conflict of interest

Authors declare no conflict of interest.

Nomenclature

ROS	reactive Oxygen Species
NETs	neutrophil extracellular traps
MSCs	mesenchymal Stem Cells
HSP	heat shock protein
TSG	tumor susceptibility gene
MVBs	multivesicular bodies
ILVs	intraluminal vesicles
ESCRT	endosomal sorting complex required for transport
mRNA	messenger RNA
miRNA	microRNA
lncRNA	long noncoding RNA
circRNA	circular RNA
piRNA	PIWI-interacting RNA
EMC	epithelial–mesenchymal communication

TECs	tubular epithelial cells
CaSR	calcium-sensing receptor
IPC	ischemic preconditioning
S1P	sphingosine 1-phosphate
BBB	blood-brain barrier
BUN	blood urea nitrogen

Author details

Maritza G. Verdugo-Molinares[1], Marco Ku-Centurion[1] and Zesergio Melo[2]*

1 Medical and Pharmaceutical Biotechnology Unit, Center for Research and Assistance in Technology and Design of the State of Jalisco, A.C. (CIATEJ), Mexico

2 CONAHCYT-Western Biomedical Research Center, IMSS, Guadalajara, Mexico

*Address all correspondence to: zcmelo@conahcyt.mx

References

[1] Kalluri R, LeBleu VS. The biology, function, and biomedical applications of exosomes. Science. 2020;**367**(6478):eaau6977

[2] Liu J, Ren L, Li S, Li W, Zheng X, Yang Y, et al. The biology, function, and applications of exosomes in cancer. Acta Pharmaceutica Sinica B. 2021;**11**(9):2783-2797

[3] Saheera S, Jani VP, Witwer KW, Kutty S. Extracellular vesicle interplay in cardiovascular pathophysiology. American Journal of Physiology. Heart and Circulatory Physiology. 2021;**320**(5):H1749-H1H61

[4] Zhang XYX, Shi H, Wu L, Qian H, Xu W. Exosomes in cancer: Small particle, big player. Journal of Hematology & Oncology. 2015;**8**(83)

[5] Anand SSM, Mathivanan S. Exomeres: A new member of extracellular vesicles family. Sub-Cellular Biochemistry. 2021;**97**:89-97

[6] Pegtel DMGS. Exosomes. Annual Review of Biochemistry. 2019;**88**:27

[7] Yuting Yang GS, Wang H, Li H, Zhang T, Tao N, Ding X. Interferometric plasmonic imaging and detection of single exosomes. PNAS. 2018;**115**(41):5

[8] Kalluri RLV. The biology, function, and biomedical applications of exosomes. Science. 2020;**7**:367

[9] Krylova SVFD. The machinery of exosomes: Biogenesis, release, and uptake. International Journal of Molecular Sciences. 2023;**24**:2

[10] Kahlert CKR. Exosomes in tumor microenvironment influence cancer progression and metastasis. Journal of Molecular Medicine (Berlin, Germany). 2013;**9**(4):7

[11] Saheera S, Potnuri AG, Krishnamurthy P. Nano-vesicle (Mis) communication in senescence-related pathologies. Cell. 2020;**9**:9

[12] Winter VH, M.T. Exploring the ESCRTing machinery in eukaryotes. Trends in Plant Science. 2006;**11**:9

[13] Chiaruttini NR-ML, Colom A, Humbert F, Lenz M, Scheuring S, Roux A. Relaxation of loaded ESCRT-III spiral springs drives membrane deformation. Cell. 2015;**163**(4):14

[14] Perez-Hernandez DG-VC, Jorge I, López-Martín S, Ursa A, Sánchez-Madrid F, Vázquez J, et al. The intracellular interactome of tetraspanin-enriched microdomains reveals their function as sorting machineries toward exosomes. The Journal of Biological Chemistry. 2013;**288**(17):13

[15] Trajkovic KHC, Chiantia S, Rajendran L, Wenzel D, Wieland F, Schwille P, et al. Ceramide triggers budding of exosome vesicles into multivesicular endosomes. Science. 2008;**29**(319):4

[16] Lau NCHY, J.W.P. From exosome biogenesis to absorption: Key takeaways for cancer research. Cancers. 2023;**15**:1992

[17] Polo S, Sigismund S, Faretta M, Guidi M, Capua MR, Bossi G, et al. A single motif responsible for ubiquitin recognition and monoubiquitination in endocytic proteins. Nature. 2002;**416**:451-455

[18] Villarroya-Beltri CG-VC, Sánchez-Cabo F, Pérez-Hernández D, Vázquez J, Martin-Cofreces N, Martinez-Herrera DJ, et al. Sumoylated hnRNPA2B1 controls the sorting of miRNAs into exosomes through binding to specific motifs. Nature Communications. 2013;**288**(17):12

[19] Ferreira JV, da Rosa Soares A, Ramalho J, Carvalho CM, Cardoso MH, Pintado P, et al. LAMP2A regulates the loading of proteins into exosomes. Science Advances. 2022;**8**(12):eabm1140

[20] Moreno-Gonzalo OF-DI, Sanchez-Madrid F. Post-translational add-ons mark the path in exosomal protein sorting. Cellular and Molecular Life Sciences. 2018;**8**:eabm1140

[21] TYYAM M. SNARE complex assembly and disassembly. Current Biology. 2018;**28**(8):R397, R401

[22] Stephan Munich AS-V, Buchser WJ, Beer-Stolz D, Vujanovic NL. Dendritic cell exosomes directly kill tumor cells and activate natural killer cells via TNF superfamily ligands. OncoImmunology. 2012;**1**(7):1074-1083

[23] Johnstone RMAM, Hammond JR, Orr L, Turbide C. Vesicle formation during reticulocyte maturation. Association of plasma membrane activities with released vesicles (exosomes). The Journal of Biological Chemistry. 1987;**262**(19):9412-9420

[24] Poliakov ASM, Dokland T, Amling CL, Mobley JA. Structural heterogeneity and protein composition of exosome-like vesicles (prostasomes) in human semen. The Prostate. 2009;**69**(2):159-167

[25] Alvarez MLKM, Kanchi Ravi R, DiStefano JK. Comparison of protein, microRNA, and mRNA yields using different methods of urinary exosome isolation for the discovery of kidney disease biomarkers. Kidney. 2012;**82**(9):1024-1032

[26] Zhang PHM, Zeng Y. Ultrasensitive microfluidic analysis of circulating exosomes using a nanostructured graphene oxide/polydopamine coating. Lab on a Chip. 2016;**16**(16):3033-3042

[27] Zhao ZYY, Zeng Y, He M. A microfluidic ExoSearch chip for multiplexed exosome detection towards blood-based ovarian cancer diagnosis. Lab on a Chip. 2016;**16**(3):489-496

[28] Dan Yu YL, Wang M, Jianmei G, Wenrong X, Cai H, Fang X, et al. Exosomes as a new frontier of cancer liquid biopsy. Molecular Cancer. 2022;**21**:56

[29] Wan YCG, Liu X, Hao SJ, Nisic M, Zhu CD, Xia YQ, et al. Rapid magnetic isolation of extracellular vesicles via lipid-based nanoprobes. Nature Biomedical Engineering. 2017;**1**:0058

[30] Tian FZS, Liu C, Han Z, Liu Y, Deng J, Li Y, et al. Protein analysis of extracellular vesicles to monitor and predict therapeutic response in metastatic breast cancer. Nature Communications. 2021;**12**(1):2536

[31] Lee KSH, Weissleder R, Lee H. Acoustic purification of extracellular microvesicles. ACS Nano. 2015;**9**(3):2321-2327

[32] Govindappa PK, Patil M, Garikipati VNS, Verma SK, Saheera S, Narasimhan G, et al. Targeting exosome-associated human antigen R attenuates fibrosis and inflammation in diabetic heart. The FASEB Journal. 2020;**34**(2):2238-2251

[33] Isola AL, Chen S. Exosomes: The messengers of health and disease.

Current Neuropharmacology. 2017;**15**(1):157-165

[34] Duan P, Tan J, Miao Y, Zhang Q. Potential role of exosomes in the pathophysiology, diagnosis, and treatment of hypoxic diseases. American Journal of Translational Research. 2019;**11**(3):1184-1201

[35] Basile DP, Anderson MD, Sutton TA. Pathophysiology of acute kidney injury. Comprehensive Physiology. 2012;**2**(2):1303-1353

[36] Lee SA, Choi C, Yoo TH. Extracellular vesicles in kidneys and their clinical potential in renal diseases. Kidney Research and Clinical Practice. 2021;**40**(2):194-207

[37] Liu X, Miao J, Wang C, Zhou S, Chen S, Ren Q, et al. Tubule-derived exosomes play a central role in fibroblast activation and kidney fibrosis. Kidney International. 2020;**97**(6):1181-1195

[38] Borges FT, Melo SA, Ozdemir BC, Kato N, Revuelta I, Miller CA, et al. TGF-beta1-containing exosomes from injured epithelial cells activate fibroblasts to initiate tissue regenerative responses and fibrosis. Journal of the American Society of Nephrology. 2013;**24**(3):385-392

[39] Dominguez JH, Liu Y, Gao H, Dominguez JM 2nd, Xie D, Kelly KJ. Renal tubular cell-derived extracellular vesicles accelerate the recovery of established renal ischemia reperfusion injury. Journal of the American Society of Nephrology. 2017;**28**(12):3533-3544

[40] Zhou X, Zhao S, Li W, Ruan Y, Yuan R, Ning J, et al. Tubular cell-derived exosomal miR-150-5p contributes to renal fibrosis following unilateral ischemia-reperfusion injury by activating fibroblast *in vitro* and *in vivo*. International Journal of Biological Sciences. 2021;**17**(14):4021-4033

[41] Lv LL, Feng Y, Wu M, Wang B, Li ZL, Zhong X, et al. Exosomal miRNA-19b-3p of tubular epithelial cells promotes M1 macrophage activation in kidney injury. Cell Death and Differentiation. 2020;**27**(1):210-226

[42] Jin M, Zhang S, Wang M, Li Q, Ren J, Luo Y, et al. Exosomes in pathogenesis, diagnosis, and therapy of ischemic stroke. Frontiers in Bioengineering and Biotechnology. 2022;**10**:980548

[43] Sonoda H, Yokota-Ikeda N, Oshikawa S, Kanno Y, Yoshinaga K, Uchida K, et al. Decreased abundance of urinary exosomal aquaporin-1 in renal ischemia-reperfusion injury. American Journal of Physiology. Renal Physiology. 2009;**297**(4):F1006-F1016

[44] Zhou C, Zhou F, He Y, Liu Y, Cao Y. Exosomes in cerebral ischemia-reperfusion injury: Current perspectives and future challenges. Brain Sciences. 2022;**12**(12):1657

[45] Zhang L, Mao L, Wang H. The neuroprotection effects of exosome in central nervous system injuries: A new target for therapeutic intervention. Molecular Neurobiology. 2022;**59**(12):7152-7169

[46] Pei X, Li Y, Zhu L, Zhou Z. Astrocyte-derived exosomes suppress autophagy and ameliorate neuronal damage in experimental ischemic stroke. Experimental Cell Research. 2019;**382**(2):111474

[47] Song Y, Li Z, He T, Qu M, Jiang L, Li W, et al. M2 microglia-derived exosomes protect the mouse brain from ischemia-reperfusion injury via exosomal miR-124. Theranostics. 2019;**9**(10):2910-2923

[48] Qian Y, Chopp M, Chen J. Emerging role of microRNAs in ischemic stroke with comorbidities. Experimental Neurology. 2020;**331**:113382

[49] Zhang D, Cai G, Liu K, Zhuang Z, Jia K, Pei S, et al. Microglia exosomal miRNA-137 attenuates ischemic brain injury through targeting Notch1. Aging (Albany NY). 2021;**13**(3):4079-4095

[50] Wan T, Huang Y, Gao X, Wu W, Guo W. Microglia polarization: A novel target of exosome for stroke treatment. Frontiers in Cell and Development Biology. 2022;**10**:842320

[51] Pluta R, Jablonski M. Exosomes in post-ischemic brain. In: Pluta R, editor. Cerebral Ischemia. Brisbane, Australia: Exon Publications; 2021

[52] Li H, Luo Y, Liu P, Liu P, Hua W, Zhang Y, et al. Exosomes containing miR-451a is involved in the protective effect of cerebral ischemic preconditioning against cerebral ischemia and reperfusion injury. CNS Neuroscience & Therapeutics. 2021;**27**(5):564-576

[53] Meng S, Su Z, Liu Z, Wang N, Wang Z. Rac1 contributes to cerebral ischemia reperfusion-induced injury in mice by regulation of Notch2. Neuroscience. 2015;**306**:100-114

[54] Lee EC, Ha TW, Lee DH, Hong DY, Park SW, Lee JY, et al. Utility of exosomes in ischemic and hemorrhagic stroke diagnosis and treatment. International Journal of Molecular Sciences. 2022;**23**(15):8367

[55] He J, Liu D, Zhao L, Zhou D, Rong J, Zhang L, et al. Myocardial ischemia/reperfusion injury: Mechanisms of injury and implications for management (review). Experimental and Therapeutic Medicine. 2022;**23**(6):430

[56] Liu N, Xie L, Xiao P, Chen X, Kong W, Lou Q, et al. Cardiac fibroblasts secrete exosome microRNA to suppress cardiomyocyte pyroptosis in myocardial ischemia/reperfusion injury. Molecular and Cellular Biochemistry. 2022;**477**(4):1249-1260

[57] Zhai TY, Cui BH, Zhou Y, Xu XY, Zou L, Lin X, et al. Exosomes released from CaSR-stimulated PMNs reduce ischaemia/reperfusion injury. Oxidative Medicine and Cellular Longevity. 2021;**2021**:3010548

[58] Halkein J, Tabruyn SP, Ricke-Hoch M, Haghikia A, Nguyen NQ, Scherr M, et al. MicroRNA-146a is a therapeutic target and biomarker for peripartum cardiomyopathy. The Journal of Clinical Investigation. 2013;**123**(5):2143-2154

[59] Johnson T, Zhao L, Manuel G, Taylor H, Liu D. Approaches to therapeutic angiogenesis for ischemic heart disease. Journal of Molecular Medicine (Berlin, Germany). 2019;**97**(2):141-151

[60] Jadli AS, Parasor A, Gomes KP, Shandilya R, Patel VB. Exosomes in cardiovascular diseases: Pathological potential of nano-messenger. Frontiers in Cardiovascular Medicine. 2021;**8**:767488

[61] Rosand O, Hoydal MA. Cardiac exosomes in ischemic heart disease-a narrative review. Diagnostics (Basel). 2021;**11**(2):269

[62] Zhang J, Zhang X. Ischaemic preconditioning-induced serum exosomes protect against myocardial ischaemia/reperfusion injury in rats by activating the PI3K/AKT signalling pathway. Cell Biochemistry and Function. 2021;**39**(2):287-295

[63] Li D, Zhao Y, Zhang C, Wang F, Zhou Y, Jin S. Plasma exosomes at the late phase of remote ischemic pre-conditioning attenuate myocardial ischemia-reperfusion injury through transferring miR-126a-3p. Frontiers in Cardiovascular Medicine. 2021;**8**:736226

[64] Ma H, Wang C, Liu X, Zhan M, Wei W, Niu J. Src homolog and collagen homolog1 isoforms in acute and chronic liver injuries. Life Sciences. 2021;**273**:119302

[65] Jiao Y, Xu P, Shi H, Chen D, Shi H. Advances on liver cell-derived exosomes in liver diseases. Journal of Cellular and Molecular Medicine. 2021;**25**(1):15-26

[66] Nojima H, Freeman CM, Schuster RM, Japtok L, Kleuser B, Edwards MJ, et al. Hepatocyte exosomes mediate liver repair and regeneration via sphingosine-1-phosphate. Journal of Hepatology. 2016;**64**(1):60-68

[67] Zhao J, Chen XD, Yan ZZ, Huang WF, Liu KX, Li C. Gut-derived exosomes induce liver injury after intestinal ischemia/reperfusion by promoting hepatic macrophage polarization. Inflammation. 2022;**45**(6):2325-2338

[68] Mendt M, Rezvani K, Shpall E. Mesenchymal stem cell-derived exosomes for clinical use. Bone Marrow Transplantation. 2019;**54**(Suppl 2):789-792

[69] Janockova J, Slovinska L, Harvanova D, Spakova T, Rosocha J. New therapeutic approaches of mesenchymal stem cells-derived exosomes. Journal of Biomedical Science. 2021;**28**(1):39

[70] Tenchov R, Sasso JM, Wang X, Liaw WS, Chen CA, Zhou QA. Exosomes horizontal line nature's lipid nanoparticles, a rising star in drug delivery and diagnostics. ACS Nano. 2022;**16**(11):17802-17846

[71] Hade MD, Suire CN, Suo Z. Mesenchymal stem cell-derived exosomes: Applications in regenerative medicine. Cell. 2021;**10**(8):1959

[72] Tian T, Zhang HX, He CP, Fan S, Zhu YL, Qi C, et al. Surface functionalized exosomes as targeted drug delivery vehicles for cerebral ischemia therapy. Biomaterials. 2018;**150**:137-149

[73] Moeinabadi-Bidgoli K, Rezaee M, Hossein-Khannazer N, Babajani A, Aghdaei HA, Arki MK, et al. Exosomes for angiogenesis induction in ischemic disorders. Journal of Cellular and Molecular Medicine. 2023;**27**(6):763-787

[74] Arabpour M, Saghazadeh A, Rezaei N. Anti-inflammatory and M2 macrophage polarization-promoting effect of mesenchymal stem cell-derived exosomes. International Immunopharmacology. 2021;**97**:107823

[75] Patil M, Saheera S, Dubey PK, Kahn-Krell A, Kumar Govindappa P, Singh S, et al. Novel mechanisms of exosome-mediated phagocytosis of dead cells in injured heart. Circulation Research. 2021;**129**(11):1006-1020

[76] Xunian Z, Kalluri R. Biology and therapeutic potential of mesenchymal stem cell-derived exosomes. Cancer Science. 2020;**111**(9):3100-3110

[77] Xu R, Bai Y, Min S, Xu X, Tang T, Ju S. In vivo monitoring and assessment of exogenous mesenchymal stem cell-derived exosomes in mice with ischemic stroke by molecular imaging. International Journal of Nanomedicine. 2020;**15**:9011-9023

[78] Kosanovic M, Milutinovic B, Kutzner TJ, Mouloud Y, Bozic M. Clinical

prospect of mesenchymal stromal/stem cell-derived extracellular vesicles in kidney disease: Challenges and the way forward. Pharmaceutics. 2023;**15**(7):1911

[79] Dabrowska S, Andrzejewska A, Lukomska B, Janowski M. Neuroinflammation as a target for treatment of stroke using mesenchymal stem cells and extracellular vesicles. Journal of Neuroinflammation. 2019;**16**(1):178

[80] Gao J, Li A, Hu J, Feng L, Liu L, Shen Z. Recent developments in isolating methods for exosomes. Frontiers in Bioengineering and Biotechnology. 2022;**10**:1100892

[81] Yakubovich EI, Polischouk AG, Evtushenko VI. Principles and problems of exosome isolation from biological fluids. Biochemistry (Moscow), Supplement Series A: Membrane and Cell Biology. 2022;**16**(2):115-126

[82] Dimik M, Abeysinghe P, Logan J, Mitchell M. The exosome: A review of current therapeutic roles and capabilities in human reproduction. Drug Delivery and Translational Research. 2023;**13**(2):473-502

[83] Adlerz K, Patel D, Rowley J, Ng K, Ahsan T. Strategies for scalable manufacturing and translation of MSC-derived extracellular vesicles. Stem Cell Research. 2020;**48**:101978

[84] Schwarzenbach H, Gahan PB. Exosomes in immune regulation. Noncoding RNA. 2021;7:1

[85] Bhatia R, Chang J, Munoz JL, Walker ND. Forging new therapeutic targets: Efforts of tumor derived exosomes to prepare the pre-metastatic niche for cancer cell dissemination and dormancy. Biomedicine. 2023;**11**(6):1614

[86] Liang Y, Duan L, Lu J, Xia J. Engineering exosomes for targeted drug delivery. Theranostics. 2021;**11**(7):3183-3195

[87] Chen S, Sun F, Qian H, Xu W, Jiang J. Preconditioning and engineering strategies for improving the efficacy of mesenchymal stem cell-derived exosomes in cell-free therapy. Stem Cells International. 2022;**2022**:1779346

[88] Batrakova EV, Kim MS. Development and regulation of exosome-based therapy products. Wiley Interdisciplinary Reviews. Nanomedicine and Nanobiotechnology. 2016;**8**(5):744-757

[89] Asadpour A, Yahaya BH, Bicknell K, Cottrell GS, Widera D. Uncovering the gray zone: Mapping the global landscape of direct-to-consumer businesses offering interventions based on secretomes, extracellular vesicles, and exosomes. Stem Cell Research & Therapy. 2023;**14**(1):111

Section 5

Renal Ischemia and Hypoxia

Chapter 11

Renal Ischemia and Hypoxia: Functional Differences and Possible Clinical and Therapeutic Consequences

Robbert Bipat, Paul Steels and Jerry Toelsie

Abstract

End stage kidney disease contributes to a huge burden on global health. Recent advances have shown that ischemic and hypoxic conditions may contribute to the progression of the disorder and that acute kidney injury may cause and aggravate the condition. Ischemia and hypoxia are two distinct conditions with different pathophysiological and structural consequences as proven in the brain and liver of rats. Until now, these differences have not been shown to exist in the kidney. In this study, we assess the possible functional differences in the outcome of ischemic and hypoxic stress on the kidney. For this purpose, we perfused isolated rabbit kidneys with their autologous blood and applied short periods of ischemia or hypoxia in separate series of experiments. The results showed that the kidneys exposed to hypoxic stress suffered more functional damage than those subjected to ischemia. This conclusion was based on a lower creatinine clearance and urine osmolality, and a higher fractional excretion of urea, sodium, and glucose in the hypoxia series of kidneys. Consequently, we recommend monitoring hypoxemic conditions closely and correcting the condition as soon as possible, since even for a short period it may already have deteriorating effects on the renal function.

Keywords: isolated perfused rabbit kidney, autologous blood, hypoxia, ischemia, renal failure, urine osmolality, acute kidney injury

1. Introduction

1.1 Ischemia or hypoxia

Ischemia and hypoxia play major roles in the pathophysiology of important diseases and conditions like stroke [1], cardiovascular disease [2], and even Alzheimer's dementia [3], but also in therapeutic procedures like the survival of organ transplants [4, 5]. Survival of organ transplants as well as patients depends on the proper function of the graft [6], while for some procedures like renal transplantation, there is an inherent period of sustained ischemia and hypoxia [7, 8].

IntechOpen

Traditionally the terms ischemia and hypoxia are mixed and often used without any distinction between these two entities [3, 9–13]. This assumption is probably based on the common molecular reactions observed in ischemia as well as hypoxia [14]. Investigators, however, have found clear distinctions in the pathophysiological consequences of these entities. For instance, a study on rats showed that experimental ischemia of the brains led to necrosis of the neurons while this consequence was absent under hypoxic conditions, even at a low perfusion pressure of 30 mmHg [15]. Another study showed that the veno-arterial difference of PCO_2 was far less under hypoxic conditions compared to ischemia in the hindlimb of dogs [16], and consequently implies that ischemia and hypoxia may follow different mechanisms of disease. In this chapter ischemia is defined as a sudden decrease in perfusion pressure of the kidney, while hypoxia is defined as a reduction in partial oxygen pressure in the blood with intact perfusion [17, 18].

In addition to the pathologic conditions mentioned above, hypoxia also plays a role in the physiological regulation of physiological processes. For instance, the process of angiogenesis is triggered by hypoxic conditions in the absence of a total ischemic shutdown of the vessels [10]. Hypoxia also plays a role in the differentiation of stem cells [19, 20]. Furthermore, the condition is involved in wound healing [21] and it is believed that mild hypoxia promotes vessel growth in the placenta during pregnancy [22].

Conditions involving hypoxia, but not ischemia include, for instance, moderate to severe anemia and diseases that limit the gas exchange in the lungs. Anemia leads to hypoxic conditions in the tissues of organs that are prone to an already low oxygen pressure under physiological conditions. These are, for example, the epithelial lining of the gut [23] and the medullary vasa recta in the kidneys [24]. Recent findings, however, demonstrate that both structural and functional changes occur because of anemia leading to hypoxia in tissues that are normally abundantly oxygenated [25]. Furthermore, tumors are especially susceptible to hypoxia in anemic states [26].

Apart from anemia, conditions that limit the diffusing capacity in the pulmonary alveoli will also lead to hypoxic conditions in other organs and tissues. For instance, hypoxic hepatitis can be the result of respiratory or cardiac failure with respiratory failure being responsible for 13–20% of the cases [27]. One of the important contributing factors to the damage seen in this disorder of the liver is hypoxemia [28]. The condition was formerly more known as “shock liver” and the change in nomenclature highlights the role that hypoxia plays in its pathophysiology [28].

Recently we saw more hypoxemic conditions with the advent of the SARS-2 COVID 19 pandemic. Even without clear signs, patients suffering from this infection show mild to moderate hypoxemia [29]. Furthermore, in the absence of direct damage caused by the virus, pathologic conditions observed in the heart, liver, and kidneys in severe conditions of this infection hint toward the involvement of hypoxic conditions in these organs [30–33]. Recently studies described the possible effect of air pollution on the development of chronic kidney disease [34]. The cause is probably the presence of specific particulate matter in the air, but it remains to be determined if a low atmospheric oxygen content may also contribute to this [35].

1.2 Kidney disease and hypoxia

The global prevalence of chronic kidney disease was estimated between 9 and 14% of the population, and the number of patients who needed kidney replacement therapy exceeded 5 million in 2017 [36, 37]. With an annual individual cost of up to

40,000 Euro [38], this easily amounts to at least 200 billion Euro and is one of the most challenging public health concerns. The main causes of chronic kidney disease are diabetes and hypertension [39]. Furthermore, acute kidney injury plays a key role in the etiology and progress of the disease [40]. For both the acute and the chronic phases of the disease, hypoxia of the medullary environment plays a role in both the initial cause and then the progression to chronic and end-stage renal disease [41–44]. The hypoxia may be the result of ischemic disease [45], nephrotoxic damage of the renal interstitial space [43, 46], or from disturbances not related to the kidney [31].

1.3 Isolated perfused kidneys

The kidney is a very intricate organ with highly coordinated activity. The experimental investigation of renal function must be separated from extrarenal and potential intrarenal regulatory mechanisms due to the interdependence of organs [47, 48]. Studies in vivo are frequently hampered by contemporaneous changes in blood pressure, circulating fluid volume, CO_2 and O_2 tensions, or neurogenic and hormonal reactions to experimental stimuli [48]. For these reasons, it is very convenient to study the function of the kidney under healthy and pathological circumstances in isolated perfused preparations of the organ. There are various methods to isolate and perfuse kidneys.

The idea to artificially perfuse organs originated in the 18th century when Le Gallois thought of a substitute for the heart to maintain any part of the body indefinitely [49], first attempts to perfuse isolated organs were not made until the 19th century by Löbell [50]. With the introduction of the isolated perfused rat kidney in 1959, the era of isolated perfused kidneys started [51] and in the following years, kidneys of various animals like dogs, rabbits, pigs, sheep, monkeys and even human kidneys have been isolated and perfused [52]. Studies concentrated on the physiology, pathophysiology, and pharmacology of renal function [53–56].

In the past 60 years, it has become clear that the function of the isolated perfused kidneys depends largely on the choice of perfusate. This varies between a completely artificial physiological buffer to autologous blood. All studies have shown that the best physiological results were achieved from preparations perfused with any kind of perfusates that contained red blood cells, preferably autologous blood [48]. Organs perfused with a low content of red blood cells always show moderate to severe degrees of necrosis in the medullary part of the kidneys [57]. For these reasons, we developed an isolated rabbit kidney model that was perfused with autologous blood [58].

1.4 Aim of the study

In this study we applied short-term ischemic and hypoxic conditions to isolated rabbit kidneys perfused with autologous blood. The goal of this was to determine whether there is a difference in effects with these two conditions since this will affect the way we think about their pathophysiologic mechanisms and possible management of these conditions in the clinical setting. Isolated kidneys perfused with blood already show structural and functional defects in the organ at 7–25 minutes of warm ischemia [59]. Consequently, we limited the ischemia and hypoxia time to 25 minutes, to keep the possibility of fast recovery of the organ after reperfusion and reoxygenation. This allowed us to establish possible functional differences between these two kinds of interventions since previous studies showed that the isolated organ worked perfectly for about 2–3 hours [58].

2. Methods

2.1 Surgery and setup

The surgery and perfusion were carried out exactly as described by Cuypers and coworkers [48, 58]. Briefly, rabbits weighing 3–4 kg had their left kidneys removed under ketamine anesthesia (3–10 mg/kg body weight), and the kidney was then perfused with a modest volume (25 ml) of the same animal's heparinized blood in a closed circuit with a pump and an oxygenator. Warm oil was dripped over the kidney surface while the entire circulatory system was kept in a bath with temperature control set at 38°C. A PowerLab 4E analog-digital converter (AD Instruments) was used to constantly monitor and record perfusion pressure (Gould Statham pressure transducer: P23 ID) and renal blood flow (RBF; Skalar Transflow 600 System, extracorporeal probe, internal diameter 3 mm). The pumping system was set to maintain the perfusion pressure at 100 mm Hg. The oxygenator was perfused with a gas mixture of either 96% O_2 and 4% CO_2 under normal conditions or 96% N_2 and 4% CO_2 to create a hypoxic condition at a perfusion rate of 300 mL/min. **Figure 1** gives an overview of this setup.

2.2 Perfusion and renal function

A ureteral catheter was used to collect urine. Continuous infusion (0.1 ml/min) was administered throughout the perfusion to make up for urine excretion. The infusion solution's composition (in mM) was as follows: 35 mM NaCl, 40 mM KCl, 7.3 mM creatinine, 133 mM urea, 3.4 mM NaH2PO4, 13.6 mM Na2HPO4, 22.6 mM NaHCO3,

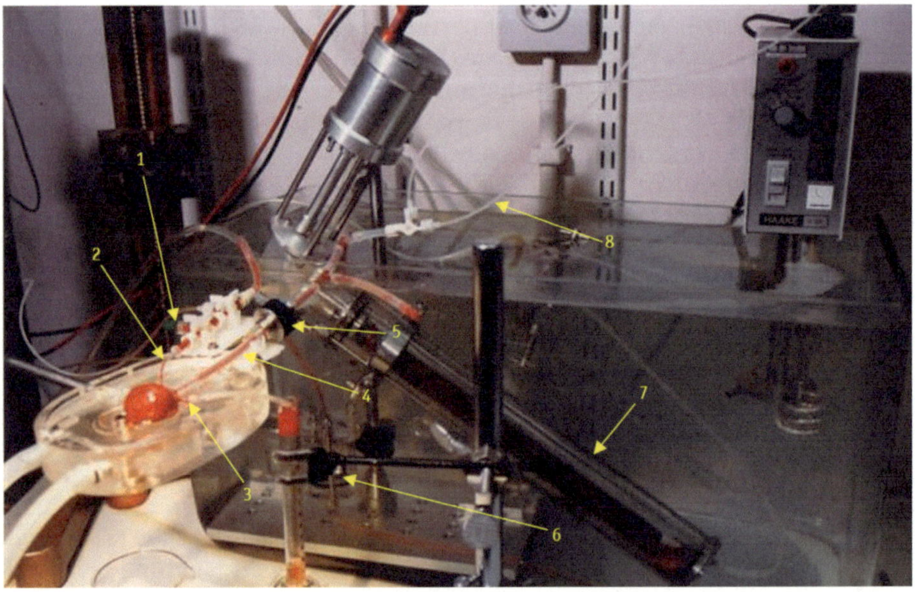

Figure 1.
The experimental setup. 1. Arterial sampling site, 2. Arterial line, 3. Ureter, 4. Venous line, 5. Flow sensor, 6. Pulsating pump in warm water bath, 7. Oxygenator in water bath, 8. Infusion lines. Taken from [48] with permission.

10 mM glutamine, and 55 mM glucose. Additionally, it had 30 IU/l of [Arg8]-vasopressin (AVP; Sigma). Additional NaCl (145–290 mM) was administered to make up for the extra urine output and osmolyte loss when urine flow (UF) surpassed 0.1 ml/min. All infusion was stopped when urine flow was zero. The hematocrit was maintained at 32–33% by replacing any blood loss through sampling and hemorrhage with an equivalent volume of whole blood. The kidneys were given at least 25 minutes to recover after the perfusion was established. After the first recovery, there were four 30-min perfusion sessions (P1–P4) during which urine was taken. At the conclusion of each period, blood samples were obtained. As a baseline, the data entered in P1 were used.

2.3 Experimental procedures

In the first series of experiments (n = 5), the perfusion of the kidney was shut down with a direct bypass of the arterial line to the venous line during the second period (P2). In P3 the perfusion was restored. The reason for keeping the blood in circulation was to prevent stagnation, which would lead to the formation of thrombotic and vasoconstrictive factors [60]. In the second series of studies (n = 5), the oxygenator's oxygen supply was stopped at the end of P1 and replaced with nitrogen (96 percent N_2, 4 percent CO_2), which was provided during P2 (25–30 min). This caused a drop in mean arterial blood PO_2 from 144 ± 36 to 11 ± 3 mm Hg (n = 5, with SD). The perfusion pressure was kept at 100 mmHg and the flow rate of gas through the oxygenator at 300 mL/min. In P3 and P4 the perfusion and oxygenation were restored (**Figure 2**).

2.4 Animals and chemicals

The highest-grade chemicals were used throughout, and they were all acquired from Sigma Belgium. White adult rabbits were housed in the university's animal facility. All institutional ethical norms and procedures were followed when handling animals.

2.5 Analyses and calculations

A Beckman Synchron Clinical System CX3 was used to perform Na+, K+, urea, and creatinine analyses on plasma and urine samples. A Knauer-Halb micro-osmometer was used to measure the osmolality of the plasma and urine. To assess the glomerular filtration rate, creatinine clearance (CCr) was computed as CCr = (UCr UF)/PCr, where UCr and PCr stand for the creatinine concentrations in the urine and plasma, respectively (GFR). With the use of a Chiron Diagnostics 238 pH/blood gas analyzer, pH, PCO2, and PO2 were measured (Bayer) [58].

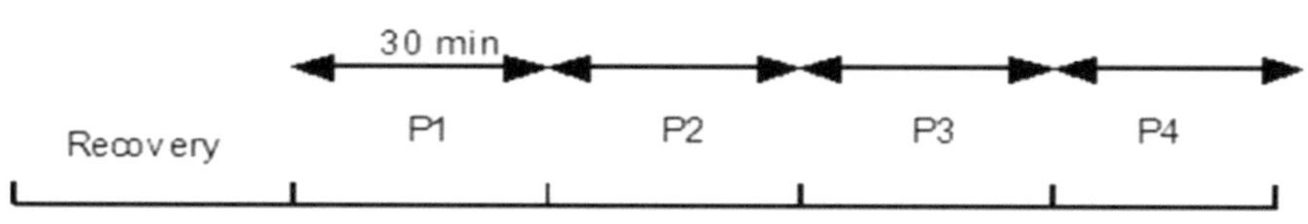

Figure 2.
Protocol of experiments.

2.6 Statistics

The data are presented as median with interquartile range and were evaluated using Student's T-test to compare the two series, and the Brown-Forsythe ANOVA test, followed by Dunnett's T3 multiple comparisons test to compare values within the series. Differences were deemed significant at $p < 0.05$.

3. Results

The main findings are summarized in **Table 1**.

The RBF increased during hypoxia in P2, but returned to the lower value in P3 and P4. **Figure 3** is a representative trace of this flow. After reperfusion, The RBF recovered in P3 and P4 in the ischemia series. The urine flow stopped in both series during the interventions in P2. In P3 and P4 it recovered in both series, but in the hypoxia series, there was a significantly higher urine flow compared to P1. The lack of urine flow in the P2 did not allow us to determine the rest of the parameters in this period. In both series the creatinine clearance (CCr) decreased in P3 and P4, but at a much lower value in the hypoxia series, despite a comparable increase of urine flow.

Urine osmolality decreased after both interventions but was significantly lower in the hypoxia series. The absolute urea excretion was significantly lower in the hypoxia

	Ischemia				Hypoxia			
	P1	P2	P3	P4	P1	P2	P3	P4
RBF (ml/min. gkw)	2.2 (1.7–2.7)	—	1.8 (1.4–2.1)	2.3 (1.8–2.8)	1.9 (1.6–3.0)	5.5 (4.5–6.5)$	2.7 (1.7–4.7)	3.0 (2.1–4.5)
PO_2 (mmHg)[†]	134 (89–189)		170 (150–221)	196 (170–262)	131 (115–180)	12 (9–14)	142 (126–204)	154 (135–194)
UF (microliter/ min.gkw)	4.0 (2.9–4.7)		3.2 (0.4–5.7)	5.6 (2.7–9.6)	3.8 (3.0–5.7)		1.7 (1.3–2.8)	9.4 (5.9–11.45)$
CCr (microliter/ min.gkw)	291 (228–438)		93 (41–113)$	149 (88–180)$	337 (248–530)		10 (6–13)$*	39 (33–51)$*
POsm (mOsm/kg)	279 (274–280)		283 (276–292)	287 (280–289)	278 (263–286)		283 (267–289)	280 (272–294)
UOsm (mOsm/kg)	690 (635–930)		430 (370–530)$	390 (320–420)$	740 (700–980)		310 (285–328)$*	310 (295–325)$*
PUrea (mmol/l)	15.7 (12.7–18.7)		21.3 (19.8–22.8)$	23.0 (22.0–30.4)$	14.2 (8.7–16.8)		20 (16.5–23)	24.8 (22.3–27.5)$
EUrea (micromole/ min.gkw)	0.69 (0.49–0.93)		0.48 (0.21–0.75)	0.96 (0.50–1.52)	0.64 (0.56–1.2)		0.11 (0.06–0.14)$*	0.54 (0.48–0.73)
FEUrea (%)	15 (12–17)		26 (23–29)$	43 (34–51)$	16 (13–27)		54 (50–66)$*	56 (50–68)$*

	Ischemia				Hypoxia			
	P1	P2	P3	P4	P1	P2	P3	P4
PNa (mmol/l)	138 (136–139)		138 (137–140)	138 (136–141)	135 (132–137)		130 (125–133)*	132 (127–136)*
ENa (micromole/ min.gkw)	0.69 (0.63–0.95)		0.39 (0.14–0.89)	0.67 (0.22–0.96)	0.93 (0.58–1.41)		0.19 (0.17–0.36)	1.12 (0.62–1.22)
FENa (%)	1.7 (1.3–2.4)		3.0 (2.5–5.6)	3.6 (2.8–8.1)	1.6 (1.2–2.6)		21.8 (18.3–23.6)$*	20 (13.1–22.6)$*
PK (mmol/l)	2.4 (2.1–2.6)		3.0 (2.5–4.0)	3.2 (2.5–5.2)	3.0 (2.4–3.8)		7.2 (6.6–7.8)$*	4.4 (3.7–4.7)
EK (micromole/ min.gkw)	0.47 (0.38–0.52)		0.17 (0.10–0.24)	0.23(0.14–0.35)	0.51 (0.34–0.60)		0.05 (0.03–0.06)*	0.24 (0.18–0.32)
PGluc (mg/100 ml)	204 (155–243)		141 (108–173)	101 (78–138)$	178 (163–244)		79 (61–102)$*	96 (55–112)$
FEGluc (%)	1.2 (1.0–29)		2.6 (1.1–5.5)	0.9 (0.5–2.9)	1.8 (1.4–4.6)		22 (12–25)$*	18 (10–25)$*

$ $p < 0.05$ versus P1.
** $p < 0.05$ versus ischemia.*
† at the end of the period, gkw: gram of kidney weight.
RBF: renal blood flow, PO2: partial oxygen pressure, UF: urine flow, CCr: creatinine clearance, POsm: plasma osmolality, UOsm: urine osmolality, PUrea: plasma urea, EUrea: absolute excretion of urea, FEUrea: fractional excretion of urea, PNa: plasma sodium, ENa: absolute excretion of sodium, FENa: fractional excretion of sodium, PK: plasma potassium, EK: absolute excretion of potassium, PGluc: plasma glucose, FEGluc: fractional excretion of glucose.

Table 1.
Renal function parameters found under ischemic and hypoxic conditions.

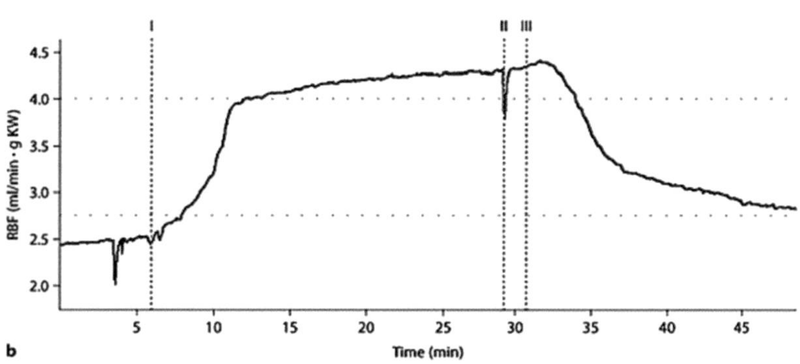

Figure 3.
Renal blood flow during hypoxia in an individual experiment. I: Start hypoxia, II: Sampling of blood, III: Reoxygenation (taken from [61] under a creative commons attribution non-commercial-No-Derivs 3.0 license. The full article is available at https://www.karger.com/article/FullText/333478).

series after reoxygenation and recovered in P4. In P3 and P4, the fractional excretion of urea was however higher in both series. The fractional excretion of sodium increased significantly higher after reoxygenation. Furthermore, the plasma potassium value was significantly higher in P3 after reoxygenation but decreased in P4 closer to the control value in P1. Finally, we found that the plasma glucose decreased significantly after reoxygenation and compared with the ischemia series, and in addition the fractional excretion of glucose was significantly higher after reoxygenation.

4. Discussion

In the present study we investigated the effects of two conditions, ischemia and hypoxia, on isolated rabbit kidneys perfused with autologous blood. Both these conditions led to acute renal failure, reflected by a significant decrease in creatinine clearance, increase of plasma urea, and decrease of urine osmolality in the presence of AVP, after reperfusion and reoxygenation, respectively. In addition, the decline in function was already observed after a short 30-minute intervention.

4.1 Renal blood flow, urine flow, and creatinine clearance

The increased renal blood flow during hypoxia is surprising since previous studies showed that hypoxemia leads to increased vascular resistance in the kidneys. Subjects who received donor kidneys had a higher vascular resistance under hypoxemic conditions, while the resistance was much lower with hyperoxia in the allograft [62]. Older studies concluded that reperfusion after ischemic injury resulted in a reduction of renal blood flow of up to 50% after reperfusion, a phenomenon called "no-reflow" [63–65]. The lower flow was not only the result of vasoconstriction but also suggestively an entrapment of red blood cells [66]. A recent study also reported a sustained lower renal blood flow in experimental ischemia in *in vivo* experiments conducted on rats [67]. We do not have any plausible explanation for the absence of significant vasoconstriction after ischemia and even the presence of vasodilatation during hypoxemia and after reoxygenation in our experiments. It may be due to the fact that the isolated organ is not under influence of other systemic influences after ischemia-reperfusion. Support for this can be found in the fact that with hypoxemia there is a generalized vasodilatation with resulting decreased perfusion pressure and renal blood flow. This induces vasoconstriction as a compensatory mechanism and is probably mediated by the renin-angiotensin aldosterone system [68]. Obviously, these mechanisms are not involved in our model.

The cessation of urine flow and consequently the creatinine clearance during ischemia is clearly the result of the absence of any perfusion pressure. However, this phenomenon is also observed during hypoxia. In previous reports, we showed that the absence of urine flow is possibly the result of a generalized swelling of oxygen-dependent cells. We found that the intratubular hydrostatic pressure increased during the hypoxic phase but remained at the control level when the infusion included mannitol. In these experiments, in the presence of mannitol, urine flow, and creatinine clearance remained reasonably good and were perhaps not due to the diuretic effect since furosemide did not produce this improvement [61, 69]. The high renal blood flow and the absence of vasoconstriction after reoxygenation argues against structural changes in the vessels.

4.2 Urine osmolality and urea excretion

The urine osmolality was significantly lower after both reperfusion and reoxygenation, but significantly less after the latter. Generally, acute renal failure is associated with lower urine osmolality values [70]. Here we observed a significantly lower urine osmolality in the case of hypoxia, to almost the plasma osmolality. This difference cannot be explained simply by the lack of energy in the thick ascending limb of the loop of Henle, since this should be the case in both experimental conditions. It is more plausible that with intact and higher blood flow in case of hypoxia, the necessary solutes for concentrating the urine are washed out in the medulla of the organ. The relatively low blood flow in the renal medulla under physiological conditions is absolutely necessary for the maintenance of this solute gradient [71]. The accompanying hypoxia will only worsen the concentrating capacity in this case [71].

We observed that the absolute excretion of urea was initially lower with hypoxia but recovered in the last period. Previous results showed that urea is necessary for the maximum concentrating capacity of these isolated perfused kidneys [72]. What we observed in the present study is that the absolute excretion of urea recovered quickly despite a very low creatinine clearance. Consequently, the fractional excretion (FEUrea) is significantly higher compared to controls, and this is more pronounced in the hypoxia series. In fact, one study suggested that a higher FEUrea is more closely associated with tubular necrosis and that a lower FEUrea reflects the possibility of prerenal failure [73]. Our findings are in line with these latter two outcomes, and this adds more evidence that the damage is more prominent in the hypoxia series compared to the ischemia series. Moreover, it was found that the FEUrea was significantly higher in persistent acute renal failure compared to the transient form that lasted up to 3 days in patients and that this parameter hence is useful as a marker for the seriousness of the condition [74]. The FEUrea can be calculated with a simple formula in a clinical setting, without determination of the GFR [1].

4.3 Sodium and potassium

Similar to the fractional excretion of urea, that of sodium (FENa) was also significantly higher in the hypoxia series compared to the ischemia after reoxygenation and reperfusion. Since the reabsorption of sodium is ATP dependent, this could mean that the high fractional excretion in the presence of sufficient energy after reoxygenation, there are already widespread functional problems after the short period of oxygen deprivation [75]. On the other hand, we also observe a high plasma potassium (PK) immediately after reoxygenation, which is immediately resolved in the last period of perfusion in the absence of a high K excretion. This means that the abundance of potassium was probably caused by exit from the intracellular space in the hypoxic state but re-entered the cells after oxygen supply was restored [61].

4.4 Glucose

The lower plasma glucose in the hypoxia series may be explained by the high energy demand to restore the intracellular potassium content as explained in the previous section [76]. In addition, it indicates that there are enough remaining cells to keep the metabolism ongoing. Furthermore, it may reflect a high utilization of glucose and ongoing glycolysis during the deprivation of oxygen. Indeed one study showed a tight coupling of the sodium-potassium ATPase to glycolysis in rat cardiomyocytes [77]. We also observed a higher fractional excretion of glucose after hypoxia compared to ischemia, which indicates that the hypoxic stress also interfered with the

---

[1] [(urine urea nitrogen/ blood urea nitrogen)/(urine creatinine/plasma creatinine)] × 100

proximal tubule function [78]. All these factors may explain the worse outcome of renal function during hypoxia compared to the ischemic state.

4.5 Clinical and therapeutic implications

The results of this study show that there is a functional difference between the outcome in conditions characterized by compromised perfusion of the kidney and a situation with intact circulation but with a low oxygen content of the blood. The outcome of the latter is worse with respect to renal functional parameters like creatinine clearance, urine osmolality, fractional excretion of urea, sodium and glucose, and escape of potassium from the intracellular space. Examples of clinical conditions accompanied by a low oxygen content in the blood are severe anemia [79], compromised diffusion of oxygen in the lungs as we have seen in COVID-19 cases [31, 80], and cardiopulmonary bypass procedures [81]. The present results accentuate that it is of paramount importance to preserve the oxygen supply to the kidneys, to prevent worsening of the organ's function in circulatory compromised situations or procedures. It is, therefore, important to monitor hemoglobin level and oxygen saturation in patients at risk, since hypoxemia may sometimes be present without clinical signs [80, 82]. In addition, we have shown that even a short period of hypoxemia may already cause functional damage to the kidney. This should be a reason to recommend that the monitoring and treatment of the hypoxemia conditions should be more vigilant [83]. Who knows, maybe there is such a condition as pulmo-renal syndrome similar to hepatorenal syndrome?

5. Conclusion

There is a clear distinction in the pathophysiological consequences of ischemia and hypoxia. In this study, we showed thathypoxemia without compromise of the circulation has a significantly worse outcome for renal function, even when present for only a short time of 30 minutes. Acute kidney disease or injury can evolve into chronic disorders or may worsen an already chronic situation. We, therefore, recommend that possible hypoxic states must be monitored closely and corrected adequately in conditions accompanied by an inherent circulatory or oxygen content deficiency.

Acknowledgements

We are indebted to Prof Dr. Yves Cuypers, who passed away in 2018. He taught us the technique of perfusing isolated kidneys with blood. Our gratitude also involves Wilfried Leyssens who passed away in 2015. They both participated in the design of and assisted to conduct the study presented here.

Conflict of interest

"The authors declare no conflict of interest." The study was carried out with funds available from the university.

DOI: http://dx.doi.org/10.5772/intechopen.1002391

Author details

Robbert Bipat[1*], Paul Steels[2] and Jerry Toelsie[1]

1 Faculty of Medicine, Department of Physiology, Anton de Kom University of Suriname, Paramaribo, Suriname

2 Faculty of Medicine, Department of Physiology, University of Hasselt, Hasselt, Belgium

*Address all correspondence to: robbert.bipat@uvs.edu

References

[1] Nour M, Scalzo F, Liebeskind DS. Ischemia-reperfusion injury in stroke. Interventional Neurology. 2012;**1**:185-199. DOI: 10.1159/000353125

[2] Semenza GL. Hypoxia-inducible factor 1 and cardiovascular disease. Annual Review of Physiology. 2014;**76**:39. DOI: 10.1146/annurev-physiol-021113-170322

[3] Salminen A, Kauppinen A, Kaarniranta K. Hypoxia/ischemia activate processing of amyloid precursor protein: Impact of vascular dysfunction in the pathogenesis of Alzheimer's disease. Journal of Neurochemistry. 2017;**140**:536-549. DOI: 10.1111/JNC.13932

[4] Zhao H, Alam A, Soo AP, George AJT, Ma D. Ischemia-reperfusion injury reduces long term renal graft survival: Mechanism and beyond. eBioMedicine. 2018;**28**:31-42. DOI: 10.1016/j.ebiom.2018.01.025

[5] Fernández AR, Sánchez-Tarjuelo R, Cravedi P, Ochando J, López-Hoyos M. Review: Ischemia reperfusion injury—A translational perspective in organ transplantation. International Journal of Molecular Sciences. 2020;**21**:8549. DOI: 10.3390/IJMS21228549

[6] Yarlagadda SG, Coca SG, Formica RN, Poggio ED, Parikh CR. Association between delayed graft function and allograft and patient survival: A systematic review and meta-analysis. Nephrology Dialysis Transplantation. 2009;**24**:1039-1047. DOI: 10.1093/NDT/GFN667

[7] Perico N, Cattaneo D, Sayegh MH, Remuzzi G. Delayed graft function in kidney transplantation. Lancet. 2004;**364**:1814-1827. DOI: 10.1016/S0140-6736(04)17406-0

[8] Rosenberger C, Eckardt KU. Oxygenation of the transplanted kidney. Seminars in Nephrology. 2019;**39**:554-566. DOI: 10.1016/j.semnephrol.2019.10.005

[9] Northington FJ, Chavez-Valdez R, Martin LJ. Neuronal cell death in neonatal hypoxia-ischemia. Annals of Neurology. 2011;**69**:743-758. DOI: 10.1002/ana.22419

[10] Semenza GL. Vascular responses to hypoxia and ischemia. Arteriosclerosis, Thrombosis, and Vascular Biology. 2010;**30**:648-652. DOI: 10.1161/atvbaha.108.181644

[11] Jiang M, Liu K, Luo J, Dong Z. Autophagy is a Renoprotective mechanism during in vitro hypoxia and in vivo ischemia-reperfusion injury. The American Journal of Pathology. 2010;**176**:1181-1192. DOI: 10.2353/AJPATH.2010.090594

[12] Douglas-Escobar M, Weiss MD. Biomarkers of hypoxic-ischemic encephalopathy in newborns. Frontiers in Neurology. 2012;**3**:144. DOI: 10.3389/

[13] Malek M, Nematbakhsh M. Renal ischemia/reperfusion injury; from pathophysiology to treatment. Journal of Renal Injury Prevention. 2015;**4**:20. DOI: 10.12861/jrip.2015.06

[14] Rosenberger C, Mandriota S, Jürgensen JS, Wiesener MS, Hörstrup JH, Frei U, et al. Expression of hypoxia-inducible factor-1α and -2α in hypoxic and ischemic rat kidneys. Journal of the American Society of Nephrology.

2002;**13**:1721-1732. DOI: 10.1097/01.asn.0000017223.49823.2a

[15] Miyamoto O, Auer RN. Hypoxia, hyperoxia, ischemia, and brain necrosis. Neurology. 2000;**54**:362-362. DOI: 10.1212/wnl.54.2.362

[16] Vallet B, Teboul JL, Cain S, Curtis S. Venoarterial CO2 difference during regional ischemic or hypoxic hypoxia. Journal of Applied Physiology. 2000;**89**:1317-1321. DOI: 10.1152/jappl.2000.89.4.1317

[17] Brezis M, Rosen S, Silva P, Epstein FH. Renal ischemia: A new perspective. Kidney International. 1984;**26**:375-383. DOI: 10.1038/ki.1984.185

[18] Abuelo JG. Normotensive ischemic acute renal failure. New England Journal of Medicine. 2007;**357**:797-805. DOI: 10.1056/NEJMra064398

[19] Hawkins KE, Sharp TV, Mckay TR. The role of hypoxia in stem cell potency and differentiation. 2013;**8**:771-782. DOI: 10.2217/rme.13.71

[20] Abdollahi H, Harris LJ, Zhang P, McIlhenny S, Srinivas V, Tulenko T, et al. The role of hypoxia in stem cell differentiation and therapeutics. Journal of Surgical Research. 2011;**165**:112-117. DOI: 10.1016/J.JSS.2009.09.057

[21] Hong WX, Hu MS, Esquivel M, Liang GY, Rennert RC, McArdle A, et al. The role of hypoxia-inducible factor in wound healing. 2014;**3**:390-399. Available from: https://homeliebertpubcom/wound. DOI: 10.1089/wound.2013.0520

[22] Stangret A, Skoda M, Wnuk A, Pyzlak M, Szukiewicz D. Mild anemia during pregnancy upregulates placental vascularity development. Medical Hypotheses. 2017;**102**:37-40. DOI: 10.1016/j.mehy.2017.03.007

[23] Arthur CM, Nalbant D, Feldman HA, Saeedi BJ, Matthews J, Robinson BS, et al. Anemia induces gut inflammation and injury in an animal model of preterm infants. Transfusion (Paris). 2019;**59**:1233-1245. DOI: 10.1111/TRF.15254

[24] Evans RG, Smith DW, Lee CJ, Ngo JP, Gardiner BS. What makes the kidney susceptible to hypoxia? The Anatomical Record. 2020;**303**:2544-2552. DOI: 10.1002/AR.24260

[25] Cahill LS, Gazdzinski LM, Tsui AK, Zhou YQ, Portnoy S, Liu E, et al. Functional and anatomical evidence of cerebral tissue hypoxia in young sickle cell anemia mice. Journal of Cerebral Blood Flow and Metabolism. 2017;**37**:994-1005. DOI: 10.1177/0271678x16649194/asset/images/large/10.1177_0271678x16649194-fig 2.jpeg

[26] Wilson MJ, van Haaren M, Harlaar JJ, Park HC, Bonjer HJ, Jeekel J, et al. Long-term prognostic value of preoperative anemia in patients with colorectal cancer: A systematic review and meta-analysis. Surgical Oncology. 2017;**26**:96-104. DOI: 10.1016/j.suronc.2017.01.005

[27] Henrion J. Hypoxic hepatitis. Liver International. 2012;**32**:1039-1052. DOI: 10.1111/J.1478-3231.2011.02655.X

[28] Waseem N, Chen PH. Hypoxic hepatitis: A review and clinical update. Journal of Clinical and Translational Hepatology. 2016;**4**:263. DOI: 10.14218/JCTH.2016.00022

[29] Fuglebjerg NJU, Jensen TO, Hoyer N, Ryrsø CK, Madsen BL, Harboe ZB. Silent hypoxia in patients with SARS CoV-2 infection before hospital discharge. International Journal of Infectious Diseases. 2020;**99**:100-101. DOI: 10.1016/J.IJID.2020.07.014

[30] Li J, Fan JG. Characteristics and mechanism of liver injury in 2019 coronavirus disease. Journal of Clinical and Translational Hepatology. 2020;**8**:13. DOI: 10.14218/JCTH.2020.00019

[31] Ahmadian E, Hosseiniyan Khatibi SM, Razi Soofiyani S, Abediazar S, Shoja MM, Ardalan M, et al. Covid-19 and kidney injury: Pathophysiology and molecular mechanisms. Reviews in Medical Virology. 2021;**31**:e2176. DOI: 10.1002/RMV.2176

[32] Chong WH, Saha BK. Relationship between severe acute respiratory syndrome coronavirus 2 (SARS-CoV-2) and the Etiology of acute kidney injury (AKI). The American Journal of the Medical Sciences. 2021;**361**:287-296. DOI: 10.1016/J.AMJMS.2020.10.025

[33] Khalil S, Collins A, Mubarak N, Khalil T. Third degree heart block and elevated troponin following acute respiratory hypoxic failure in a COVID-19 recovered patient in the absence of coronary artery disease. Journal of Cardiology Case Reports. 2020;**4**:1-3

[34] Tsai HJ, Wu PY, Huang JC, Chen SC. Environmental pollution and chronic kidney disease. International Journal of Medical Sciences. 2021;**18**:1121. DOI: 10.7150/IJMS.51594

[35] Al-Aly Z, Bowe B. Air pollution and kidney disease. Clinical Journal of the American Society of Nephrology. 2020;**15**:301. DOI: 10.2215/CJN.16031219

[36] Cockwell P, Fisher LA. The global burden of chronic kidney disease. The Lancet. 2020;**395**:662-664. DOI: 10.1016/S0140-6736(19)32977-0

[37] Lv JC, Zhang LX. Prevalence and disease burden of chronic kidney disease. In: Liu B-C, Lan H-Y, Lv L-L, editors. Renal Fibrosis: Mechanisms and Therapies. Vol. 1165. New York LLC: Springer; 2019. pp. 3-15. DOI: 10.1007/978-981-13-8871-2_1/COVER

[38] Sánchez-Escuredo A, Alsina A, Diekmann F, Revuelta I, Esforzado N, Ricart MJ, et al. Economic analysis of the treatment of end-stage renal disease treatment: Living-donor kidney transplantation versus Hemodialysis. Transplantation Proceedings. 2015;**47**:30-33. DOI: 10.1016/J.TRANSPROCEED.2014.12.005

[39] Levey AS, Coresh J. Chronic kidney disease. The Lancet. 2012;**379**:165-180. DOI: 10.1016/S0140-6736(11)60178-5

[40] Venkatachalam MA, Griffin KA, Lan R, Geng H, Saikumar P, Bidani AK. Acute kidney injury: A springboard for progression in chronic kidney disease. American Journal of Physiology. Renal Physiology. 2010;**298**:1078-1094. DOI: 10.1152/ajprenal.00017.2010/asset/images/large/zh20051058870007.jpeg

[41] Ullah MM, Basile DP. Role of renal hypoxia in the progression from acute kidney injury to chronic kidney disease. Seminars in Nephrology. 2019;**39**:567-580. DOI: 10.1016/j.semnephrol.2019.10.006

[42] Nangaku M. Hypoxia and Tubulointerstitial injury: A final common pathway to end-stage renal failure. Nephron Experimental Nephrology. 2004;**98**:e8-e12. DOI: 10.1159/000079927

[43] Heyman SN, Khamaisi M, Zorbavel D, Rosen S, Abassi Z. Role of hypoxia in renal failure caused by Nephrotoxins and hypertonic solutions. Seminars in Nephrology. 2019;**39**:530-542. DOI: 10.1016/j.semnephrol.2019.10.003

[44] Fu Q, Colgan SP, Shelley CS. Hypoxia: The force that drives chronic

kidney disease. Clinical Medicine & Research. 2016;**14**:15-39. DOI: 10.3121/cmr.2015.1282

[45] Textor SC, Lerman LO. The role of hypoxia in ischemic chronic kidney disease. Seminars in Nephrology. 2019;**39**:589-598. DOI: 10.1016/J.SEMNEPHROL.2019.10.008

[46] Li ZL, Liu BC. Hypoxia and renal Tubulointerstitial fibrosis. Advances in Experimental Medicine and Biology. 2019;**1165**:467-485. DOI: 10.1007/978-981-13-8871-2_23/COVER

[47] Gong R, Dworkin LD. Brenner and Rector's the Kidney. Philadelphia: Saunders Elsevier; 2008

[48] Bipat R. Renal function-study performed on an isolated rabbit kidney perfused with autologous blood [thesis] University of Hasselt. 2004

[49] Le Gallois MJJC. Experiments on the principle of life, and particularly on the principle of the motions of the heart, and on the seat of this principle.... Experiments on the Principle of Life, and Particularly on the Principle of the Motions of the Heart, and on the Seat of This Principle... 2012. DOI: 10.1037/13894-000.

[50] Hierholzer K, Ullrich KJ. History of renal physiology in Germany during the 19th century. American Journal of Nephrology. 1999;**19**:243-256. DOI: 10.1159/000013458

[51] Weiss C, Passow H, Rothstein A. Autoregulation of flow in isolated rat kidney in the absence of red cells. 1959;**196**:1115-1118. DOI: 10.1152/ajplegacy.1959.196.5.1115

[52] Nizet A. The isolated perfused kidney: Possibilities, limitations and results. Kidney International. 1975;7:1-11. DOI: 10.1038/KI.1975.1

[53] Marques AAM, da Silva CHF, de Souza P, de Almeida CLB, Cechinel-Filho V, Lourenço ELB, et al. Nitric oxide and Ca2+—activated high-conductance K+ channels mediate nothofagin-induced endothelium-dependent vasodilation in the perfused rat kidney. Chemico-Biological Interactions. 2020;**327**:109182

[54] Pool MBF, Vos J, Eijken M, van Pel M, Reinders MEJ, Ploeg RJ, et al. Treating ischemically damaged porcine kidneys with human bone marrow-and adipose tissue-derived mesenchymal stromal cells during ex vivo normothermic machine perfusion. Stem Cells and Development. 2020;**29**:1320-1330

[55] Huijink TM, Venema LH, Posma RA, de Vries NJ, Westerkamp AC, Ottens PJ, et al. Metformin preconditioning and postconditioning to reduce ischemia reperfusion injury in an isolated ex vivo rat and porcine kidney normothermic machine perfusion model. Clinical and Translational Science. 2021;**14**:222-230

[56] Pool MBF, Hartveld L, Leuvenink HGD, Moers C. Normothermic machine perfusion of ischaemically damaged porcine kidneys with autologous, allogeneic porcine and human red blood cells. PLoS One. 2020;**15**:e0229566

[57] Lieberthal W, Stephens GW, Wolf EF, Rennke HG, Vasilevsky ML, Valeri CR, et al. Effect of erythrocytes on the function and morphology of the isolated perfused rat kidney. Kidney & Blood Pressure Research. 1987;**10**:14-24. DOI: 10.1159/000173109

[58] Cuypers Y, Vandenreyt I, Bipat R, Toelsie J, Van Damme B, Steels P. The functional state of the isolated rabbit kidney perfused with autologous blood. Pflügers Archiv. 2000;**440**:634-642. DOI: 10.1007/s004240000320

[59] Harper SJF, Hosgood SA, Waller HL, Yang B, Kay MD, Goncalves I, et al. The effect of warm ischemic time on renal function and injury in the isolated hemoperfused kidney. Transplantation. 2008;**86**:445-451. DOI: 10.1097/tp.0b013e31817fe0cd

[60] Nizet A, Cuypers Y, Deetjen P, Kramer K. Functional capacity of the isolated perfused dog kidney. Pflügers Archiv für die Gesamte Physiologie des Menschen und der Tiere. 1967;**296**:179-195. DOI: 10.1007/BF00363758

[61] Bipat R, Steels P, Cuypers Y, Toelsie JR. Mannitol reduces the hydrostatic pressure in the proximal tubule of the isolated blood-perfused rabbit kidney during hypoxic stress and improves its function. Nephron Extra. 2011;**1**:201-211. DOI: 10.1159/000333478

[62] Sharkey RA, Mulloy EMT, O'Neill SJ. Acute effects of hypoxaemia, hyperoxaemia and hypercapnia on renal blood flow in normal and renal transplant subjects. European Respiratory Journal. 1998;**12**:653-657. DOI: 10.1183/09031936.98.12030653

[63] Thiel G, Rougemont D de, Kriz W, Mason J, Torhorst J, Wolgast M. The role of reduced medullary perfusion in the genesis of acute ischemic renal failure. Nephron 1982;31:321-323. DOI: 10.1159/000182674.

[64] Mason J, Torhorst J, Welsch J. Role of the medullary perfusion defect in the pathogenesis of ischemic renal failure. Kidney International. 1984;**26**:283-293. DOI: 10.1038/KI.1984.171

[65] Johnston WH, Latta H. Glomerular mesangial and endothelial cell swelling following temporary renal ischemia and its role in the no-reflow phenomenon. The American Journal of Pathology. 1977;**89**:153

[66] Hellberg POA, Kallskog O, Wolgast M. Red cell trapping and postischemic renal blood flow. Differences between the cortex, outer and inner medulla. Kidney International. 1991;**40**:625-631. DOI: 10.1038/KI.1991.254

[67] Freitas F, Attwell D. Pericyte-mediated constriction of renal capillaries evokes no-reflow and kidney injury following ischaemia. eLife. Cardiology Case Reports. 2020;**4**:1-26 DOI: 10.7554/elife.74211

[68] Huet F, Semama DS, Gouyon JB, Guignard JP. Protective effect of Perindoprilat in the hypoxemia-induced renal dysfunction in the Newborn rabbit. Pediatric Research. 1999;**45**:138-142. DOI: 10.1203/00006450-199901000-00023

[69] Bipat R, Toelsie J, Steels P, Cuypers Y. Mannitol in contrast to furosemide, reduces tubular obstruction and improves renal function during and after hypoxic stress in the isolated rabbit kidney perfused with autologous blood. Abstract presented in the form of a poster at the meeting of the 'Belgian Society for Fundamental and Clinical Physiology and Pharmacology', Brussels (Belgium) 17th of November 2001

[70] Bagshaw SM, Langenberg C, Wan L, May CN, Bellomo R. A systematic review of urinary findings in experimental septic acute renal failure. Critical Care Medicine. 2007;**35**:1592-1598. DOI: 10.1097/01.CCM.0000266684.17500.2F

[71] Brezis M, Rosen S. Hypoxia of the renal medulla—Its implications for disease. New England Journal of Medicine. 1995;**332**:647-655

[72] Steels P, Toelsie J, Cuypers Y, Bipat R. Urea is important for the urinary

concentration capacity of the isolated blood perfused rabbit kidney. In: ASN Renal Week 2010, Denver. Journal of the American Society of Nephrology. 2010;**21**:484A

[73] Carvounis CP, Nisar S, Guro-Razuman S. Significance of the fractional excretion of urea in the differential diagnosis of acute renal failure. Kidney International. 2002;**62**:2223-2229. DOI: 10.1046/J.1523-1755.2002.00683.X

[74] Dewitte A, Biais M, Petit L, Cochard JF, Hilbert G, Combe C, et al. Fractional excretion of urea as a diagnostic index in acute kidney injury in intensive care patients. Journal of Critical Care. 2012;**27**:505-510. DOI: 10.1016/J.JCRC.2012.02.018

[75] Steiner RW. Interpreting the fractional excretion of sodium. The American Journal of Medicine. 1984;**77**:699-702. DOI: 10.1016/0002-9343(84)90368-1

[76] Pirahanchi Y, Jessu R, Aeddula NR. Physiology, Sodium Potassium Pump. Treasure Island (FL), USA: StatPearls; 2022

[77] Sepp M, Sokolova N, Jugai S, Mandel M, Peterson P, Vendelin M. Tight coupling of Na+/K+-ATPase with glycolysis demonstrated in Permeabilized rat Cardiomyocytes. PLoS One. 2014;**9**:e99413. DOI: 10.1371/journal.pone.0099413

[78] Bishop JH, Green R, Thomas S. Free-flow reabsorption of glucose, sodium, osmoles and water in rat proximal convoluted tubule. The Journal of Physiology. 1979;**288**:331-351. DOI: 10.1113/jphysiol.1979.sp012698

[79] Greenburg AG. Pathophysiology of anemia. The American Journal of Medicine. 1996;**101**:7S-11S. DOI: 10.1016/S0002-9343(96)00161-1

[80] Nouri-Vaskeh M, Sharifi A, Khalili N, Zand R, Sharifi A. Dyspneic and non-dyspneic (silent) hypoxemia in COVID-19: Possible neurological mechanism. Clinical Neurology and Neurosurgery. 2020;**198**:106217. DOI: 10.1016/J.CLINEURO.2020.106217

[81] Lankadeva YR, Cochrane AD, Marino B, Iguchi N, Hood SG, Bellomo R, et al. Strategies that improve renal medullary oxygenation during experimental cardiopulmonary bypass may mitigate postoperative acute kidney injury. Kidney International. 2019;**95**:1338-1346. DOI: 10.1016/J.KINT.2019.01.032

[82] Swenson KE, Ruoss SJ, Swenson ER. The pathophysiology and dangers of silent hypoxemia in COVID-19 lung injury. Annals of the American Thoracic Society. 2021;**18**:1098-1105. DOI: 10.1513/annalsats.202011-1376cme/suppl_file/disclosures.pdf

[83] Shenoy N, Luchtel R, Gulani P. Considerations for target oxygen saturation in COVID-19 patients: Are we under-shooting? BMC Medicine. 2020;**18**:1-6. DOI: 10.1186/S12916-020-01735-2/FIGURES/1